Atlas of
Aesthetic
Face & Neck
Surgery

Atlas of
Aesthetic
Face & Neck
Surgery

Gregory Stephen LaTrenta, MD
Clinical Associate Professor of Surgery (Plastics)
The Joan and Sanford Weill Medical College of Cornell University
Associate Attending Surgeon
The New York Presbyterian Hospital
Attending Surgeon
Manhattan Eye, Ear, and Throat Hospital
New York, New York

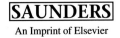

SAUNDERS
An Imprint of Elsevier

SAUNDERS
An Imprint of Elsevier

The Curtis Center
Independence Square West
Philadelphia, PA 19106

ATLAS OF AESTHETIC FACE & NECK SURGERY   ISBN 0-7216-8572-2

Library of Congress Cataloging-in-Publication Data

LaTrenta, Gregory S.
   Atlas of aesthetic face and neck surgery/Gregory LaTrenta.—1st ed.
     p. ; cm.
   ISBN 0-7216-8572-2
     1. Surgery, Plastic—Atlases. 2. Neck—Surgery—Atlases. 3. Face—Surgery—Atlases. I.
   Title.
     [DNLM: 1. Face—surgery—Atlases. 2. Neck—surgery—Atlases. 3. Surgery,
     Plastic—methods—Atlases. WE 17 L362a 2004]
     RD118.L36 2004
   617.5'20592—dc21   2003045652

Editor-in-Chief: Richard Lampert
Acquisitions Editor: Peter McEllhenney
Project Manager: Linda Van Pelt

Printed in China
Last digit is the print number: 9 8 7 6 5 4 3 2 1

For Linda, Lucas, and Alexandra,
Your sweet dreams soften
the bright midnight light
emitted from my computer,
illuminating this journey.

—Gregg LaTrenta

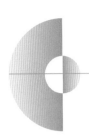

Preface

Major shifts in cosmetic plastic surgery techniques do not arrive with the new year, but rather with the passage of decades. This *Atlas of Aesthetic Face & Neck Surgery* follows the second edition of *Aesthetic Plastic Surgery*, which I published with my mentor, Dr. Thomas Rees, almost a decade ago. This *Atlas* has been written in the spirit of that text; it is primarily designed for residents and for the younger surgeon embarking on his or her career in plastic surgery. I've selected the tried-and-true procedures over the exotic, since the tried-and-true are the workhorse techniques by which we satisfy our patients' ever-growing cosmetic needs. Newer techniques that are noteworthy and practical, however, are also detailed. I hope these prove helpful to the reluctant seasoned veteran. The atlas format was chosen over the academic text format because of its simplicity and reader-friendliness.

Although brief and succinct, this *Atlas of Aesthetic Face & Neck Surgery* provides a comprehensive review of pertinent facial cosmetic procedures. The opening section offers a practical discussion of facial and neck anatomy, followed by information on recent research in facial aging, and it finishes with how to take a prospective patient from first visit to the operating room. The technical, middle section reviews surgery of the forehead and brow regions, elucidating the advantages and disadvantages of traditional open versus closed endoscopic approaches. The heart of the book is devoted to aesthetic surgery of the midface and neck, which includes the classic one-layer operation, the independent two-layer SMAS-platysmal lift, the extended and/or composite lift, and the minimal incision lift. The last section discusses the male patient, as well as adjunctive techniques, such as chin implants and laser resurfacing. The atlas concludes with a practical review of complications and untoward sequelae.

The younger surgeon should begin on the book's opening page. The more experienced surgeon may want to start with the final chapters. My hope is that you find this atlas useful and enjoyable and that it assists you in your desire to offer your patients the best possible outcome.

—Gregg LaTrenta, MD

Contents

1
THE AESTHETIC ANATOMY OF THE FACE — 2

Fat — 2
The Retaining Ligaments — 8
Superficial Musculoaponeurotic System
  and Facial Fascia — 16
The Facial Nerve — 28
The Facial Muscles — 36
Arterial Supply — 42
Sensory Supply — 44

2
THE AGING FACE — 46

Theories of Aging — 46
Wrinkles — 48
Facial Soft Tissue Foundations — 52
The Areolar Planes — 58
Regional Anatomy — 62

3
SURGICAL APPROACHES TO THE FOREHEAD AND BROW — 68

Indications — 72
Anatomical Considerations — 78
Aesthetic Considerations — 80
Techniques — 82

4
ONE-LAYER APPROACHES TO THE FACE AND NECK — 118

Indications — 119
Operative Strategies — 120
Technique — 148

5
TWO-LAYER APPROACHES TO THE MIDFACE AND NECK — 186

The Superficial Musculoaponeurotic
  System and the Platysma — 187
One-Layer Versus Two-Layer
  Techniques — 188
Indications — 190
Techniques — 200
Anterior Approaches — 254

6
THE MALE PATIENT; ADJUNCTIVE TECHNIQUES; COMPLICATIONS AND UNTOWARD SEQUELAE — 288

The Male Patient — 288
Adjunctive Techniques — 312
Complications and Untoward
  Sequelae — 326

Index — 341

Atlas of
Aesthetic
Face & Neck
Surgery

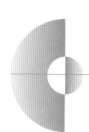

CHAPTER ONE

The Aesthetic Anatomy of the Face

We've all heard the dictum for buying real estate: "location, location, location." An analogous dictum applies for performing facial cosmetic procedures: "anatomy, anatomy, anatomy." Paramount to a successful outcome is a thorough understanding of the anatomical building blocks, neurocircuitry, and blood supply of the human face and neck. This chapter reviews the basic anatomy of the face and neck in practical and simple fashion, omitting burdensome and obscure detail of no relevance. The basic building blocks—fat, the superficial musculoaponeurotic system (SMAS) and facial fascia, and the retaining ligament system—are covered first, followed by discussions of the facial nerve and the facial muscles and then sections on the vascular supply and the sensory nerve supply. Artistically inspired illustrations, along with photographs of fresh anatomical dissections, are presented to clarify concepts of normal anatomy and aging-related changes. In addition, key points are provided after each subsection for the busy surgeon who prefers a "quick read."

FAT

Fat, along with its carrier, the fascia superficialis of the head and neck, forms the basic contours of the human face. Although bone, muscle, and skin are the other key structural ingredients, fat and fascia superficialis constitute the sine qua non for contour. This fact is dramatically illustrated in patients suffering from facial lipodystrophy secondary to treatment with human immunodeficiency virus (HIV) protease inhibitors. In these patients, subcutaneous atrophy of fat in the face can range in degree from minor to severe and occasionally can result in near-complete collapse of facial contour (Fig. 1-1). Cadaveric investigations have demonstrated that 80% of fat in the face and neck is above the lower border of the mandible and only 20% between the lower border of the mandible and the clavicles. Much of the beauty of the human face as well as the uniqueness of each person's physical appearance is better appreciated with a thorough knowledge of the role of fat in defining facial volume and contour.

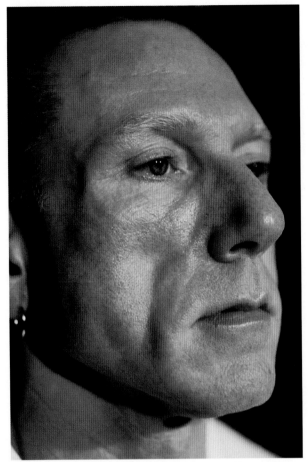

Figure 1-1 *Facial atrophy secondary to treatment with protease inhibitors. Contour loss in the face, due solely to atrophy of subcutaneous fat, can be severe.*

Subcutaneous fat in the face and neck is separated into superficial and deep layers by the fascia superficialis or the SMAS (Fig. 1-2). This fascia superficialis is called the *temporoparietal fascia* and *galea* in the temporal region and forehead and the *SMAS* in the midface and neck. The SMAS splits in the midface and neck to envelop the majority of midfacial musculature and the platysma muscle. Cadaveric investigations have revealed that fat that is superficial to the SMAS is distributed in small yellow lobules densely interwoven by thick nests of fibrous septa connecting the SMAS to the dermis. This weave of superficial fat within the superficial fascia is tightest in the forehead, temporal, and mental regions, with progressive loosening on descending into the midface, cheek, and neck regions. Fat superficial to the SMAS comprises 56% of total fat in the human face. This superficial layer of fat is continuous yet nonuniform in the face and neck. The superficial fat is densest in the cheek, especially around the nasolabial folds and jowls, in the premental and glabella regions, and in the anterior neck regions (Fig. 1-3).

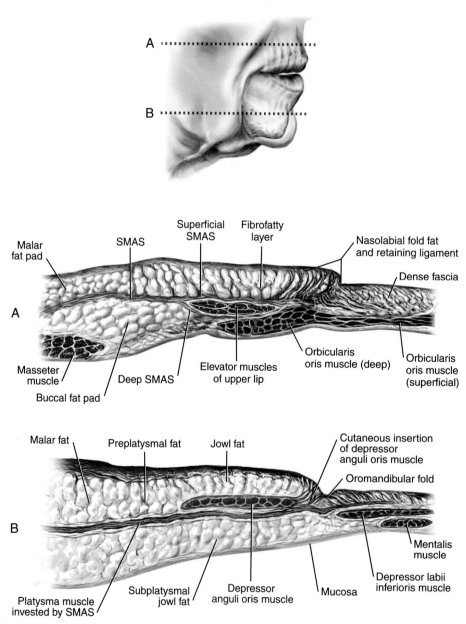

Figure 1-2 *Cross-sectional anatomy of the face at the level of the nasolabial* **(A)** *and oromandibular* **(B)** *folds. Fat superficial to the SMAS consists of small lobules tightly woven into fibrous septa that connect the SMAS to the dermis. Fat deep to the SMAS consists of large lobules interspersed between the structures of the facial mimetic musculature and not divided by fibrous septa.*

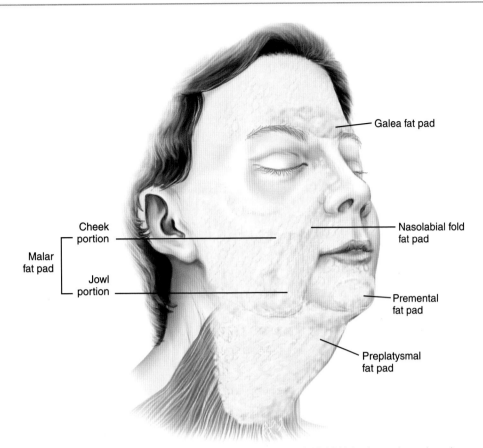

Figure 1-3 *Fat superficial to the SMAS is densest in the cheek, nasolabial fold, jowl, anterior neck, and premental regions. Superficial fat is sparse in the forehead, glabella, temporal, orbital, perioral, and posterior neck triangle regions.*

Fat deep to the SMAS is less abundant and comprises 44% of total facial fat. Unlike superficial fat, deep fat is discontinuous and distributed in large white lobules divided by a sparse network of thin fibrous septa. Deep fat is densest in the temporal, periocular, anterior and middle cheek, and submental regions (Fig. 1-4). In the temporal region, the deep fat pad consists of the superficial temporal fat pad and the temporal extension of the deep fat pad of Bichat. In the periocular region, the deep fat pad consists of the periorbital fat pads deep to the orbital septum and the suborbicularis oculi fat pad (SOOF). The SOOF is the supraperiosteal submuscular fat pad situated over the lower portion of the zygomatic body. The SOOF is separated from the periorbital fat pads by the orbital septum. In the cheek, the deep fat pad is densest in the anterior cheek region interspersed within fibers of the facial mimetic musculature. In the middle cheek region, the deep fat pad consists of the buccal and pharyngeal extensions of the deep fat pad of Bichat. In the neck, the subplatysma fat pad is densest directly under the chin and comprises 35% of total neck fat. Deep fat is sparse in the forehead, upper temporal, lateral cheek, and middle and lateral neck regions. A face entirely bereft of superficial and deep fat is truly cadaveric in appearance (Fig. 1-5*A-C*).

KEY POINTS

1) Eighty percent of fat is in the face and only 20% in the neck.

2) Fifty-six percent of fat in the face and neck is above the superficial fascia; this superficial fat is densely intertwined within a network of fascia.

3) Forty-four percent of fat in the face and neck is deep to the superficial fascia; this deep fat is very loosely held by a honeycomb of fascia.

4) The superficial fat layer is continuous and densest in the cheek, especially around the nasolabial fold and jowls, in the premental and glabella regions, and in the anterior neck regions.

5) The deep fat layer is discontinuous and densest in the temporal, periocular, anterior and middle cheek, and submental regions.

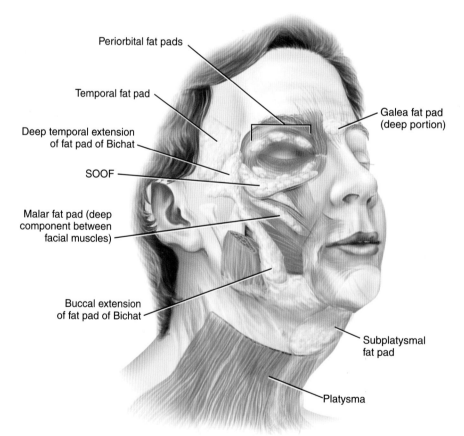

Periorbital fat pads

Temporal fat pad

Deep temporal extension of fat pad of Bichat

SOOF

Malar fat pad (deep component between facial muscles)

Buccal extension of fat pad of Bichat

Galea fat pad (deep portion)

Subplatysmal fat pad

Platysma

Figure 1-4 *Fat deep to the SMAS is densest in the temporal, suborbicularis oculi, anterior and middle cheek, and submental regions. Deep fat is sparse in the lateral cheek and lateral neck regions and almost nonexistent in the forehead, upper temporal, glabella, mental, and perioral regions. SOOF, suborbicularis oculi fat.*

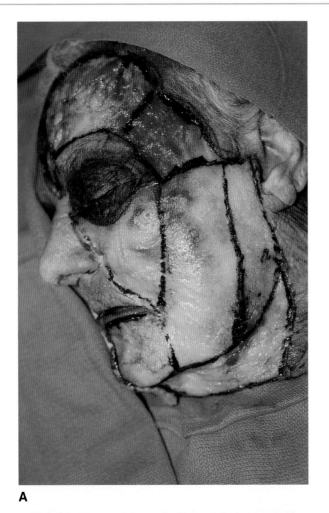

A

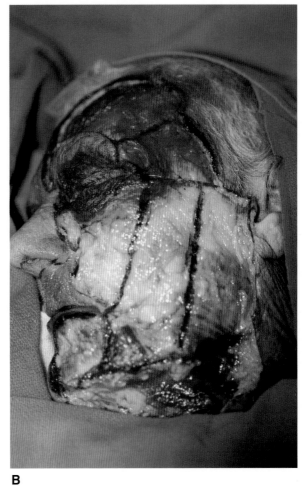

B

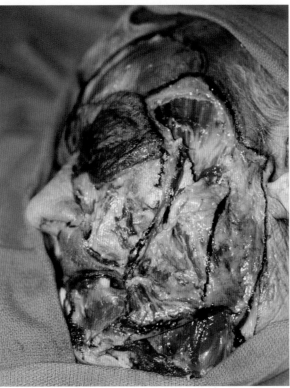

C

Figure 1-5 *Clinical cadaveric study. **A**, The skin has been removed, revealing the continuous yellow layer of fat superficial to the SMAS. Superficial fat comprises 56% of total facial fat. Note that superficial fat is densely adherent to the dermis in the forehead, temporal, and premental regions. **B**, The skin, superficial fat, and SMAS have been removed, revealing the discontinuous white layer of large deep fat lobules, densest in the anterior and middle cheek regions. Deep fat comprises 44% of total facial fat. **C**, The skin, SMAS, and superficial and deep layers of fat, including the fat pad of Bichat, have been removed, demonstrating the near-complete loss of contour evident in faces bereft of fat.*

THE RETAINING LIGAMENTS

Aponeurotic condensations of fibrous connective tissue that weave between the soft tissue layers of the face and neck and anchor the soft tissue to the underlying skeleton are called the *retaining ligaments*. These ligaments can be divided into true retaining ligaments, which anchor the skin to the periosteum at key bony sutural interfaces, and false retaining ligaments, which anchor the intervening fascial tissue layers to each other (Fig. 1-6).

True Retaining Ligaments

True retaining ligaments are short, stout, tight fibrous tissue attachments of the dermis to the periosteum. The true retaining ligaments of the face are found in four locations: orbital, zygomatic, mandibular, and buccal-maxillary (Fig. 1-7).

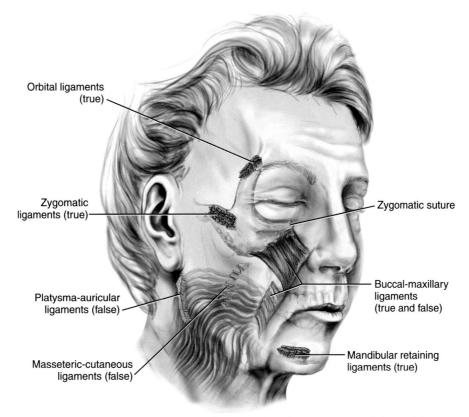

Orbital ligaments (true)

Zygomatic ligaments (true)

Zygomatic suture

Platysma-auricular ligaments (false)

Buccal-maxillary ligaments (true and false)

Masseteric-cutaneous ligaments (false)

Mandibular retaining ligaments (true)

Figure 1-6 *The true and false retaining ligament system of the face. Note that the false retaining ligaments are in the anterior, middle, and posterior cheek regions.*

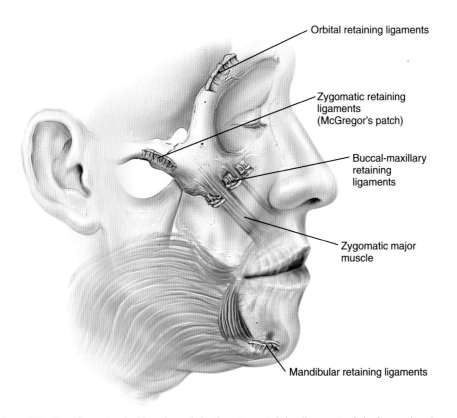

Orbital retaining ligaments

Zygomatic retaining ligaments (McGregor's patch)

Buccal-maxillary retaining ligaments

Zygomatic major muscle

Mandibular retaining ligaments

Figure 1-7 *Specific anatomical locations of the three true retaining ligaments of the face and neck.*

The orbital retaining ligaments are 6 to 8 mm in length and centered over the zygomaticofrontal suture (Fig. 1-8). Several firm, taut white fibers are contiguous with the temporal crest. A small artery, a sensory nerve, and several large veins are evident coursing through the area. These structures are subject to injury when subperiosteal dissection is performed during temporal and endoscopic forehead lifts. When these veins are encountered, it is far better to perform hemostasis before their dissection than after their division.

The zygomatic retaining ligaments, found in a grouping termed *McGregor's patch*, are approximately 1.0 cm in length and extend along the inferior surface of the anterior third of the zygomatic arch and the posterior half of the zygomatic body along the zygomaticotemporal and intrazygomatic sutures. The zygomatic retaining ligaments extend directly from the periosteum into the dermis. Several groupings are occasionally evident. A typical grouping is a bundle of white firm fibers 3 mm in width and 0.5 mm in thickness (Fig. 1-9*A* and *B*). An artery and a sensory nerve course to the skin through one of these bundles. One of the rami of the zygomatic branch of the facial nerve courses deep and inferior to the ligament. On encountering this ligament, extra care must be exercised to achieve a superficial plane of dissection in order to avoid facial nerve injury.

The mandibular retaining ligament is a short, thick, stout ligament arising on the anterior third of the inferior mandibular border at an intramandibular suture. The ligament is 3 to 4 mm in thickness and arises anterior to the origin of the depressor anguli oris muscle (Fig. 1-10). The ligament forms an osseous anchor between the periosteum of the anterior mandible, extending through the anterior fibers of the platysma and locking into the skin anterior to the jowl. An artery and a vein are encountered adjacent to the ligament. Therefore, the ligament should be electrocoagulated before its division; otherwise, a difficult-to-visualize and nasty bleeder will need to be cauterized afterward.

The buccal-maxillary retaining ligaments are unique in that they have both true ligament and false ligament components. The true component of the buccal-maxillary retaining ligaments is the upper portion, the maxillary ligaments (see Fig. 1-10*B*; see also cross-sectional anatomy in Fig. 1-36). The maxillary retaining ligaments are approximately 3 to 5 mm in thickness and 1.0 to 1.5 cm in length and are composed of thick, dense fibroelastic tissue. The maxillary ligaments arise from the periosteal surface along the zygomaticomaxillary suture, in a manner very similar to the way in which the orbital and zygomatic ligaments arise along the other zygomatic sutural interfaces. The maxillary retaining ligaments form an anterior "fence" of suspension for the cheek. The true portion of the buccal-maxillary ligaments extends as far superiorly as the orbital rim along the line of the zygomaticomaxillary suture.

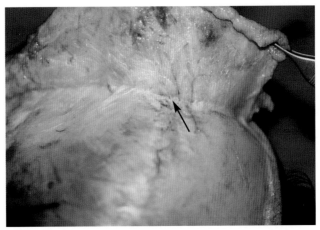

Figure 1-8   *Orbital retaining ligaments at the zygomaticofrontal suture.*

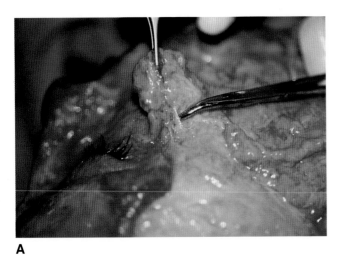

A

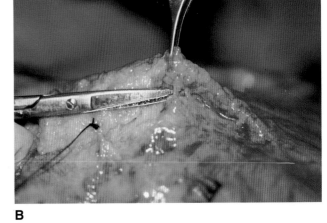

B

Figure 1-9   ***A*** *and* ***B****, Zygomatic retaining ligaments at McGregor's patch.*

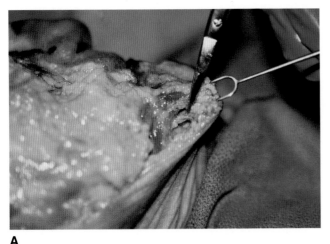

A

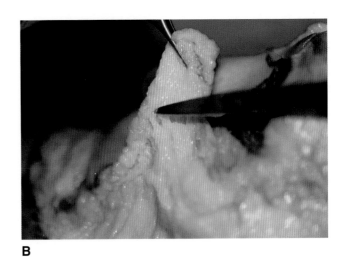

B

Figure 1-10   ***A****, Mandibular retaining ligament at the anterior mandibular border.* ***B****, Maxillary (upper) component of the buccal-maxillary retaining ligaments.*

False Retaining Ligaments

The false retaining ligaments are tendrils of connective tissue that attach the superficial facial fascia to the deep facial fascia. The false retaining ligaments are broadly based and function like sheets of Velcro in connecting tissues superficial to the superficial facial fascia to tissues deep to the deep facial fascia. The false retaining ligaments are located primarily in the cheek in three key locations: (1) platysma-auricular ligaments, located over the angle of the mandible in the posterior cheek, (2) masseteric-cutaneous ligaments, located anterior to the masseter muscle in the middle cheek, and (3) buccal-maxillary ligaments, located in a broad fencelike arrangement lateral to the nasolabial groove in the anterior cheek (see Fig. 1-6).

The platysma-auricular ligaments form a thick fascial aponeurosis that intimately attaches the posterosuperior border of the platysma and the lobule of the ear to the SMAS and skin overlying the angle of the mandible (Fig. 1-11A). This aponeurosis provides a dissection plane that leads directly to the external surface of the platysma (Fig. 1-11B). The surgical significance of this sheet of ligaments is evident during the development of platysma rotation flaps for neck rejuvenation. The great auricular nerve is located immediately posterior to the ligament and is subject to injury or division when dissection becomes deep or misdirected. This aponeurosis provides a warning that branches of the great auricular nerve are nearby.

The masseteric-cutaneous ligaments are a thin picket fence–like extension of epimysium fibers emanating from the entire anterior border of the masseter muscle, which inserts into the dermis of the middle cheek of the face (Fig. 1-12). These ligaments are easily demonstrated during sub-SMAS facialplasty dissections. If the SMAS is elevated anterior to the parotid, the areolar plane between superficial and deep facial fascias is entered. This is a clear plane until the masseteric-cutaneous ligaments are encountered along the entire anterior border of the masseter muscle. The masseteric-cutaneous ligaments provide support to the soft tissue medial cheek and are responsible for the submalar hollow that is a characteristic feature of the facial aging process.

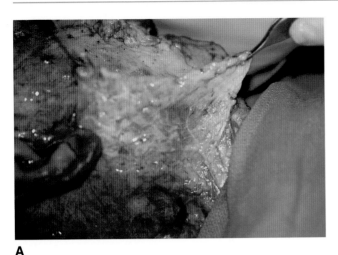
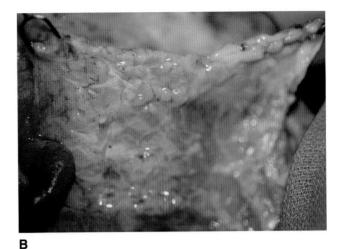

A   B

Figure 1-11   **A** *and* **B**, *The broad sheet of platysma-auricular ligaments, which extend in a wide swathe between the lobule of the ear and the platysma muscle.*

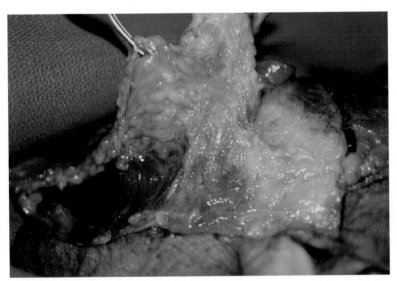
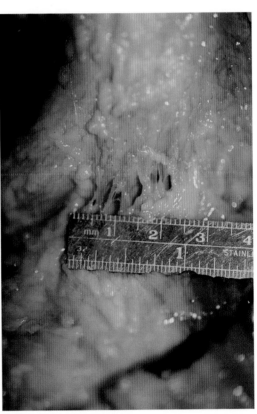

A   B

Figure 1-12   **A**, *Masseteric-cutaneous ligaments.* **B**, *Close-up view.*

The buccal-maxillary ligaments (Fig.1-13) provide soft tissue support in the region of the face most susceptible to facial aging: the anterior cheek adjacent to the nasolabial fold. The buccal or lower component of these fascial ligaments forms a series of long (1.0 to 2.0 cm), thick (3 to 6 mm), loose condensations of highly elastic fibrous tissue that supports the dense fat of the superficial and deep anterior cheek. The buccal retaining ligaments arise from the fibrofascial covering of the upper buccal mucosa and extend superolaterally in an oblique direction into the SOOF and anterior cheek (see cross-sectional anatomy in Fig. 1-36). They are densely adherent to the large adipose globules within the deep fat compartment of the nasolabial region. They also, like the upper maxillary component, extend into the superficial fat loosely held by the SMAS of the anterior cheek. Because the SMAS in the anterior cheek is thin and discontinuous, these ligaments are very difficult to demonstrate clinically unless one chooses a buccal approach for the midfacial cheek lift. The buccal-maxillary ligaments are the weakest retaining ligaments of the face because (1) they originate over the highly mobile, hollow, and extensible buccal mucosal recess of the maxilla and (2) they have the highest composition of elastic fibers of all the retaining ligaments. These structural features account for why the anterior cheek region is so susceptible to sagging with aging.

KEY POINTS

1) The retaining ligaments are aponeurotic condensations of fibrous connective tissue that weave between the soft tissue layers of the face and neck, anchoring the soft tissue to deeper structures.
2) The true retaining ligaments anchor dermis to periosteum and are located over the zygomaticofrontal suture, over the zygomatic arch–body suture, over the anterior mandibular body suture, and over the zygomaticomaxillary suture.
3) The false retaining ligaments anchor the superficial fascia to the deep fascia and are located in the anterior, middle, and posterior cheek.

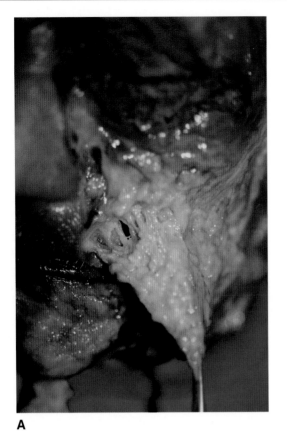 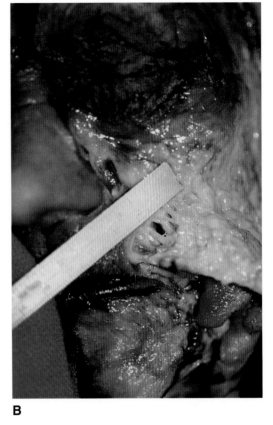

A **B**

Figure 1-13 *Buccal-fascial ligaments.*

SUPERFICIAL MUSCULOAPONEUROTIC SYSTEM AND FACIAL FASCIA

The anatomy of the SMAS and its application in facial cosmetic surgery have been studied extensively. The original concept was that the SMAS is a fibromuscular network running deep to the dermis and superficial to the facial motor nerves, extending from the superficial temporal musculature above to the platysma musculature below (Fig. 1-14*A* and *B*). Recent research on facial anatomy has provided the modern concept that the SMAS is actually composed of several layers that split to invest the superficial mimetic musculature and that the facial nerve, while deep to the peripheral SMAS, pierces the central SMAS to innervate the facial muscles. Although much of our understanding may have changed, the SMAS still serves us best as a surgical vehicle for safely "lifting" the key components of the face and neck—the skin, the superficial fat, and the platysma muscle.

The SMAS is thickest and most uniform in the parotid-masseteric region, where it is attached to the parotid sheath. The SMAS is thinnest with significant discontinuity in the anterior cheek region. The SMAS is also quite thick in the temporoparietal region of the forehead, where it is called the temporoparietal fascia, and in the scalp, where it is called the galea. Otherwise, the SMAS is thin and variable in thickness throughout the face. Although the SMAS derives its surgical significance as a vehicle for safely lifting the fat and subcutaneous tissue of the face and neck, functionally the SMAS acts as a distributor and amplifier of facial muscular activity. These functions are performed chiefly through the SMAS's complex web of attachments to nearly all components of the face: skin, fat, muscle, periosteum, and mucosa.

Facial soft tissue architecture is best understood if we think of it as an onion. The facial soft tissues are composed of a concentric lamellar arrangement of layers. From superficial to deep, these layers consist of skin, superficial fat, SMAS, mimetic musculature and intervening deep fat, the deep facial fascia, and the planes containing the facial nerve, parotid duct, and buccal fat pad. This unique relationship of facial structural anatomy is best appreciated if we perform a superficial to deep layered dissection of the face and neck using the approach commonly utilized for rhytidectomy, as follows.

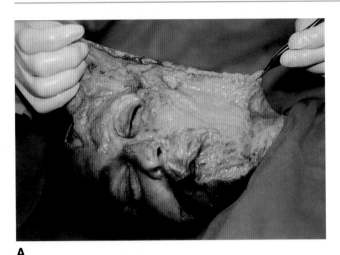
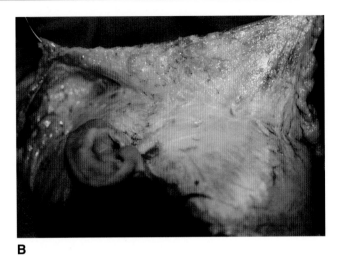

A **B**

Figure 1-14 *The SMAS is a fibrofatty and muscular network located deep to the dermis and superficial to the facial motor nerves, extending from the temporal and scalp region above and investing the platysma musculature below.* **A,** *Medial view;* **B,** *lateral view.*

Following dissection of skin and superficial fat, the superficial layer of SMAS is evident extending throughout the face and neck region (Fig. 1-15). This is the approach commonly used for supra-SMAS "lifts." Above the zygomatic arch, the superficial SMAS is abundant and is referred to as the temporoparietal fascia (Fig. 1-16). The surgical significance of the temporoparietal fascia is that the frontal branch of the facial nerve crosses over the superficial surface of the midportion of the zygomatic arch and traverses the temporal region on the undersurface of this layer. The frontal branch of the facial nerve, which often has more than one branch, traverses the temporal region to innervate the frontalis, corrugator, procerus, and depressor supercilii musculature. The frontal branch of the superficial temporal artery parallels and is superior to the nerve within the temporoparietal fascia. Below the zygomatic arch, the superficial SMAS forms the superficial fascial covering of the orbicularis oculi, the zygomaticus major and minor, and the platysma musculature. The SMAS truly invests these muscles with a superficial and a deep layer. The true retaining ligaments provide the primary support for the facial subcutaneous tissues through the complex interconnections of the SMAS. These ligaments anchor the dermis to the underlying periosteum of the facial skeleton at several key locations. The true retaining ligaments are most evident within the SMAS over McGregor's patch, which exists along the inferior border of the anterior zygomatic arch and zygomatic body posterior to the origin of the zygomaticus minor. The false retaining ligaments represent a coalescence of superficial and deep facial fascias, and provide a secondary weaker system of support for the cheeks. The false retaining system fixes the superficial SMAS to the deeper fascia and weakly tethers the covering dermis through the attachments of the SMAS to superficial fat and dermis. The false retaining system is densest in the anterior cheek 1 to 2 cm lateral to the nasolabial crease—the buccal-maxillary suspensory ligaments. This fencelike arrangement of false retaining ligaments helps to account for the almost universal appearance of the nasolabial fold in the face.

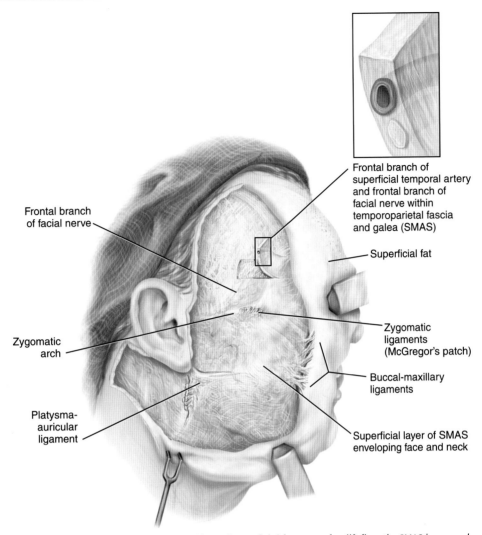

Frontal branch of
superficial temporal artery
and frontal branch of
facial nerve within
temporoparietal fascia
and galea (SMAS)

Frontal branch
of facial nerve

Superficial fat

Zygomatic
ligaments
(McGregor's patch)

Zygomatic
arch

Buccal-maxillary
ligaments

Platysma-
auricular
ligament

Superficial layer of SMAS
enveloping face and neck

Figure 1-15 *Following dissection of the skin and superficial fat onto a facelift flap, the SMAS is exposed. Note the frontal branch of the facial nerve within the temporoparietal fascia. See text for details.*

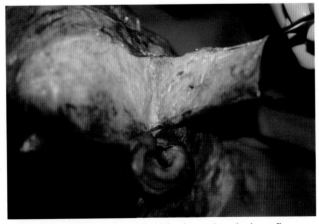

Figure 1-16 *The temporoparietal fascia can be raised as a flap.*

Following dissection of the skin, superficial fat, and superficial SMAS, the sub-SMAS anatomy is evident (Fig. 1-17). Because the frontal branch of the facial nerve runs within the temporoparietal fascia from the midportion of the zygomatic arch to its insertion in the forehead musculature, the main bulk of the frontal branch is well within the facial flap when the sub-SMAS anatomy is encountered. Above the zygomatic arch, as the temporoparietal fascia is lifted with the flap, the superficial layer of the deep temporal fascia is exposed. If a small incision is made in the lower part of the superficial layer of deep temporal fascia, the superficial temporal fat pad is exposed. Along the upper lateral orbit over the zygomaticofrontal suture, the orbital retaining ligaments are encountered. The orbital retaining ligaments are true retaining ligaments for the upper face and midface. Below the zygomatic arch, the superficial surface of the orbicularis oculi, zygomaticus major and minor, and platysma muscles is exposed. These mimetic muscles are innervated on their deep surfaces by branches of the facial nerve. The body and tail of the parotid gland are exposed anterior and inferior to the auricle. The SMAS is densely adherent to the capsule of the parotid, which accounts for its relative thickness in this region. Several false retaining ligaments are notable in the midface: the thick sheetlike platysma-auricular suspensory ligaments at the angle of the jaw and the picket fence–like arrangement of the masseteric-cutaneous suspensory ligaments along the anterior border of the masseter muscle. Also evident in the lower anterior cheek anterior to the superficial jowl fat pad are the mandibular retaining ligaments. These are short, stout true retaining ligaments, representing dermal to periosteal attachment along the anterior third of the mandibular body about 1 cm above the border of the jaw. The broad swathe of platysma muscle is evident obliquely crossing the midface from the angle of the mandible and weaving into the superficial perioral musculature with several fascicles of the risorius muscle and depressor anguli oris. The thickness, size, and extent of the platysma muscle are highly variable.

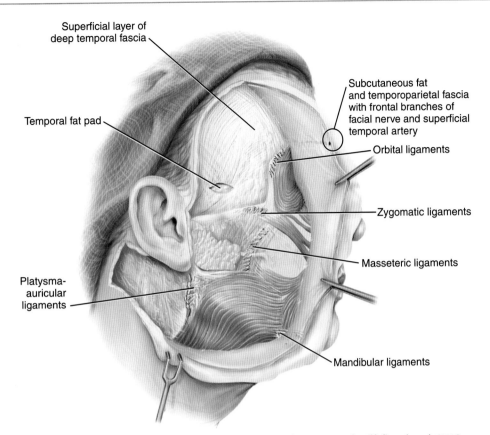

Superficial layer of
deep temporal fascia

Temporal fat pad

Subcutaneous fat
and temporoparietal fascia
with frontal branches of
facial nerve and superficial
temporal artery

Orbital ligaments

Zygomatic ligaments

Masseteric ligaments

Platysma-
auricular
ligaments

Mandibular ligaments

Figure 1-17 *Following dissection of the skin, superficial fat, and SMAS onto a facelift flap, the sub-SMAS mimetic musculature anatomy—the orbicularis oculi, zygomaticus major and minor, and platysma muscles—is evident. The frontal branch of the facial nerve is within the facelift flap. See text for details.*

Following dissection of the skin, superficial fat, SMAS, and superficial mimetic musculature, the sub-mimetic musculature anatomy and deep layer of SMAS become evident (Fig. 1-18). Above the zygomatic arch, the temporal fat pad is encountered. The temporal fat pad is situated between the superficial and deep layers of the deep temporal fascia. If a small slit is made in the superior part of the deep temporal fascia near the temporal line of fusion, the temporalis muscle is encountered. If a small slit is made in the deep temporal fascia just above the zygomatic arch and anterior to the temporal fat pad, the temporal component of the fat pad of Bichat, or deep temporal fat pad, is encountered. Below the zygomatic arch and anterior to the parotid gland, the deep fascia over the masseter muscle is notable. This deep, thin, translucent layer of SMAS continues into the face and is called the *parotidomasseteric fascia* (Fig. 1-19). The surgical significance of this layer is that the facial nerve branches, the parotid duct, and the facial artery and vein lie deep to the parotidomasseteric fascia (Fig. 1-20).

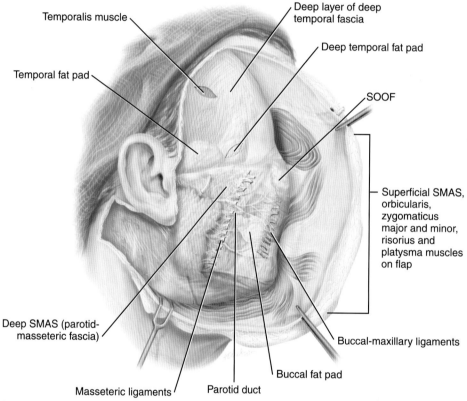

Figure 1-18 *Following dissection of the skin, superficial fat, SMAS, and superficial mimetic musculature onto the facelift flap, the sub-mimetic musculature and deep fascial anatomy are evident. The temporal fat pad is evident above the zygomatic arch, and the parotid-masseteric fascia is evident anterior to the parotid with intervening masseteric-cutaneous ligaments. See text for details.*

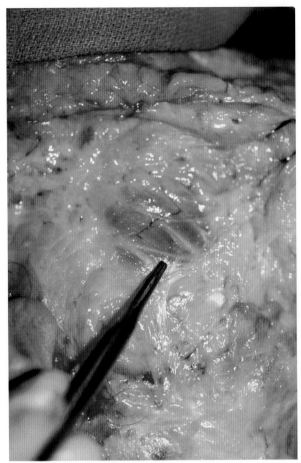

Figure 1-19 *The thin, filmy, translucent parotid-masseteric fascia, with facial nerve branches evident underneath.*

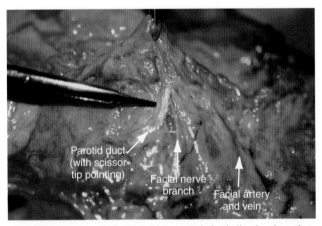

Figure 1-20 *Beneath the parotid-masseteric fascia lies the plane that includes the parotid duct, the facial nerve branches, and the facial artery and vein.*

Great care must be exercised in dissecting superficial to the parotidomasseteric fascia for two reasons: (1) the parotidomasseteric fascia is thin and fragile, and (2) the facial nerve branches pierce the parotidomasseteric fascia medially to become more superficial as they begin to innervate the superficial mimetic musculature (Fig. 1-21). Also encountered anterior to the masseter and deep to the deep fascia is the buccal portion of the buccal fat pad of Bichat (Fig. 1-22*A* and *B*). With gentle traction, this portion of the buccal fat pad can easily be extracted during rhytidectomy in selected patients with "fat cheeks." Anteriorly, the buccal-maxillary retaining ligaments are noted, which become contiguous with the upper buccal mucosa and the periosteum over the zygomaticomaxillary suture. Below the orbicularis oculi muscle in the upper midface is the SOOF. The SOOF is localized below the orbital rim and separated from the orbital fat pads by the thin orbital and malar septa (Fig. 1-23). The SOOF is primarily responsible for the formation of malar bags, which appear inferolateral to the more commonly situated lower eyelid bags.

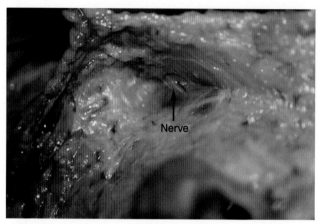

Figure 1-21   *Marginal mandibular facial nerve branch piercing the parotid masseteric fascia to innervate the platysma muscle.*

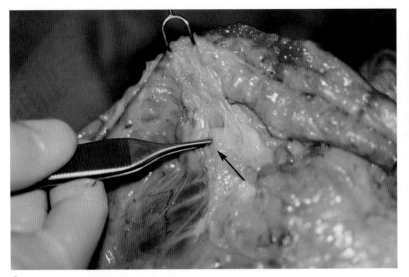

A

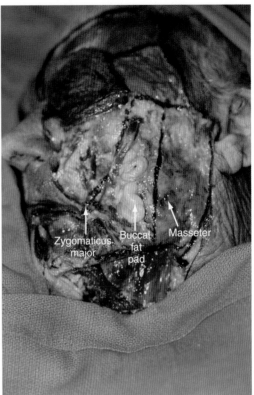

B

Figure 1-22 **A**, *The buccal extension of the fat pad of Bichat is deep to the masseteric-cutaneous ligaments. The facial nerve branches are superficial to the buccal fat pad.* **B**, *The buccal extension of the fat pad of Bichat is anterior to the masseter muscle and posterior to the zygomaticus major muscle.*

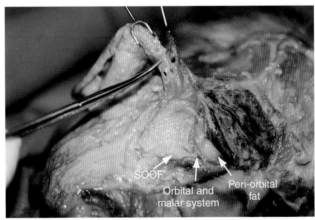

Figure 1-23 *The SOOF is localized below the widely fanned-out orbicularis oculi and inferior to the orbital rim. The SOOF is separated from the orbital fat pads by the thin orbital and malar septa. The scissors point to the zygomatic retaining ligaments, which are coalesced within the SMAS covering the orbicularis oculi.*

Following dissection of the skin, superficial fat, superficial SMAS, superficial mimetic musculature, and deep layer of SMAS, the deep facial structures and facial nerve become evident (Fig. 1-24). Above the zygomatic arch, the temporalis muscle and the temporal component of the fat pad of Bichat are noted. The bulk of the deep temporal fat pad can be noted behind the lateral wall of the orbit and zygomatic arch. The stump of the frontal branch of the facial nerve is evident below the midportion of the zygomatic arch, where it pierces the deep SMAS. The distal segment of the frontal branch is within the temporoparietal fascia on the facial flap. The main bundle of the frontal branch of the facial nerve is subject to violation and injury above the zygomatic arch in the temporal region as it traverses this region within the temporoparietal fascia. The facial nerve–free safe zone of dissection is noted over the inferior portion of the anterior zygomatic arch and zygomatic body. The deeper perioral musculature is evident within this plane, including the deeply situated levator anguli oris, the buccinator, and the mentalis. These muscles are innervated by the facial nerve along their superficial surfaces. The facial nerve branches are superficial to the plane that encompasses the buccal fat pad, the parotid duct, and the facial artery and vein.

KEY POINTS

1) The facial soft tissue architecture is in a concentric lamellar arrangement of layers consisting of skin, superficial fat, superficial SMAS, mimetic musculature with intervening deep fat, deep SMAS, and the plane containing the facial nerve, parotid duct, facial artery and vein, and buccal fat pad.

2) The SMAS is a fibromuscular network that lies deep to the dermis and superficial to the facial motor nerves, extending from the superficial temporal musculature above to the platysma musculature below.

3) The SMAS is significant as a functional distributor and amplifier of facial muscular activity, as well as a structural vehicle for safely lifting the subcutaneous tissues of the face and neck through its complex network of attachments to the skin, fat, muscle, periosteum, and mucosa.

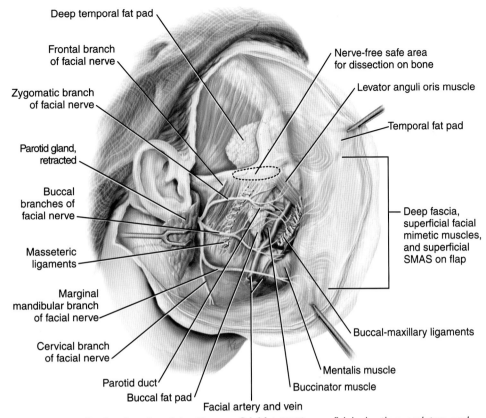

Deep temporal fat pad

Frontal branch
of facial nerve

Zygomatic branch
of facial nerve

Parotid gland,
retracted

Buccal
branches of
facial nerve

Masseteric
ligaments

Marginal
mandibular branch
of facial nerve

Cervical branch
of facial nerve

Parotid duct

Buccal fat pad

Facial artery and vein

Nerve-free safe area
for dissection on bone

Levator anguli oris muscle

Temporal fat pad

Deep fascia,
superficial facial
mimetic muscles,
and superficial
SMAS on flap

Buccal-maxillary ligaments

Mentalis muscle

Buccinator muscle

Figure 1-24 *Following dissection of the skin, superficial fat, SMAS, superficial mimetic musculature, and deep facial fascia onto the facelift flap, the deep subfascial anatomy is evident. The main trunk and branches of the facial nerve are evident below the zygomatic arch within the plane that includes the buccal fat pad, the parotid duct, and the facial artery and vein. See text for details.*

THE FACIAL NERVE

The main trunk and branches of the facial nerve are evident below the zygomatic arch within the plane that includes the buccal fat pad, the parotid duct, and the facial artery and vein (see Fig. 1-24). The main trunk of the facial nerve, which usually bifurcates into temporal and cervical divisions (or, rarely, trifurcates), is encased between the superficial and deep lobes of the parotid gland. The facial nerve becomes more superficial after it bifurcates. The divisions and branches pass along the superficial surface of the masseter muscle deep to the parotidomasseteric fascia. Anterior to the masseter muscle, the nerve branches lie deep to the deep layer of the SMAS, and interconnections cease. The terminal branches then rapidly become superficial to innervate the mimetic musculature and, subsequently, become subject to injury.

The temporal division has five to seven branches and many interconnections within its own branches—one to the frontal region, two to the orbital region, three to the zygomatic region, and two to the buccal region. The zygomatic branch is the largest and most important functionally. The frontal branch is the smallest and has the least number of interconnections and is a terminal branch in the vast majority of patients.

The cervical division is smaller and consists of three to five branches with many interconnections between branches—one to the buccal region, three to the mandibular region, and one to the cervical region. Connections between the major divisions occur in 75% to 90% of patients. The marginal mandibular branch is delicate and interconnects with other branches of the cervical division in only 10% to 15% of patients.

The zygomatic and buccal branches of the facial nerve form the bulk of the facial nerve and traverse the cheek superficial to the buccal fat pad on their way to innervate the periocular and perioral facial mimetic musculature. Distal to the masseter muscle they become more superficial as they penetrate the parotidomasseteric fascia to innervate the mimetic musculature. The zygomatic and buccal branches can be injured in any of several ways: by direct pressure from plication sutures carried through the parotidomasseteric fascia; by direct injury from aggressive surgical dissection of the SMAS anterior to the parotid gland, especially in patients with scant subcutaneous tissue or small, short parotid glands; or by indirect pressure from deeply situated hematomas within the buccal fat pad space.

The frontal branch of the temporal division and the marginal mandibular branch of the cervical division are the branches most liable to injury during rhytidectomy and are considered separately.

The frontal branch leaves the parotid gland below the zygomatic arch and penetrates the gland at almost a right angle to cross the midportion of the arch along the superficial surface (Fig. 1-25). The frontal branch courses within the temporoparietal fascia (superficial temporal fascia) through the temporal region and crosses the sentinel vein at approximately halfway through its course (Fig. 1-26). The frontal branch enters the frontalis muscle and the deep portion of the orbicularis muscle above the level of the superior orbital rim. The frontal

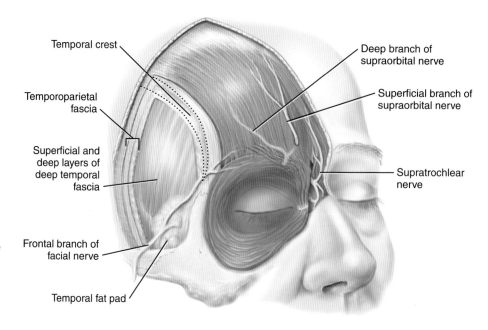

Temporal crest

Temporoparietal fascia

Superficial and deep layers of deep temporal fascia

Frontal branch of facial nerve

Temporal fat pad

Deep branch of supraorbital nerve

Superficial branch of supraorbital nerve

Supratrochlear nerve

Figure 1-25 *Anatomy of the temporal and forehead region. Note the path of the frontal branch of the facial nerve and its relationship to the zygomatic arch and orbital rim.*

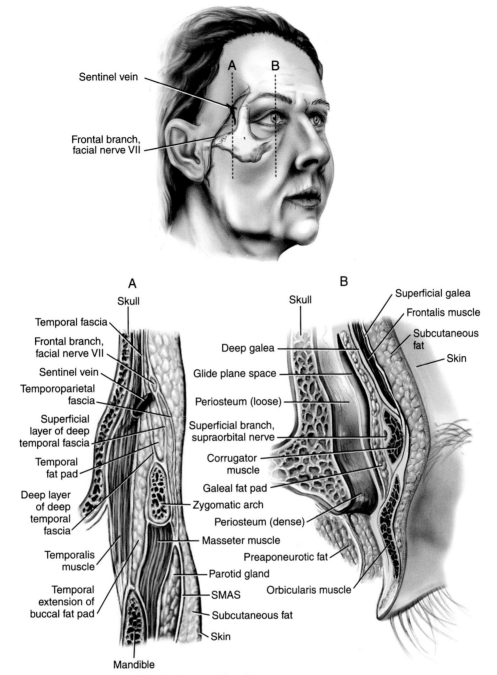

Figure 1-26 *Temporal and forehead cross-sectional anatomy.*

branch of the superficial temporal artery also parallels the course of the nerve and lies directly superior to it (see Fig. 1-15). The sentinel vein and the frontal branch of the superficial temporal artery are good surface landmarks for approximating the subcutaneous position of the nerve.

The cross-sectional anatomy of the temporal region and that of the central brow are illustrated in Figure 1-26*A* and *B*. From a clinical standpoint, the temporal region is the triangle formed by the zygomatic arch, the temporal crest, and the first inch or two of the anterior hairline. The temporal region consists of three layers below the skin and superficial fat.

The frontal branch of the facial nerve courses along the deep surface of the most superficial of the three temporal layers, the temporoparietal fascia. The temporoparietal fascia is continuous with the SMAS of the face and the superficial galea of the brow. Deep to the temporoparietal fascia is the loose areolar plane, which separates the temporoparietal fascia from the deep temporal fascia. This loose areolar plane, or subaponeurotic plane, is the plane easily entered in performing a temporal brow lift. Clinically, the frontal branch of the facial nerve can easily be injured in performing a temporal lift through the loose areolar plane because of the vulnerable location of the nerve; excessive trauma with scissor dissection directed superficially in performing a temporal lift should be avoided at all costs!

The middle layer in the temporal region is the superficial temporal fat pad, which is situated between the superficial and deep layers of the deep temporal fascia. Anterior to the temporal line of fusion, both superficial and deep layers of deep temporal fascia join to become the deep galea. The clinical significance of the deep galea in the brow region is that the galea fat pad and the glide plane space of the forehead are situated deep to the deep galea—hence, if a temporal approach to the forehead is chosen, it is far safer to dip into a subperiosteal plane. The superficial temporal fat pad extends from the temporal line of fusion down to the zygomatic arch and as far forward as the lateral orbital walls (Fig. 1-27).

The third and deepest layer in the temporal region is the temporal extension of the buccal fat pad (Figs. 1-28 and 1-29). This begins between 2 and 4 cm above the zygomatic arch, separates the arch from the temporalis muscle, and extends into the buccal and retropharyngeal spaces to join with other extensions of the fat pad of Bichat.

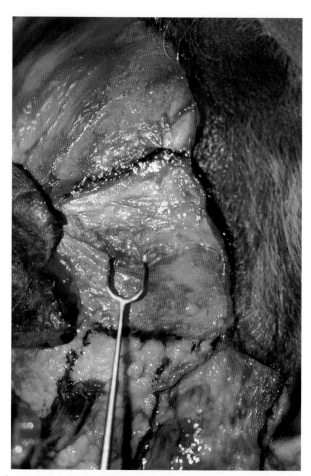

Figure 1-27 Temporal fat pad. Note that the superficial temporal fat pad is between the superficial and deep layers of the deep temporal fascia and extends from the temporal line of fusion down to the zygomatic arch and forward as far as the lateral orbital walls.

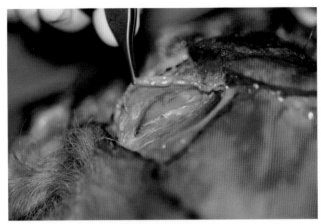

Figure 1-28 *Temporal extension of the buccal fat pad of Bichat. This portion of the fat pad is below the deep temporal fascia. Note that the temporal fat pad is on the flap retracted by the forceps.*

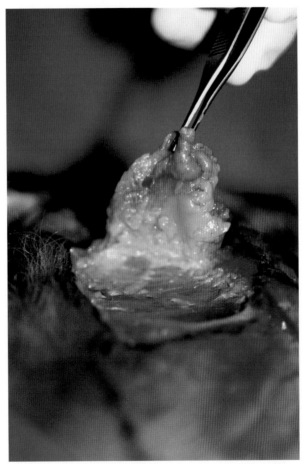

Figure 1-29 *Temporal extension of the buccal fat pad of Bichat. Note that this portion of the fat pad is superficial to the temporalis muscle.*

The marginal mandibular branch always enters the platysma muscle along its deep surface (Fig. 1-30). During rhytidectomy after elevation of the superficial SMAS and fat off the face and neck, the broad swathe of the platysma muscle is evident (Fig. 1-31). The wide depressor anguli oris muscle is evident superficial to the platysma, with many of its fibers virtually indistinguishable from platysma fibers. Other pertinent anatomy in the region below the mandibular border includes the external jugular vein and the greater auricular nerve. The external jugular vein can be injured if dissection is carried too deep over the fascia covering the sternocleidomastoid muscle. If injured, the vein should be transected and ligated. The greater auricular nerve exits the deep cervical fascia and crosses the sternocleidomastoid fascia 6.5 cm below the lobule. If injured, the greater auricular nerve should be repaired, preferably by microneurovascular technique. If this repair is not performed, permanent numbness of the ear is more than likely.

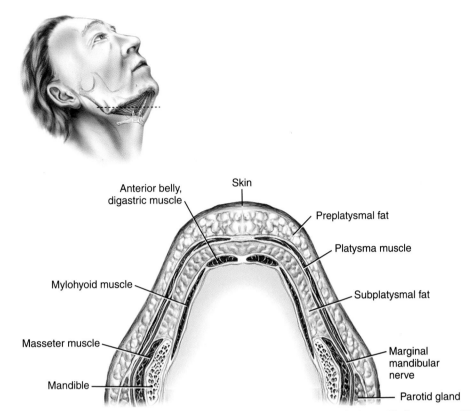

Figure 1-30 *Cross-sectional anatomy of the neck. Note the path of the marginal mandibular nerve and its relationship to the SMAS and platysma in the neck.*

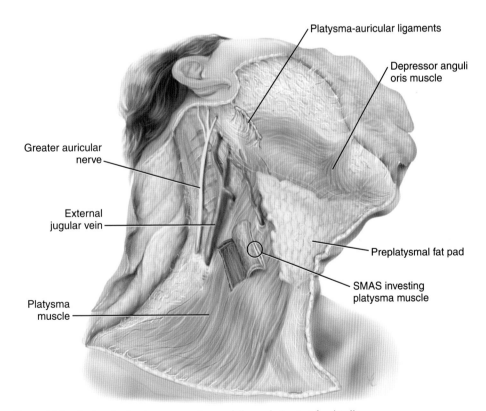

Figure 1-31 *Regional subcutaneous anatomy of the neck. See text for details.*

The mandibular branch of the facial nerve is liable to injury by a variety of methods once the platysma muscle has been elevated (Fig. 1-32). During dissection of the parotid platysma ligament for elevation of platysma rotation flaps, the main body of the marginal mandibular nerve can be transected. Cadaver studies have found that the marginal mandibular branch is above the inferior portion of the mandible posterior to the facial artery in 81% of cases, and within 1 to 2 cm below the mandible in 19% of cases. Clinical studies, however, have shown that the mandibular branch is at least 1 to 2 cm below the lower portion of the mandible in almost every instance, and in some patients with lax and atrophic tissues, the nerve is 3 to 4 cm below the mandible. In older patients or those with atrophic, thin, or split platysma musculature, and in patients with previous SMAS or platysma muscle surgery, the nerve may be superficially situated between several platysma muscle fibers as it courses over the face. This makes the marginal mandibular branch vulnerable to injury by deep ligatures, electrocoagulation, plication sutures, or even forceps and clamps. Head position during surgery also influences the position of the nerve relative to the inferior mandibular border. If the patient's neck is extended during surgery, the nerve descends lower. Clinical studies have shown that 15% of patients have a connection between the mandibular division and the buccal division of the facial nerve; therefore, in these cases, considerable recovery of function may be expected if the mandibular nerve is transected. In the remainder of cases, injury to this nerve may leave a permanent deficit. This deficit will be conspicuous if the entire mandibular division is injured; however, it may be subtle if only the distal branches to the platysma muscle are affected.

KEY POINTS

1) The main trunk and branches of the facial nerve are evident below the zygomatic arch within the plane that includes the buccal fat pad, the parotid duct, and the facial artery and vein.

2) Anterior to the masseter muscle, the facial nerve branches lie deep to a discontinuous deep SMAS layer, interconnections cease between branches, and terminal nerve fibers become superficial and subject to injury.

3) The zygomatic and buccal branches of the facial nerve form the bulk of the facial nerve and traverse the cheek superficial to the buccal fat pad on their way to innervate the vast majority of the periocular and perioral mimetic musculature.

4) The frontal branch of the facial nerve is the smallest, has the least number of interconnections, and is a terminal branch in the vast majority of patients.

5) The marginal mandibular branch of the facial nerve lies deep to the platysma muscle and interconnects with other branches of the cervical division in only 10% to 15% of patients.

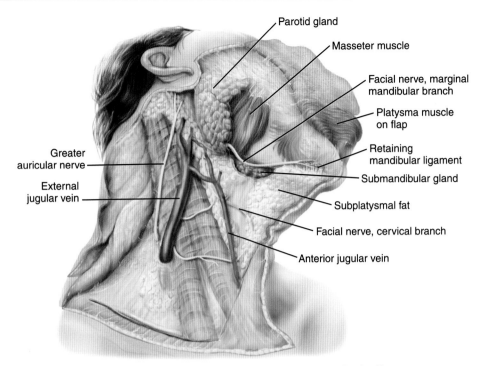

Parotid gland

Masseter muscle

Facial nerve, marginal
mandibular branch

Platysma muscle
on flap

Retaining
mandibular ligament

Submandibular gland

Subplatysmal fat

Facial nerve, cervical branch

Anterior jugular vein

Greater
auricular nerve

External
jugular vein

Figure 1-32 *Subfascial and subplatysmal anatomy of the neck. See text for details.*

THE FACIAL MUSCLES

The surgeon performing modern-day facial rejuvenation techniques requires an intimate knowledge of the musculature of the brow, midface, mouth, and neck. The facial muscles work in synchronous groups; when one group contracts, others pull in the opposite direction. Each muscle is made up of 75 to 150 fibrils, with each fibril "hardwired" into a filament of the facial nerve. Each fibril can contract independently and create facial movement. Over the years, repeated muscle action thrusts the skin into mimetic folds known as *Langer's lines*. The facial muscles are layered and interwoven into the superficial and deep facial fascias. Fibrous strands arising from the SMAS go to the skin surface and attach to the dermis, thereby allowing muscular contraction to create the myriad variations in facial expression.

The Periocular Muscles

The periocular muscles consist of the elevators and depressors of the eyebrow and forehead (Fig. 1-33). Eyelid musculature and anatomy are reviewed separately elsewhere.

The frontalis muscles are centrally situated in the forehead between the temporal lines of fusion within the superficial and deep planes of the galea. The skin of the forehead is firmly fixed to the dermis through multiple fibrous septa that pass from the epimysium of the muscle through the superficial fat in a tight honeycomb pattern. The frontalis muscle is the primary elevator of the eyebrow; when this muscle is hypertrophied, transverse forehead lines result. The frontalis muscle is innervated by the frontal branch of the facial nerve, which enters the muscle above the level of the superior orbital rim.

The corrugator supercilii muscles, along with the lateral orbicularis oculi muscles, antagonize the action of the frontalis muscles and are the primary depressors of the eyebrow. The corrugator muscles originate from the frontal bone near the superomedial orbital rim lateral to the origin of the procerus muscles (Fig. 1-34). The corrugator muscles insert into the dermis of the forehead skin above the middle third of the eyebrow. The corrugator passes through the galea fat pad and pierces the frontalis and orbicularis oculi en route to its dermal insertion. The corrugators are looped by the superficial and deep branches of the supraorbital nerve. The corrugators inferomedially depress the eyebrows, pull the eyebrows together, and pull the lateral aspect of the eyebrow into a more ptotic position. The corrugator muscles are considered to be the major determinant of vertical glabellar furrows. The motor nerve supply is a branch of the frontal branch of the facial nerve that enters the corrugator muscles before it pierces the frontalis muscles.

The procerus muscles originate in a paramedian location over the nasal bones considerably inferior and medial to the origin of the corrugator supercilii muscles (see Fig. 1-33). Like the corrugator and frontalis, the procerus is innervated by the frontal branch of the facial nerve. The procerus muscles have fibers that splay over the nasal dorsum. The procerus muscles are primarily responsible for the snarl expression, which heaps up the medial glabella and dorsal nasal skin. The procerus muscles also cause transverse glabella and root-of-the-nose furrows and lines. Similar to the corrugators, the procerus muscles are nearly looped by the superficial and deep branches of the supratrochlear nerve.

The orbicularis oculi muscle is a complex muscle with tarsal, palpebral, and orbital components. Whereas the tarsal and palpebral components close the eyelids, the orbital component depresses the eyebrows and elevates the lower eyelids, as during the protective eyelid reflex. The orbital component, along with the corrugator supercilii, antagonizes the action of the frontalis muscle and directly contributes to eyebrow ptosis, especially in the lateral temporal region. The innervation of the orbicularis oculi is complex and includes the frontal and zygomatic branches of the facial nerve.

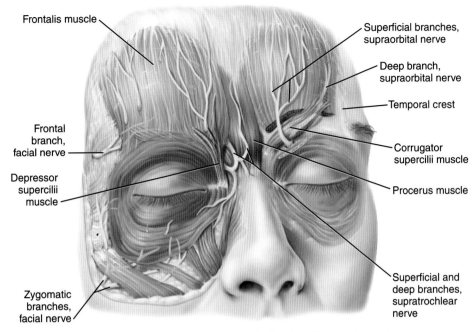

Figure 1-33 *Regional neuromuscular anatomy of the forehead and brow: external view.*

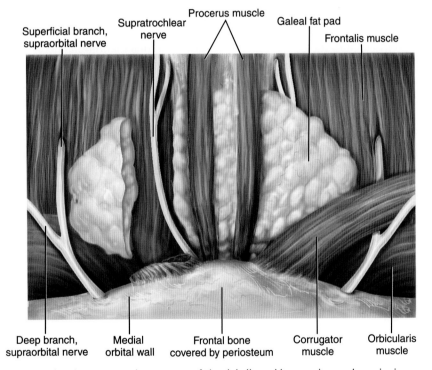

Figure 1-34 *Regional neuromuscular anatomy of the glabella and brow region: endoscopic view.*

The Perioral Muscles

The perioral muscles consist of elevators of the upper lip, elevators and depressors of the corner of the mouth, and depressors of the lower lip (Figs. 1-35 and 1-36). The cutaneous insertions of the four primary lip elevators—the zygomaticus major and minor and levator anguli oris and levator labii superioris muscles—form the nasolabial crease. The labiomandibular crease is determined primarily by the depressor anguli oris muscle, with minor contribution from the platysma.

The superficial perioral mimetic musculature includes the risorius, zygomaticus major, zygomaticus minor, platysma, depressor anguli oris, and the superficial head of the orbicularis oris. These muscles are invested by SMAS—that is, they have SMAS located on both their superficial and deep surfaces. The superficial perioral muscles are innervated along their deep surfaces by the zygomatic, buccal, marginal mandibular, and cervical branches of the facial nerve.

The zygomaticus major and zygomaticus minor are long thin muscles that arise from the body of the zygoma and insert into the musculature of the lateral portion of the upper lip. The zygomaticus major arises lateral to the minor on the zygoma and inserts into the extreme lateral recess of the upper lip. The zygomaticus minor is a shorter muscle and inserts into the midsection of the upper lip. These muscles, along with the levator anguli oris, when contracted produce the dominant zygomatic smile—the most common smile. The zygomaticus major and minor can be injured during deep-plane rhytidectomy procedures as a result of their superficial location in the cheek. These muscles are innervated primarily by the zygomatic branches of the facial nerve.

The risorius is a thin flat muscle that occasionally is just a continuation of the platysma. Because of the direction of the muscle fibers, the risorius can easily be confused with the zygomaticus major. It originates from the parotid fascia and inserts into the skin of the corner of the mouth. This muscle retracts the corner of the mouth laterally to produce a sardonic expression and allows "seal" in the corners of the mouth.

The platysma muscle is a large fan-shaped muscle arising from the cervical fascia in the upper deltoid and pectoral regions and inserting on the lower cheek and corner of the mouth along with the depressor musculature. The platysma and depressor labii inferioris are derived from the primitive sphincter coli muscles and have a common insertion on the modiolus of the mouth. The platysma musculature demonstrates tremendous anatomical variation and, when well developed, can be a strong depressor of the corner of the lower lip. The muscle is constantly active during talking, chewing, and swallowing and in facial expression. This muscle is also primarily responsible for the formation of neck bands and the common "turkey gobbler" deformity in the neck. This muscle is supplied mainly by the cervical branch of the facial nerve; however, not infrequently, branches from the marginal mandibular nerve supply the anterior portion of the platysma.

The depressor anguli oris is a large triangular-shaped muscle arising from the anterior mandibular border lateral to the mandibular ligaments and inserting on the modiolus at the corner of the mouth and lateral part of the lip. The fibers of this muscle are continuous with those of the orbicularis and risorius muscles. This muscle draws down the lower lip during facial expressions conveying sadness or exasperation.

THE PERIORAL MUSCLES

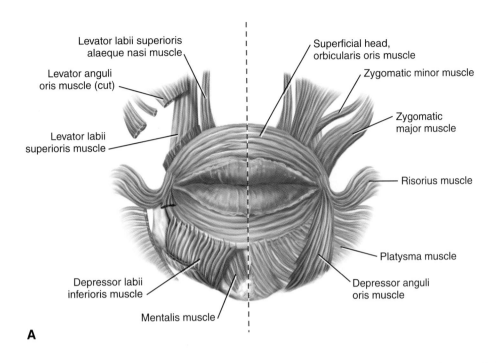

Levator labii superioris
alaeque nasi muscle

Levator anguli
oris muscle (cut)

Levator labii
superioris muscle

Superficial head,
orbicularis oris muscle

Zygomatic minor muscle

Zygomatic
major muscle

Risorius muscle

Platysma muscle

Depressor labii
inferioris muscle

Depressor anguli
oris muscle

Mentalis muscle

A

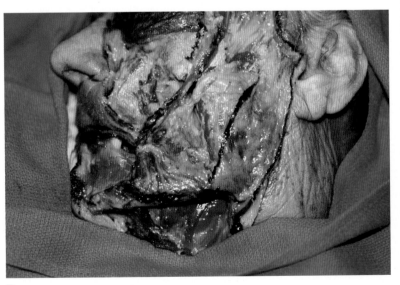

B

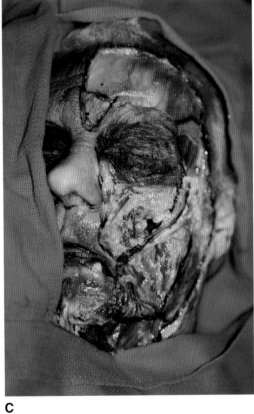

C

Figure 1-35   *Perioral musculature.* **A**, *Anterior view showing the layered relationship of the deep and superficial musculature. The superficial and deep layers account for the myriad movements of the lips.* **B** *and* **C**, *Photographs from cadaveric dissection with fat removed, revealing superficial and deep facial musculature.*

The orbicularis oris is a complex muscle with both superficial and deep portions. The superficial portion is a sling-shaped muscle superficial to the other muscles converging on the mouth. The superficial portion compresses the lips against the teeth. The deeper fibers are derived from the buccinator, thereby acting primarily to move the lips away from the teeth. The orbicularis oris is supplied by the buccal branch of the facial nerve and the marginal mandibular branch.

The deep perioral mimetic musculature includes the levator labii superioris, levator anguli oris, levator labii nasalis, depressor labii inferioris, the deep portion of the orbicularis oris, the buccinator, and the mentalis. These muscles are innervated along their superficial surfaces by the zygomatic, buccal, and marginal mandibular branches of the facial nerve.

The deep levator musculature of the upper lip includes the levator labii superioris, the levator anguli oris, and the levator labii superioris alaeque nasi. These muscles arise from the maxilla above the canine teeth and insert into the midportion of the upper lip. They exert a nearly vertical vector of pull on the upper lip. This action causes the canine smile—a smile that peaks over the canine teeth. The levator muscles are innervated primarily by the zygomatic and buccal branches of the facial nerve.

The depressor labii inferioris originates from the oblique line of the mandible and inserts with the orbicularis oris on the skin of the lower lip. The depressor labii inferioris lies deep and medial, and its fibers are nearly perpendicular to those of the depressor anguli oris. The depressor labii inferioris draws the lower lip down and laterally to evert the vermilion border of the lower lip.

The buccinator muscle is intertwined with the deeper fibers of the orbicularis oris. The buccinator muscle acts with the deep head of the orbicularis oris to move the lips away from the teeth but works primarily to compress the cheeks toward the teeth—the mechanism of suction. The buccal fat pad is deep to the buccinator and masseter muscle bellies. The orbicularis oris is supplied by the buccal branch of the facial nerve and the marginal mandibular branch.

The mentalis muscle arises from the mandible below the incisors and inserts into the skin of the chin. Contraction of the mentalis muscle protrudes the lower lip and wrinkles the skin of the chin.

KEY POINTS

1) The facial muscles are layered and interwoven into the superficial and deep facial fascias.
2) The facial muscles work in synchronous groups; when one group contracts, others pull in the opposite direction.
3) The periocular muscles consist of the elevators and depressors of the eyebrow and forehead: the frontalis, the corrugator supercilii, the procerus, and the orbital component of the orbicularis oculi.
4) The perioral muscles consist of elevators of the upper lip, elevators and depressors of the corner of the mouth, and depressors of the lower lip: the risorius, zygomaticus major, zygomaticus minor, platysma, depressor anguli oris, and the superficial and deep heads of the orbicularis oris, the levator labii superioris, levator anguli oris, levator labii nasalis, depressor labii inferioris, the buccinator, and the mentalis.

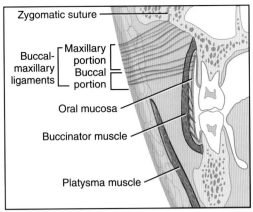

Zygomatic suture

Buccal-maxillary ligaments
Maxillary portion
Buccal portion

Oral mucosa

Buccinator muscle

Platysma muscle

Relationship between skin and oral mucosa via the buccal-maxillary ligaments

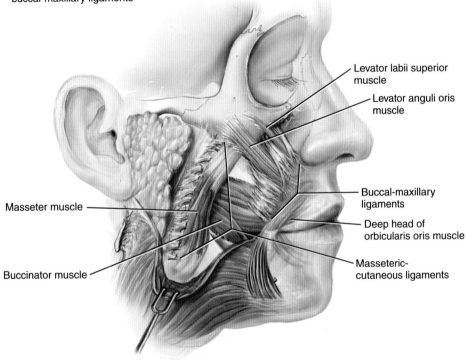

Levator labii superior muscle

Levator anguli oris muscle

Buccal-maxillary ligaments

Deep head of orbicularis oris muscle

Masseteric-cutaneous ligaments

Masseter muscle

Buccinator muscle

Figure 1-36   *Perioral musculature: lateral view. The cross-sectional anatomy of the buccal-maxillary retaining ligaments is shown in the inset.*

ARTERIAL SUPPLY

The arterial blood supply to the face and neck is provided by the external carotid artery. The arterial supply is arbitrarily divided into three zones based on anatomical landmarks (Fig. 1-37). The outer zone is the region lateral to a line drawn between the zygomaticofrontal suture and the mandibular notch. The central zone is medial to a line drawn between the supraorbital foramen and the maxillary first molar. The middle zone is between the outer and central zones.

The outer zone consists of the frontal branch of the superficial temporal, zygomatico-orbital, transverse facial, and masseteric arteries. The middle zone consists of the supraorbital, infraorbital, facial, submental, and middle and posterior jugal arteries. The central zone consists of the supratrochlear, dorsal nasal, angular, mental, and superior and inferior labial arteries.

Depending on the technique chosen, the facelift flap is supplied in large measure by sparsely populated fasciocutaneous perforating arteries. The areas of the facelift flap that are undermined routinely during rhytidectomy procedures correspond to the vascular territories supplied by the transverse facial, submental, facial, and superficial temporal arteries. The cutaneous location of the transverse facial artery is roughly 3 cm lateral and 4 cm inferior to the lateral canthus. This location corresponds to McGregor's patch. The cutaneous location of the submental artery is roughly 5.5 cm inferior and 3 cm lateral to the oral commissure. The cutaneous location of the frontal branch of the superficial temporal artery is 1 cm anterior to the root of the helix. The cutaneous location of the facial artery corresponds to the mandibular notch.

A majority of rhytidectomies performed worldwide involve subcutaneous and SMAS undermining. Subcutaneous elevation of the midface flap requires division of the zygomatic ligaments with consequent division of the transverse facial arterial contribution to the facelift flap. When undermining is extensive in the central facial region, the cutaneous contribution of the submental arteries is violated as well. Some surgeons also routinely ligate the superficial temporal arteries during the performance of the upper portion of the facial dissection. If the patient is a nonsmoker and subcutaneous dissection of the facelift flap is generous without being too thin, routine division of the transverse facial, submental, and frontal branch of the superficial temporal arterial contributions to the facelift flap can be carried out without consequent postauricular or preauricular skin flap necrosis. Adequate vascular supply is assured because of extensive collateralization from the central zone. The main contribution to the central zone is from the facial artery, which should not be encountered during routine SMAS rhytidectomy unless the dissection plane is inadvertently carried deep to the parotidomasseteric fascia. The facial vessels should never be ligated when the transverse facial, submental, and superficial temporal vessels have been divided, because the entire vascular supply to the facelift flap in these cases is derived from retrograde fill through the central zone contributions of the facial artery.

Of primary importance, choice of surgical rhytidectomy technique should be based on the anatomical defect intended to be corrected and not primarily on vascular considerations. A thorough knowledge of the vascular supply to the facelift flap is necessary, especially for procedures in patients who smoke, have vascular disorders, or have previously undergone facialplasty.

KEY POINTS

1) The arterial supply of the face and neck is divided into three zones: the outer zone is the region lateral to a line drawn between the zygomaticofrontal suture and the mandibular notch; the central zone is medial to a line drawn between the supraorbital foramen and the maxillary first molar; and the middle zone is between the outer and central zones.

2) The outer zone consists of the frontal branch of the superficial temporal, zygomatico-orbital, transverse facial, and masseteric arteries.

3) The middle zone consists of the supraorbital, infraorbital, facial, submental, and middle and posterior jugal arteries.

4) The central zone consists of the supratrochlear, dorsal nasal, angular, mental, and superior and inferior labial arteries.

5) Choice of surgical rhytidectomy technique should be based on the anatomical defect intended to be corrected and not primarily on vascular considerations.

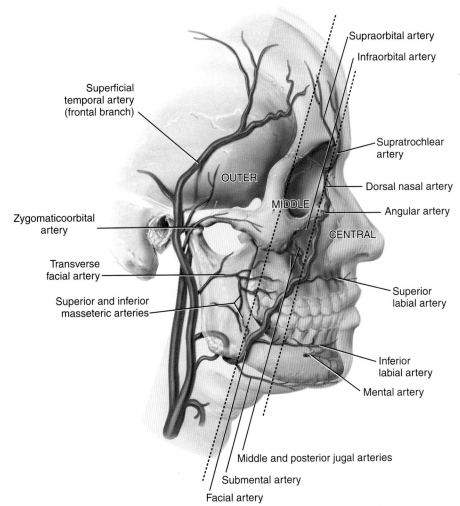

Figure 1-37 *The three zones of arterial anatomy of the face: central, middle, and outer.*

SENSORY SUPPLY

The sensory supply of the face and neck is primarily through branches of the trigeminal nerve and the cervical plexus (Fig. 1-38).

The trigeminal nerve (cranial nerve V) has three divisions. V1 terminates in five cutaneous branches: the supraorbital (superficial and deep), the supratrochlear and infratrochlear, and the external nasal and the lacrimal branches. V2 terminates in three cutaneous branches: the infraorbital, the zygomaticofacial, and the zygomatico-temporal. V3 terminates in three cutaneous branches: the mental, the buccal, and the auriculotemporal. The greater auricular nerve and the transverse cervical nerves are terminal cutaneous branches of C2 and C3, providing sensation to the auricle and anterior triangle of the neck, whereas the lesser occipital branches provide sensation to the posterior triangle of the neck.

The sensory supply of the face and neck is a rich network of communicating nerves that sprouts a nearly complete new network within several weeks to months after rhytidectomy, especially if the trunks of sensory nerve branches are preserved. Delayed return of sensory nerve function beyond 6 months after rhytidectomy is most commonly noted in the lateral cheek immediately anterior to the lobule of the ear, but not within the lobule of the ear. This region of the face is in a watershed zone between the territories provided by the zygomaticofacial, buccal, greater auricular, and transverse cervical nerve branches. Therefore, sensory return in this region of the face will take the longest after rhytidectomy.

The cutaneous landmark for the location of the greater auricular nerve is 6.5 cm directly inferior to the external acoustic meatus crossing the sternocleidomastoid muscle in an upwardly oblique direction. This nerve can be injured during undermining of the subcutaneous neck or platysma flap if the dissection violates the cervical fascia. If the greater auricular nerve is transected, repair should be performed; otherwise, permanent loss of sensation to the lobule and posterior auricle will result.

KEY POINTS

1) The sensory supply of the face and neck is primarily through branches of the trigeminal nerve and the cervical plexus.
2) If the greater auricular nerve is transected, repair should be performed immediately; otherwise, permanent sensory reduction in the lobule and posterior auricle will ensue.

Key References

Aiache A, Ramirez O: The suborbicularis oculi fat pads: Anatomic and clinical study. Plast Reconstr Surg 95:37, 1995.

Baker DC, Conley J: Avoiding facial nerve injuries in rhytidectomy. Plast Reconstr Surg 64:781, 1979.

Barton F, Gyimesi I: Anatomy of the nasolabial fold. Plast Reconstr Surg 100:1276, 1997.

Furnas D: The retaining ligaments of the face. Plast Reconstr Surg 83:11, 1989.

LaTrenta G, Raskin E: Why do we age in our cheeks? Presented at the 28th Annual Meeting of the American Society of Aesthetic Plastic Surgery, Las Vegas, May 27th, 2001.

Mitz V, Peyronie M: The superficial musculoaponeurotic system (SMAS) in the parotid and cheek area. Plast Reconstr Surg 58:80, 1976.

Pessa J, Garza P, Love V, et al: The anatomy of the labio-mandibular fold. Plast Reconstr Surg 101:482, 1998.

Rubin L: The anatomy of the nasolabial fold: The keystone of the smiling mechanism. Plast Reconstr Surg 103:687, 1999.

Stuzin J, Wagstrom L, Kawamoto H, Wolfe SA: Anatomy of the frontal branch of the facial nerve: The significance of the temporal fat pad. Plast Reconstr Surg 83:265, 1989.

Stuzin J, Baker T, Gordon H: The relationship of the superficial and deep facial fascias: Relevance to rhytidectomy and aging. Plast Reconstr Surg 89:441, 1992.

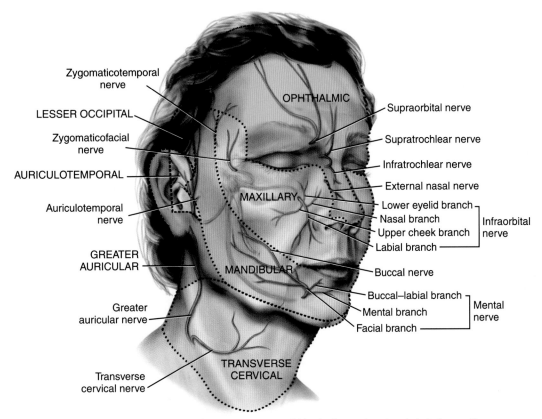

Figure 1-38 *The watershed zones of sensory anatomy within the face and neck: ophthalmic, maxillary, mandibular, and transverse cervical.*

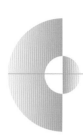

CHAPTER TWO

The Aging Face

Beauty is more than skin deep. And in the human face, aging, unfortunately, is as well. As plastic surgeons entering the second century of growth and development within our field, we have inherited powerful methods and tools to reverse the effects of aging. Yet as students entering the infancy of a new millennium of study, we are just beginning to understand what actually happens when someone ages. The fact that everyone ages in predictable patterns suggests that there are certain fundamental truths about anatomy we need to unravel before we embark upon our mission to restore a youthful appearance to our patients. And the simple question of why certain regions of the face and neck are genetically prone to aging is another we must answer. For in order to re-create beauty in the human face, we must grapple with its demise.

THEORIES OF AGING

The most commonly held theory is that facial aging is the result of *progressive gravimetric soft tissue descent.* Over time, the soft tissues of the face simply sag off the bones of the face, forming the distinctive wrinkles, furrows, folds, and eventual tissue redundancy of the aged face. Gravimetric soft tissue descent is complex, however, and encompasses several distinct processes.

One of the most important of these processes is *actinic damage or solar elastosis.* The net effect of extensive sun damage is that aging-type changes become evident in many women as early as their mid-20s, especially when there is a genetic or environmental predisposition. Wrinkles become apparent in a woman's skin in her mid-30s as estrogen levels begin to decline from their peak. The dermis begins to lose collagen and elastin, especially if the woman smoked or sunbathed without

sunscreen protection for much of her early life. By the latter half of her fourth decade, a woman's rate of renewal of skin cells begins to slow down. As a result, the epidermis becomes looser, and skin creases become organized in patterns perpendicular to the lines of muscle action. Mimetic lines and skin furrows result, especially if actinic damage continues unabated and skin care is poor. Eventually a thin, inelastic, and wrinkled skin envelope is produced. This aged skin sags when subjected to the push-pull forces of rapid weight gains and losses, which inevitably occur with pregnancy and with life's stresses. With the onset of menopause, as estrogen levels drop precipitously and relative levels of androgen increase, the dermis thins further, the epidermis becomes very irregular, and the hypodermal fat layer atrophies in later life. Blood flow to the dermis diminishes, contributing to further loosening of the epidermis and roughening of the texture of the skin. The skin inevitably begins to lose the ability to repair itself, becoming still drier and more brittle, and thinning even further. Redundancy, or the presence of skin folds, is the net result, and age spots develop when the capacity for self-repair diminishes.

In the fourth decade of life, the basal metabolic rate crests; thereafter, it begins to slow down by 4% to 5% a decade. This decreased metabolism makes it easier for a woman to put on weight, even if she maintains the same healthy diet and exercise regimen of her 20s. *Proportionate fat increases* occur in the face, along with the weight gain in the entire body, beginning around the fourth decade. Fatty tissue accumulation occurs in regions of the body called "depots," which are deep to the superficial fascia. These depots are in the abdomen, hips, thighs, and flanks. In the face and neck, similar depots are located around and under the eyes, in the anterior and middle cheeks, and under the chin.

Fat, unlike muscle, is supported solely by fascial ligaments. After years of being pulled and stretched, these fascial ligaments never regain their tautness. *Progressive fascial and ligamentous laxity* is an interrelated process that occurs with the proportionate fat increase to hasten the aging effect. Fat, along with its carrier of fascia, begins its long-dreaded sagging around the fourth decade in most women. As estrogen levels dwindle in the late 40s and plummet in the 50s and 60s, fat concentrates in deeply placed depots, yet it is paradoxically sacrificed in the hypodermis. The net result is thin, frail, lax skin that sags easily when subjected to the heavy drag and inferior descent of the laden deep fat pockets. Unlike the torso, which more often than not is shielded from actinic damage, the face and neck are the first to succumb. Sagging of all of the elements of the soft tissue, therefore, dominates the landscape.

Another, less obvious process that contributes to aging in the face and neck is *glandular tissue shrinkage.* The face and neck have the highest concentrations of glandular and lymphatic tissue in the body. Glandular tissue accounts for much of the firmness of the youthful face. With age, the glandular tissues of the face and neck shrink and shrivel, and the soft tissues subsequently lose their firmness. This effect becomes especially apparent when estrogen levels fall at around the time of menopause.

Photoaging; progressive laxity and ptosis of the facial fat, fascia, musculature, and ligaments; and glandular shrinkage combine to produce the constellation of subcutaneous soft tissue redundancy we recognize as the "aged" face. Specific regions of the face and neck age in predictable patterns because of the uniqueness of their anatomical relationships. For example, ptosis of the midfacial fat pads, combined with laxity of the midface retaining ligaments and actinic elastosis of and photodamage to the midfacial skin envelope, causes cheek folds, jowls, a deep nasolabial fold, and a submalar hollow. Ptosis and progressive lengthening of the orbicularis oculi musculature from repeated squinting, actinic elastosis of and photodamage to the periorbital skin envelope, and progressive laxity of the orbital retaining ligaments and septa cause "crow's feet," lower eyelid

"bags," and festoons. Ptosis and progressive lengthening and attenuation of the platysma musculature, loss of mandibular ligamentous support, solar elastosis and photodamage in the neck, and accumulation of submental fat cause the familiar-appearing "turkey gobbler neck" deformity with its distinctive neck folds, platysma bands, and "waddy," floppy soft tissue.

Another less obvious and more insidious process that can contribute to facial aging is *skeletal resorption* of the anterior facial skeleton. Skeletal resorption is primarily the result of progressive osteoporosis—the loss of a third or more of bone density. Half of all women older than the age of 50 suffer from osteoporosis. Skeletal resorption of the anterior maxilla and mandible is a common manifestation of osteoporosis, which also is a leading cause of loss of dentition. Skeletal resorption in the pyriform region of the maxilla leads to the commonly observed decrease in the nasolabial angle and the dreaded "droopy nose" of aging. Skeletal resorption in the inferior orbital rim, especially in men, lengthens and sags the rim inferolaterally. This contributes to the commonly observed "aged orbit," with its clinical manifestations of lateral orbital tear-trough, lateral canthal bowing, and inferior and lateral scleral show.

KEY POINTS

1) Facial aging is the result of progressive gravitational descent of soft tissue.
2) Aging becomes apparent in a woman's skin in her mid-30s as the dermis loses collagen and elastin from progressive actinic damage and solar elastosis.
3) With the onset of menopause, as estrogen levels decrease and androgen levels increase, the dermis thins, the epidermis becomes quite irregular, the hypodermal fat layer atrophies, and the deep fat layer hypertrophies.
4) Fat, unlike muscle, is supported solely by fascial ligaments, which after years of being pulled and stretched never regain their tautness.
5) Much of the firmness of the youthful face is caused by a high concentration of glandular tissue, which shrinks and shrivels with aging.
6) Skeletal resorption of the anterior facial skeleton, especially in the pyriform and inferior orbital rim regions, contributes to the appearance of the aged face.

WRINKLES

Textural changes in the skin have been classified (Fig. 2-1). Fine superficial lines in the skin are commonly referred to as *wrinkles*. Superficial lines are discrete at first and then, over time, become grouped and multidirectional. When wrinkles become associated with textural changes in the surface of the skin from photodamage and repeated facial and neck muscular contraction, they are called *mimetic lines*. When mimetic creasing extends into the dermis, *skin furrows* become apparent. When skin becomes overlapped and redundant from all of these processes, *skin folds* become apparent.

The primary causes of wrinkles are *dermal elastosis* and *repeated facial and neck muscular contraction*. Wrinkles can become mimetic when they develop perpendicular to the direction of a dominant underlying facial muscle. Glabellar wrinkles result from repeated frowning through contraction of the underlying corrugator supercilii and procerus muscles. Periorbital wrinkles and crow's feet result from repeated squinting through contraction of the underlying orbicularis oculi and zygomaticus major and minor muscles. Dermal elastosis has both an extrinsic cause—actinic damage—and an intrinsic cause—genetic inheritance. Wrinkles are the sine qua non for aging.

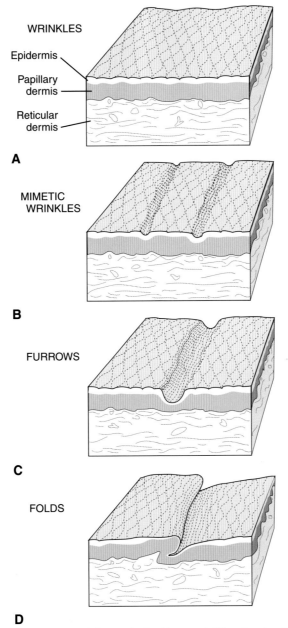

WRINKLES

Epidermis

Papillary
dermis

Reticular
dermis

A

MIMETIC
WRINKLES

B

FURROWS

C

FOLDS

D

Figure 2-1 *Textural changes in the skin:* ***A,*** *wrinkling;* ***B,*** *mimetic wrinkles;* ***C,*** *skin furrows;* ***D,*** *skin folds.*

Wrinkles have been classified according to location, depth, and severity (Fig. 2-2). Transverse lines in the forehead perpendicular to the frontalis muscle are called "worry lines." Oblique lines in the glabella perpendicular to the corrugator muscle and transverse lines at the root of the nose perpendicular to the procerus muscle are called "frown lines." Lateral periorbital lines perpendicular to the orbicularis oculi muscle are commonly referred to as "crow's feet." The dominant "smile" line in the anterior cheek, which is perpendicular to the zygomaticus muscles, is called the nasolabial line. Oblique lines in the anterior and middle cheek that run parallel to the nasolabial line are called "cheek lines." Oblique lines in the lateral cheek that are anterior to the ear and perpendicular to the platysma muscle are called "preauricular lines." Lines in the upper and lower lip that run perpendicular to the orbicularis oris muscle and bleed into the vermilion of the lip are called "lip lines." Lines running from the corner of the mouth down into the jowl are called "marionette lines." These lines parallel the depressor anguli oris muscle and run perpendicular to the platysma muscle. More commonly, however, small lines in the corner of the mouth, called "commissural lines," are noted. Curvilinear lines in the labiomental crease perpendicular to the mentalis muscle are called "chin lines." Half-moon slivers running nearly halfway around the neck perpendicular to the platysma muscle are called "transverse neck lines."

Skin folds are overlapped subcutaneous tissue. Skin folds have numerous causes. Progressive gravitational descent of genetically prone facial and neck soft tissues can make a line or a furrow into a skin fold. Rapid weight gain or loss, which stretches the subcutaneous fascial system beyond its elastic capacity and thereby creates tissue laxity, also contributes to the creation of skin folds. Excessive muscle tone may also produce skin folds, as is commonly seen when frontalis muscle hypertrophy dominates the forehead, creating the "corrugated" forehead. Paradoxically, poor muscle tone also creates skin folds. This phenomenon is commonly noted in patients with long, stretched-out sheets of platysma muscle in the neck, which band and double over on themselves, creating the turkey gobbler neck deformity. Excessive anterior maxillary and pyriform bone loss, especially coupled with lengthened and ptotic orbicularis oris muscles and thinned upper lip skin, also creates perioral and commissural skin folds.

From a therapeutic standpoint it is important to differentiate lines and furrows from skin folds. Mimetic lines and furrows respond well to multimodality therapy. Techniques include use of injectable fillers (e.g., collagen or fat), botulinum toxin injections, selective muscle interruption (e.g., corrugator and procerus muscle division or resection), and laser resurfacing. Mimetic lines and furrows do not respond well to laser resurfacing alone. Skin folds, however, demand surgical tightening procedures, such as blepharoplasty, brow lift, and facelift, for optimal therapy. Selective use of alloplastic augmentation, with occasional bone grafting or osteotomy, is also advisable when periocular and perioral skin folds predominate on the basis of bone loss. Wrinkles, mimetic wrinkles, skin furrows, and skin folds are simultaneously present in the majority of patients who seek facial and neck rejuvenation. Hence, a combination of surgical and nonsurgical therapy is advisable in most patients to achieve optimal results.

KEY POINTS

1) Fine superficial lines in the skin are commonly referred to as wrinkles.
2) Deep wrinkles that are perpendicular to the line of repeated facial and neck muscular contraction are called mimetic lines.
3) Skin furrows are mimetic lines that extend into the papillary dermis.
4) When mimetic lines and furrows extend into deep dermis and the skin becomes overlapped and redundant, they are called skin folds.
5) Wrinkles, mimetic lines, and skin furrows require multimodality therapy.
6) Skin folds require surgical tightening procedures, such as blepharoplasty, brow lift, and facelift.

WRINKLES

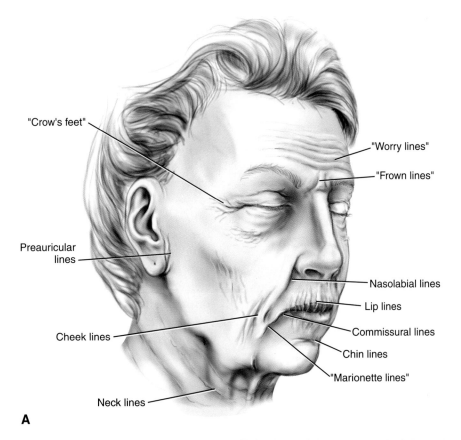

"Crow's feet"

"Worry lines"

"Frown lines"

Preauricular lines

Nasolabial lines

Lip lines

Commissural lines

Cheek lines

Chin lines

"Marionette lines"

Neck lines

A

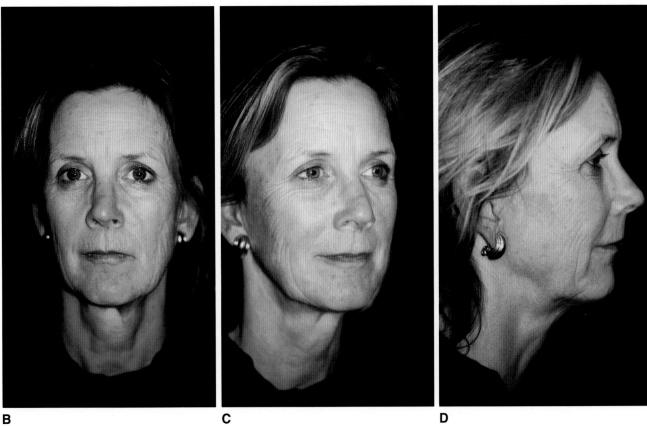

B **C** **D**

Figure 2-2   A, The commonly seen facial wrinkles. B–D, The various types of wrinkles as seen in a 54-year-old prospective patient.

FACIAL SOFT TISSUE FOUNDATIONS

The facial soft tissues sag from the foundations of the craniofacial skeleton in a very specific manner. The craniofacial skeleton is a broad and mostly smooth surface of bone. A thick netting of periosteum covers the craniofacial skeleton. This periosteum is tightly adherent to the craniofacial skeleton at specific sites—the sutural interfaces. The facial subcutaneous tissue and fascia should be thought of as an extremely intricate extension of this netting, supported primarily through condensations of the netting at the sutural interfaces. This system of suspension is called the *true retaining ligament* system.

The craniofacial skeleton has several intricate and finely chiseled cavities etched into its ornate surface. Besides the orbit and nasal cavities, there is the complex oral cavity. Unlike the orbit, which is filled by the globe and its supporting network of ligaments, muscles, and soft tissue, the oral cavity is an essentially hollow structure. This hollowness is necessary for the oral cavity to perform the vital functions of speech, mastication, respiration, and facial expression. The soft tissue covering of the oral cavity includes two major facial aesthetic subunits: the lips and the cheeks. The lips are supported primarily by strong periosteal tethers along the pyriform apertures and the mandibular ridge. The cheeks, however, are supported primarily by condensations of the superficial to the deep facial fascias. This weaker system of facial soft tissue suspension is called the *false retaining ligament* system and accounts in large measure for the clinical manifestations of facial aging.

The true and false retaining ligament systems form the soft tissue foundations of the face and neck and are the keys to understanding facial aging. The true retaining ligaments are fibrous strands no greater than 1 cm^2 in cross section that run from the dermis through to the periosteum of the craniofacial skeleton. The true retaining ligaments represent the masonry columns of support for the subcutaneous tissues of the face and neck (Fig. 2-3). As discussed in the previous chapter, the true retaining ligaments are located at four key locations: the zygomaticofrontal suture for suspension of the forehead and eyebrow, the zygomaticotemporal suture for suspension of the lateral and middle face, the juncture of the anterior and middle thirds of the mandibular body for suspension of the lower face and upper neck, and the zygomaticomaxillary suture for suspension of the anterior face.

SOFT TISSUE FOUNDATIONS
The four true ligaments –
Greek pillars of strength

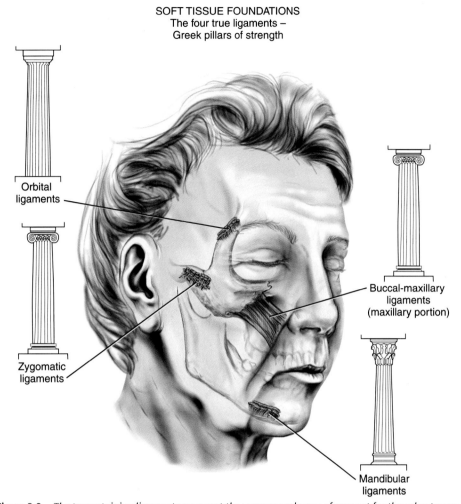

Orbital ligaments

Zygomatic ligaments

Buccal-maxillary ligaments (maxillary portion)

Mandibular ligaments

Figure 2-3   *The true retaining ligaments represent the masonry columns of support for the subcutaneous tissues of the face.*

The false retaining ligaments are arranged much like "fences"—broad swathes of superficial to deep fascial attachment similar to Velcro patches. As noted in Chapter 1, the false retaining ligaments are located at three key locations. In the anterior cheek, the "fence" is parallel and lateral to the nasolabial fold—the buccal-maxillary ligaments. In the middle cheek, the "fence" is parallel to the anterior border of the masseter muscle—the masseteric-cutaneous ligaments. In the posterior cheek, the "fence" is parallel to the angle of the mandible—the platysma-auricular ligaments.

The fascial supports of the cheek have various properties (Fig. 2-4). The posterior platysma-auricular ligaments are strong and broad, resembling a stone wall more than a fence. The platysma-auricular ligaments provide the cheeks with a broad band of strong lateral fixation to the underlying parotid gland and mandible. This "stone wall" is especially evident during subcutaneous rhytidectomy, when one encounters an unusual amount of skin adherence in the soft tissue dissection around the lobule of the ear, as well as during elevation of the lateral portion of the platysma muscle in performing a lateral platysmaplasty. The midcheek masseteric-cutaneous ligaments are multiple and knifelike, resembling a picket fence. The masseteric-cutaneous ligaments hold the middle cheek tightly to the masseter muscle and provides the soft tissue support necessary for mastication. This "picket fence" is especially evident during extended superficial musculoaponeurotic system (SMAS) rhytidectomy, when one encounters the parotidomasseteric fascia anterior to the parotid gland. The anterior buccal-maxillary ligaments are long, loose, and elastic, resembling a chain link fence. This anterior "fence" is extensible, allowing for the subtle glide and fine motor movements of facial expression and speech. This "chain link fence" is especially evident during the intraoral portion of a subperiosteal rhytidectomy, when one places intraoral sutures for fixation of the midface to the temporal fascia.

SOFT TISSUE FOUNDATIONS
False Ligaments

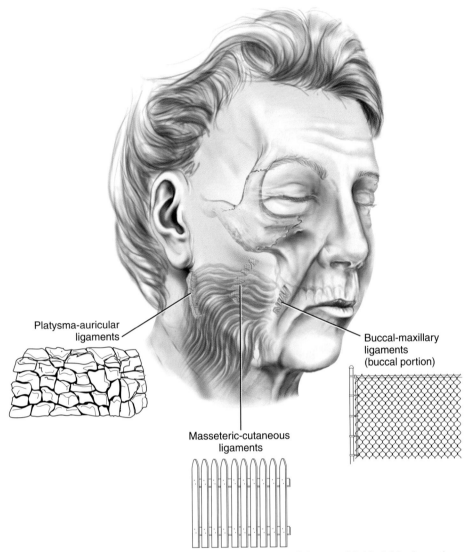

Platysma-auricular
ligaments

Masseteric-cutaneous
ligaments

Buccal-maxillary
ligaments
(buccal portion)

Figure 2-4 *The false retaining ligaments represent a coalescence of the superficial facial fascias to the deep facial fascias in the midface. They are arranged like walls or fences, each with its own unique properties.*

Studies have shown that the cheek has the highest concentration of fat in the face and neck, accounting for roughly half of total facial and neck fat. Most of this fat is located in the anterior and middle cheek regions—a full one third of total facial and neck fat. The cheeks are hollow structures, with skin, fat, and superficial fascia secured primarily to the deep fascia by the weaker false retaining system that exists within its confines. Along its borders, the cheeks are also secondarily secured to the craniofacial skeleton at the stronger true retaining ligaments through guidewire SMAS tethers. This cheek suspensory system resembles a trampoline, whose center sags significantly away from the supporting bars at the periphery (Fig. 2-5)—the greater the amount of solar elastosis, progressive fascial and ligamentous laxity, and proportionate fat increase in the cheeks, the worse the sagging. And when this sagging soft tissue is subjected to the force of gravity, the nagging signs of aging—a deep nasolabial groove and heavy nasolabial fold, cheek lines, jowls, flaccid cheeks and a turkey gobbler neck line—become painfully obvious.

With aging, the false retaining ligaments, like Cooper's ligaments in the breast, get stretched and pulled beyond their elastic potential. Under gravity's force, the clinical signs of progressive fascial laxity become most evident in the anterior cheeks. The primary cause is laxity of the anterior buccal-fascial ligaments and, to a lesser extent, the midcheek parotid-masseteric ligaments. The characteristic inferolateral descent of facial soft tissues then becomes evident, with anterior bunching of fat lateral to the nasolabial and oromandibular grooves, development of cheek lines, and jowl formation.

KEY POINTS

1) The facial subcutaneous tissues and fascia are extensions of an extremely intricate netting that is suspended from the periosteal covering of the craniofacial skeleton at the three key sutural interfaces called true retaining ligaments.
2) The cheeks, which are hollow and cover the oral cavity, are supported primarily by condensations of the superficial to deep facial fascias at three key locations called false retaining ligaments.
3) The true retaining ligaments, located in the upper, middle, and lower face, represent the masonry columns of support for the subcutaneous tissues in the face and neck.
4) The false retaining ligaments, located in the anterior, middle, and posterior cheek, are broad, fencelike attachments of the superficial to the deep fascia.

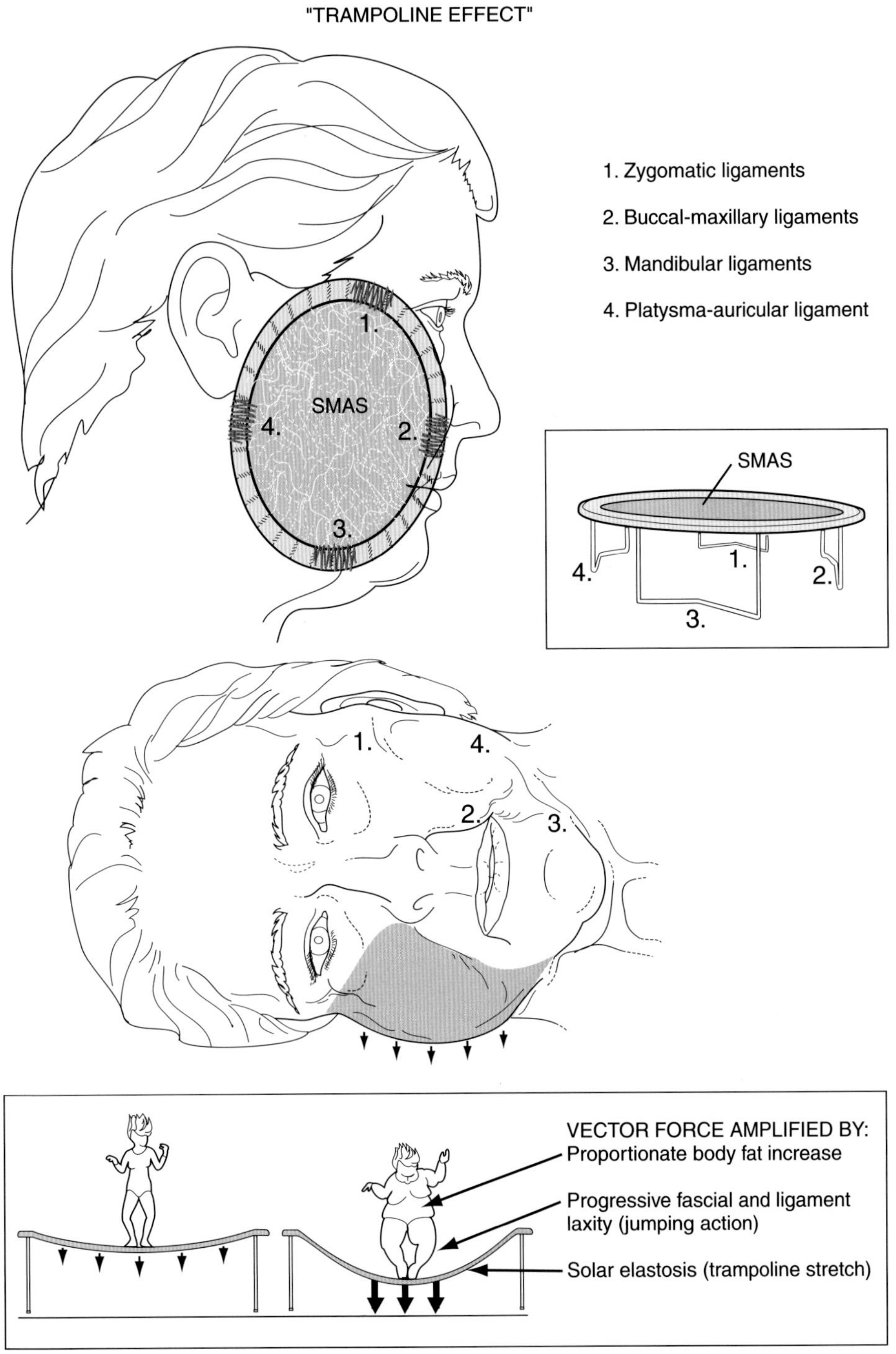

"TRAMPOLINE EFFECT"

1. Zygomatic ligaments

2. Buccal-maxillary ligaments

3. Mandibular ligaments

4. Platysma-auricular ligament

SMAS

SMAS

VECTOR FORCE AMPLIFIED BY:
Proportionate body fat increase

Progressive fascial and ligament laxity (jumping action)

Solar elastosis (trampoline stretch)

Figure 2-5 *The trampoline effect of midfacial aging. The soft tissues of the midface and cheek can be thought of as the elastic netting of a trampoline that is suspended from the bones of the face by four main supporting legs. The more the trampoline is subjected to the effects of solar skin elastosis, progressive fascial and ligamentous laxity, and proportionate fat increases, the more the trampoline of the midface sags.*

THE AREOLAR PLANES

Why do the face and neck sag so reproducibly in predictable patterns? Much of the answer to this question lies in the fact that the subcutaneous tissues in the face and neck, and in much of the human body for that matter, are composed of both superficial and deep layers of fascia. This double layering allows for a more tightly held and uniform exterior layer of superficial fat and a more loosely held and extensible interior layer of deep fat. The relationship between these two layers of fascia is complex over various regions of the body. Over joints and bony prominences, especially where sutures are located, the superficial and deep fascias are densely adherent to one another, as evidenced by the tight adherence of skin and subcutaneous tissues in these regions. In contrast, over broad periosteal surfaces and broad sheets of muscle and fascia, the superficial and deep fascias are loosely adherent, allowing for the elasticity of movement. Loosely adherent fascial separations are called *areolar planes*. The clinical significance of areolar planes is that the overlying soft tissues preferentially become ptotic over areas characterized by loosely adherent areolar planes, especially when the overlying subcutaneous tissues in these regions is heavily laden with deep fat collections.

In the forehead and brow region, this areolar plane has been termed the glide plane space (Fig. 2-6). The glide plane space is filled with loose areolar tissue and exists within subdivisions of the deep galea planes. The deep galea planes become adherent and fixed to periosteum at the level of the superior orbital rims and nasofrontal junction. This zone of adherence obliterates the glide plane space of the forehead, but, more important, becomes a cantilever type of support for the glabella, eyebrows, and forehead soft tissue. With progressive gravitational descent of the forehead, the eyebrows literally pivot and bunch up on themselves at this level. This accounts for what is commonly called *brow ptosis*. A similar process also occurs in the glabella and lateral eyebrow regions, although at a lower level relative to the superior orbital rims. In the glabella region, the glide plane space becomes obliterated, and periosteum becomes adherent at the level of the nasofrontal junction. This accounts for the fact that with progressive gravitational descent of the forehead and glabella tissue, glabella excess becomes apparent as a soft tissue bulge between the superior half of the orbits. In the lateral brow region, the orbital retaining ligaments confer strong adherence of the dermis to the lateral orbital rim at the zygomaticofrontal interface. These retaining ligaments also support the temporal soft tissue mass. The glide plane space obliteration and periosteal adherence follows the downward curvature of the lateral orbital rim level. With progressive gravitational descent of the temporal, lateral eyebrow, and forehead soft tissues, a canopy effect on the lateral eyebrow develops. This effect can easily be confused with hooded upper eyelid skin if one is not careful. In some cases, this lateral eyebrow ptosis becomes so dominant that the affected tissues abut the lower eyelid; when combined with a generous skin fold in the upper eyelid, this can obscure the superior field of vision.

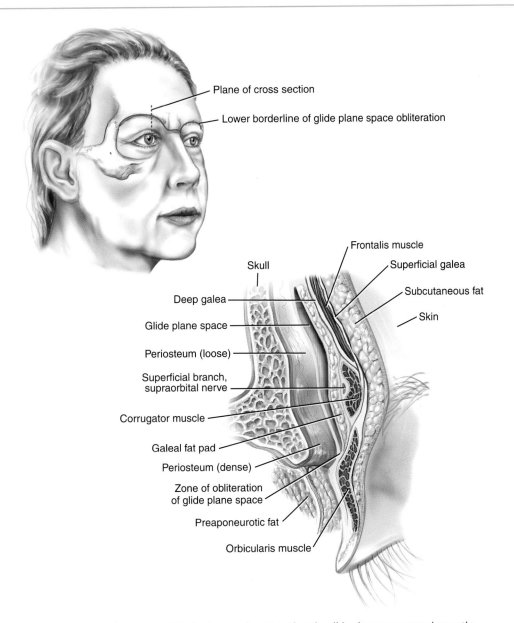

Plane of cross section

Lower borderline of glide plane space obliteration

Frontalis muscle

Superficial galea

Subcutaneous fat

Skin

Skull

Deep galea

Glide plane space

Periosteum (loose)

Superficial branch, supraorbital nerve

Corrugator muscle

Galeal fat pad

Periosteum (dense)

Zone of obliteration of glide plane space

Preaponeurotic fat

Orbicularis muscle

Figure 2-6   *The areolar planes of the forehead region. Note that the glide plane space extends over the glabella, forehead, and eyebrows and is obliterated at the level of the superior orbital rims and nasofrontal junction.*

In the temporal region, a broad and well-defined areolar plane exists between the temporoparietal fascia and the superficial layer of deep temporal fascia (Fig. 2-7). This plane extends over the entire temporal region, inferiorly as far as the zygomatic arch and anteriorly as far as the temporal line of fusion. With progressive gravitational descent of the temporal soft tissues, the weight and mass of soft tissue become evident as a lateral bunching of the periorbital "crow's feet," ptosis of the lateral eyebrows, and upper eyelid pseudoptosis and hooding (Fig. 2-8*A–D*). In extreme cases, temporal hollowing even becomes evident.

In the lower orbital and cheek regions, an areolar plane exists between the superficial fascia (SMAS) and the deep fascia (parotidomasseteric fascia) (see Fig. 2-7). This areolar plane becomes ill defined along the anterior border of the masseter muscle, where the facial nerve branches penetrate through the masseteric-cutaneous ligaments to innervate the perioral musculature. With progressive gravitational descent of the overlying lower orbital and cheek compartments, the clinical signs of aging become apparent: malar and eyelid bags, skeletonization of the zygoma, submalar hollowing, and anterior cheek bunching of soft tissues anterior to the nasolabial fold and in the jowls (see Fig. 2-8*A–D*).

In the neck region, an areolar plane exists between the platysma muscle and the underlying deep cervical investing fascia (see Fig. 2-7). The subplatysmal plane is a broad areolar plane extending anteriorly as far as the medial border of the platysma muscle, superiorly almost to the midcheek level, and inferiorly over the clavicles. With progressive gravitational descent and dragging of the heavy overlying preplatysmal fat and soft tissue compartments, the clinical signs of lower face and neck aging become apparent: jowl formation, platysma banding, and submental and neck transverse creasing (see Fig. 2-8*A–D*).

KEY POINTS

1) The subcutaneous tissues of the face and neck, and of much of the human body, are composed of both superficial and deep layers of fascia.
2) Over joints and bony prominences, especially where sutures are located, the superficial and deep fascias are densely adherent to one another.
3) Over broad periosteal surfaces and over broad sheets of muscle and fascia, the superficial and deep fascias are loosely adherent.
4) Soft tissues preferentially become ptotic in regions of the body characterized by loosely adherent areolar planes, especially when these overlying regions of subcutaneous tissue are heavily laden with superficial and deep fat collections.
5) Areolar planes exist in specific locations of the lower forehead and eyebrow regions, in the temporal region, in the anterior and middle cheek, and in the subplatysmal region of the lower face and neck.

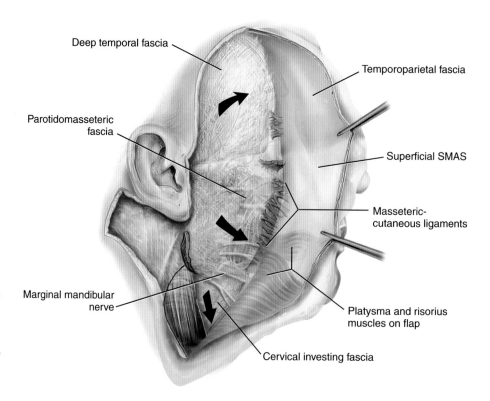

Figure 2-7   *The areolar planes of the temporal, midface, and neck regions. In the temporal region, the areolar plane exists between the temporoparietal fascia and the deep temporal fascia. In the midface, the areolar plane exists between the superficial SMAS and the parotidomasseteric fascia. In the neck, the areolar plane exists between the cervical investing fascia and the platysma.*

Deep temporal fascia

Temporoparietal fascia

Parotidomasseteric fascia

Superficial SMAS

Masseteric-cutaneous ligaments

Marginal mandibular nerve

Platysma and risorius muscles on flap

Cervical investing fascia

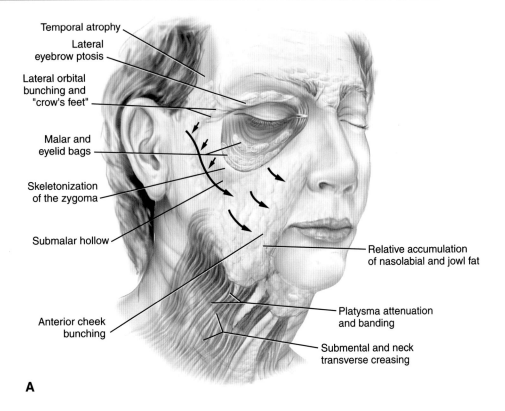

Temporal atrophy

Lateral eyebrow ptosis

Lateral orbital bunching and "crow's feet"

Malar and eyelid bags

Skeletonization of the zygoma

Submalar hollow

Anterior cheek bunching

Relative accumulation of nasolabial and jowl fat

Platysma attenuation and banding

Submental and neck transverse creasing

A

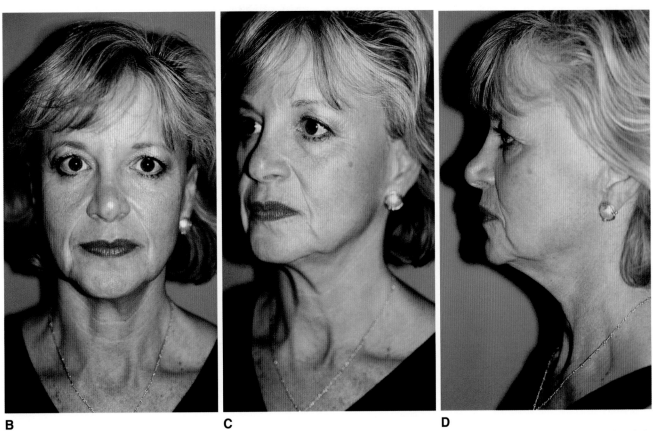

B   **C**   **D**

Figure 2-8   **A,** *Progressive gravitational descent of soft tissues in the face and neck.* **B–D,** *Many of the characteristic features are evident in this 55-year-old prospective patient.*

REGIONAL ANATOMY

From a surgical perspective, aging is best understood when the face and neck are divided into three regions: (1) the upper face, consisting of the forehead, glabella, temporal, eyebrow, and upper eyelid regions; (2) the midface, consisting of the lower eyelid, anterior, middle, and posterior cheek, and upper lip regions; and (3) the lower face and neck, consisting of the lower lip and chin, submental, and anterior neck regions. Anatomical concepts of aging in these three regions is best understood when commonly used or "lay" descriptions—such as "crow's feet" and "marionette lines"—are contrasted against the subcutaneous, muscular, and ligamentous forces responsible for their creation—in these cases, orbicularis oculi lengthening and midfacial fat ptosis, respectively (Figs. 2-9 to 2-11).

The Upper Face

Several anatomical forces are directly responsible for production of the characteristic features of the aged upper face (see Fig. 2-9A, B). Frontalis muscle lengthening and thickening cause "worry lines" or horizontal forehead lines, which can range from minor mimetic lines to deeply corrugated furrows and even skin folds. Procerus or corrugator muscle hypertrophy causes "frown lines," which can be oriented in an oblique (corrugator) or a transverse (procerus) direction. As with horizontal forehead lines, glabellar lines can range from minor mimetic wrinkles to deep furrows and folds that can extend into the reticular dermis. In the upper periorbital region, orbicularis muscle and orbital septum attenuation and ptosis along with resultant orbital fat pad pseudo-herniation cause "crow's feet," hooding of the eyelids, and upper eyelid "bags."

The etiology of brow ptosis is complex. In the upper two thirds of the forehead, a fibrous connective tissue bond exists between the deep galea and the subgalea periosteum, inhibiting soft tissue descent. The lower third of the forehead, which includes the eyebrows, does not have this bond. The result is greater lower forehead mobility. The lower forehead skin, including the eyebrows, galea fat pad, and inferior frontalis muscle, descends over time, especially if the patient is a "frowner"—depressor muscle tone (corrugator and procerus muscles) exceeds elevator muscle tone (frontalis muscle). Reciprocally, the antagonist elevator musculature of the brow (frontalis muscle) works overtime in an effort to raise the descended eyebrows, with resultant hypertrophy, especially if the patient is a "worrier." This causes transverse forehead furrows. Gravitational descent of the unsupported temporal tissue mass over the temporalis fascia contributes to lateral eyebrow ptosis, pseudoexcess of upper eyelid skin, upper eyelid skin hooding, and bunching of lateral orbital skin along the lines of the "crow's feet." Finally, in cases of extreme aging, descent of the superficial and deep temporal fat pads results in upper temporal hollowing.

KEY POINTS

1) Frontalis muscle lengthening and thickening cause "worry lines" or horizontal forehead lines.

2) Procerus or corrugator muscle hypertrophy causes "frown lines," which can be oriented in either an oblique (corrugator) or a transverse (procerus) direction.

3) Orbicularis muscle and orbital septum attenuation and ptosis, along with orbital fat pad pseudoherniation, cause "crow's feet," hooding of the eyelids, and upper eyelid "bags."

4) The tissue of the lower forehead, which includes the eyebrows, galea fat pad, and inferior frontalis muscle, is loosely adherent and descends when depressor muscle tone (corrugator and procerus muscles) overwhelms elevator muscle tone (frontalis muscle).

5) Gravitational descent of the unsupported temporal tissue mass over the temporalis fascia contributes to lateral eyebrow ptosis, pseudoexcess of upper eyelid skin, upper eyelid skin hooding, and bunching together of lateral orbital skin along the lines of the "crow's feet."

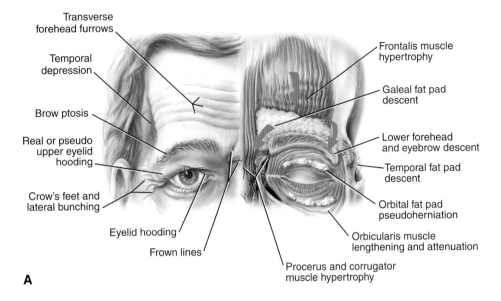

Transverse forehead furrows

Temporal depression

Brow ptosis

Real or pseudo upper eyelid hooding

Crow's feet and lateral bunching

Eyelid hooding

Frown lines

Procerus and corrugator muscle hypertrophy

Frontalis muscle hypertrophy

Galeal fat pad descent

Lower forehead and eyebrow descent

Temporal fat pad descent

Orbital fat pad pseudoherniation

Orbicularis muscle lengthening and attenuation

A

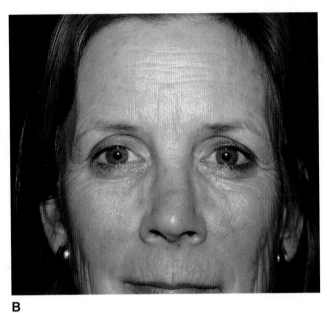

B

Figure 2-9   *Regional anatomy of the aged upper face. **A,** Anatomical concepts of facial and neck aging are contrasted with the subcutaneous, muscular, and ligamentous forces responsible for their creation. **B,** Many of the characteristic changes are evident in this 54-year-old prospective patient.*

The Midface

Several anatomical forces are directly responsible for production of the characteristic features of the aged midface (see Fig. 2-10A–C). In the lower periorbital region, orbicularis muscle, lower canthus, and orbital septum, attenuation and lengthening cause ptosis and pseudoherniation of the orbital fat pads and the sub-orbicularis oculi fat pad (SOOF). This results in lower canthal bowing, lower eyelid "bags" and wrinkles, and malar "bags." Malar bags, or festoons, can be differentiated from eyelid bags because they occur below the level of the inferior orbital rim. Malar bags represent ptosis of the SOOF.

Loss of midfacial retaining ligament cheek support results in anteroinferior descent of midface subcutaneous fat. This causes a relative accumulation of anterior and inferior cheek fat and relative loss of lateral and superior cheek fat. Because fat does not cross the nasolabial line as a result of the dense fascia-to-dermis adherence within the fold, the net effect of midface fat descent is (1) a deep nasolabial groove, (2) a heavy nasolabial fold, (3) multiple folds of cheek skin lateral to the nasolabial fold, (4) a "skeletonized" appearance of the cheekbone, and (5) a submalar hollow.

Attenuation and lengthening of the major circumferential perioral muscle, the orbicularis oris muscle, occur with aging, just as they occur with the major circumferential periorbital muscle, the orbicularis oculi muscle.

Coupled with upper lip dermal atrophy from photoaging and repeated muscular contraction, especially if the patient is a smoker, vertical lengthening of the upper lip results, along with upper lip lines. Upper lip lines can range from minor indents above the white roll to multiple vertical and oblique drapery-like lines that can extend from the vermilion of the lip nearly to the alar and nasolabial grooves. Upper lip lengthening is exacerbated by anterior maxillary and pyriform thinning from osteoporosis, as well as loss of maxillary dentition. This results in clockwise or downward rotation of the lip relative to the cranial base of the craniofacial skeleton.

KEY POINTS

1) In the lower periorbital region, orbicularis muscle, lower canthus, and orbital and malar septum, attenuation and lengthening cause ptosis and pseudoherniation of the orbital fat pads and the SOOF, resulting in lower canthal bowing, "crow's feet," and lower eyelid and malar "bags" and wrinkles.

2) Loss of midfacial retaining ligament cheek support results in anteroinferior descent of midface subcutaneous fat, causing (1) a deep nasolabial groove, (2) a heavy nasolabial fold, (3) cheek folds, (4) a "skeletonized" appearance of the cheekbone, and (5) a submalar hollow.

3) Attenuation and lengthening of the upper orbicularis oris muscle, coupled with upper lip dermal atrophy from photoaging and repeated muscular contraction, result in lengthening of a vertically lined upper lip.

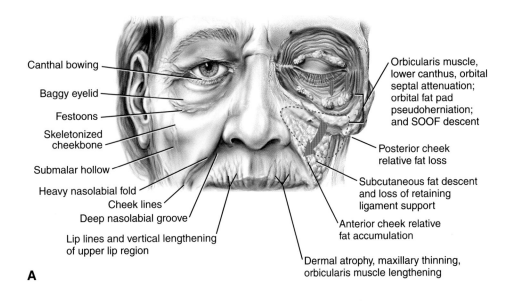

Canthal bowing

Baggy eyelid

Festoons

Skeletonized cheekbone

Submalar hollow

Heavy nasolabial fold

Cheek lines

Deep nasolabial groove

Lip lines and vertical lengthening of upper lip region

Orbicularis muscle, lower canthus, orbital septal attenuation; orbital fat pad pseudoherniation; and SOOF descent

Posterior cheek relative fat loss

Subcutaneous fat descent and loss of retaining ligament support

Anterior cheek relative fat accumulation

Dermal atrophy, maxillary thinning, orbicularis muscle lengthening

A

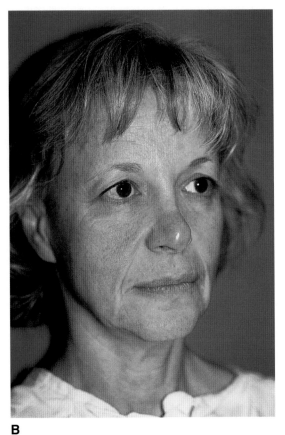

B

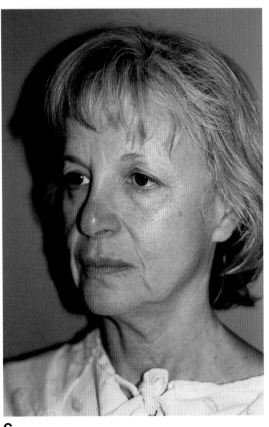

C

Figure 2-10   *Regional anatomy of the aged middle face.* **A,** *Anatomical concepts of facial and neck aging are contrasted with the subcutaneous, muscular, and ligamentous forces responsible for their creation.* **B** *and* **C,** *Many of the characteristic changes are evident in this 55-year-old prospective patient.*

The Lower Face and Neck

Several anatomical forces are directly responsible for production of the characteristic features of the aged lower face and neck (see Fig. 2-11*A–D*). In the lower perioral region, anteroinferior midfacial and lower facial fat and soft tissue descent occurs, leading eventually to the downwardly cast "sad" mouth, commissural lines, lower cheek lines, jowls, and "marionette lines." Attenuation and lengthening of the lower orbicularis oris and depressor anguli oris muscles from smoking and overuse (as in patients without lip seal, such as those with microgenia, bimaxillary protrusion, or long face syndrome), dermal atrophy from photoaging, and anterior mandibular bone loss from osteoporosis or loss of dentition also cause signs of lower perioral aging, contributing mainly to lines in the lower lip, commissures, and chin. Lower lip lines are rarely as numerous or as deep as upper lip lines.

Midfacial fat also descends and settles behind the mandibular retaining ligaments, much like leaves in the drain pipes of a gutter. This migration of fat creates the all-too-familiar "jowls." In many patients, jowls extend well below the lower mandibular border. Because much of the fat in the lower anterior region of the face is superficial to the platysma and the superficial fascia, jowls can extend a considerable distance below the mandibular border, but they never extend anterior to the mandibular retaining ligaments. Jowls are accentuated in patients with ptotic submandibular glands, which can easily be confused with excess subcutaneous fat.

In the neck, the "turkey gobbler" deformity is commonly observed. With aging, the platysma muscle attenuates, lengthens, and even dehisces, causing platysmal banding. Many patients gain weight as they age, and the neck has a rich subplatysmal fat pad, much as in the hips and flanks. This subplatysmal fat can "herniate" through platysmal dehiscences, contributing to a thickened, waddy appearance of the neck with loss of the cervicomental angle. Subcutaneous jowl fat can also descend well below the mandibular border and into the neck. With aging, the hypodermal preplatysmal fat layer actually shrinks and shrivels. Along with solar elastosis, as the neck is nearly always exposed to the sun, multiple hemicircular submental skin folds, cobblestone rhytides, and platysma bands become obvious in the skin of the neck.

> **KEY POINTS**
>
> 1) Midfacial fat descent, along with attenuation and lengthening of the lower orbicularis oris and depressor anguli oris muscles, creates lower lip, commissural, and chin lines, the downwardly cast "sad" mouth, oromandibular grooves, and "marionette lines."
> 2) Midfacial fat descent settles behind the mandibular retaining ligaments and creates "jowls," which often extend below the mandibular border.
> 3) The "turkey gobbler neck" is caused by platysma muscle attenuation, lengthening, and dehiscence, along with subplatysmal fat accumulation and pseudoherniation, hypodermal fat shrinkage, and solar elastosis of neck skin.

Key References

Knize D: An anatomically based study of the mechanism of eyebrow ptosis. Plast Reconstr Surg 97:1321, 1996.

Lemperle G, Holmes R, Cohen S, Lemperle S: A classification of facial wrinkles. Plast Reconstr Surg 108:1735, 2001.

Pessa J: An algorithm of facial aging. Plast Reconstr Surg 106:479, 2000.

Pessa J, Garza P, Love V, et al: The anatomy of the labiomandibular fold. Plast Reconstr Surg 101:482, 1998.

Rubin L: The anatomy of the nasolabial fold: The keystone of the smiling mechanism. Plast Reconstr Surg 103:687, 1999.

Stuzin J, Baker T, Gordon H: The relationship of the superficial and deep facial fascias: Relevance to rhytidectomy and aging. Plast Reconstr Surg 89:441, 1992.

Yousif N, Gosain A, Matloub H, et al: The nasolabial fold: An anatomic and histologic reappraisal. Plast Reconstr Surg 93:60, 1994.

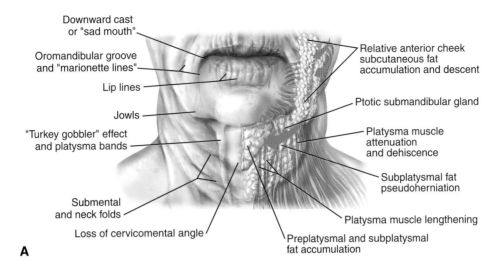

Downward cast
or "sad mouth"

Oromandibular groove
and "marionette lines"

Lip lines

Jowls

"Turkey gobbler" effect
and platysma bands

Relative anterior cheek
subcutaneous fat
accumulation and descent

Ptotic submandibular gland

Platysma muscle
attenuation
and dehiscence

Subplatysmal fat
pseudoherniation

Platysma muscle lengthening

Submental
and neck folds

Loss of cervicomental angle

Preplatysmal and subplatysmal
fat accumulation

A

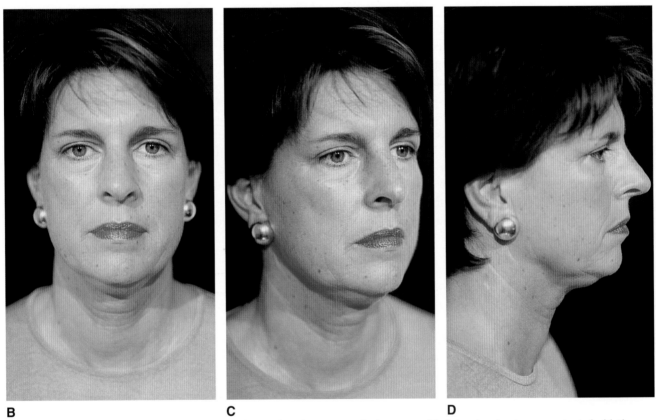

B　　　　　　　　**C**　　　　　　　　**D**

Figure 2-11　*Regional anatomy of the aged lower face and neck. **A,** Anatomical concepts of facial and neck aging are contrasted with the subcutaneous, muscular, and ligamentous forces responsible for their creation. **B** to **D,** Many of the characteristic changes are evident in this 51-year-old prospective patient.*

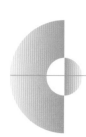

CHAPTER THREE

Surgical Approaches to the Forehead and Brow

The cosmetic concerns of patients are far easier to understand when we divide the face into three "surgical units": the upper face, the middle face, and the anterior neck (Fig. 3-1). The aging of these surgical units proceeds along anatomically guided patterns sketched out in the previous chapters. Although dividing the face into surgical units may seem arbitrary, patients invariably prioritize their complaints along these lines. Sitting with a patient in front of a mirror, the plastic surgeon will often hear "I look so tired lately [i.e., brow ptosis] I can't even see my eyes anymore," or "These lines [i.e., nasolabial folds] and this [i.e., jowls] are making me look so much older than I am," or "In the past few years I've lost my jawline and developed this waddle [i.e., platysma bands] and this stuff [i.e., submental fat] under my chin."

Each surgical unit is subdivided into the classic aesthetic subunits. It is extremely helpful to keep several copies of a schematic drawing of the aesthetic subunit of concern (see Fig. 3-1) in each patient's chart. The first copy is used during the initial consultation to prioritize a prospective patient's complaints and to document physical findings. A second, duplicate copy is then used during the preoperative consultation to tighten up and denote the techniques that have been decided on with the patient. A third and final copy is used on the day of surgery to document the surgical treatments that were actually used and to make some personal notes about technique. Along with review of the patient's preoperative and postoperative photographs, this is a terrific learning tool for the surgeon.

THE THREE SURGICAL UNITS OF THE FACE

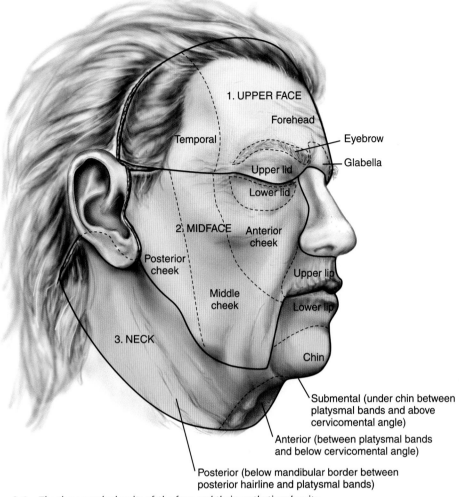

Figure 3-1 *The three surgical units of the face and their aesthetic subunits.*

Pinpointing and prioritizing the patient's complaints according to the surgical unit principle also assist the surgeon to make decisions about the sequencing of surgery (Figs. 3-2 and 3-3). Anatomical principles of facial aging have demonstrated that superficial subcutaneous tissues sag to a far greater extent than that noted to occur with deeper subcutaneous tissues. Although the superficial skin flaps are mobilized prior to deeper subcutaneous tissue mobilization when two-flap techniques are used, aesthetic results can be enhanced if the sequencing for fixation of these flaps follows a certain order. Sequencing for fixation is optimal when the order is reversed for the superficial and the deep tissues—that is, deep subcutaneous tissue fixation is best begun in the upper face, should then proceed to the middle face, and should end in the neck, whereas superficial skin flap fixation is best begun in the neck, should then proceed to the middle face, and should end in the temporal flap. The deeper tissues of the forehead and brow should be set initially so that they are not fought against and dragged down by midfacial tissues that have been prematurely locked into position. In addition, the deeper subcutaneous tissues of the midface should have a solid foundation from which they can be suspended. Likewise, the deeper

subcutaneous tissues of the midface should be set before the deeper tissues of the neck so that they are not fought against and dragged down by neck tissues that have been prematurely locked into position. In addition, the deeper subcutaneous tissues in the neck need a solid foundation from which they can be suspended. The sequencing for fixation of the skin flaps is reversed in order to avoid pleat formation and bunching. The skin flap in the neck should be tightened and fashioned before the midfacial skin flap, and likewise the midfacial skin flap should be tightened and fashioned before the temporal flap.

KEY POINTS

1) The face is divided into three surgical units: the upper face, the middle face, and the neck.
2) Patients invariably prioritize their aging concerns along the lines of these surgical units, which assists the surgeon in deciding about the sequencing for surgery.
3) The sequencing for setting the surgical units is reversed for the superficial and the deep tissues—deep tissue fixation begins in the upper face, then proceeds to the middle face, and ends in the neck, whereas skin flap fixation begins in the neck, then proceeds to the midface, and ends in the temporal region.

SKIN TIGHTENING SEQUENCING AND SKIN FLAP VECTORS

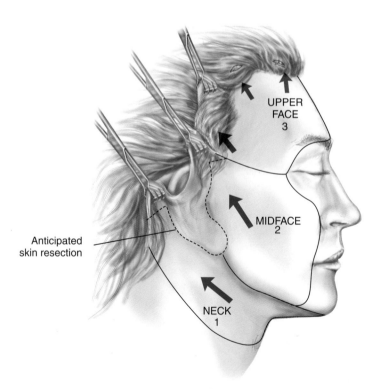

Anticipated skin resection

UPPER FACE 3

MIDFACE 2

NECK 1

Skin tightening begins in the neck, proceeds to the midface, and ends in the temporal region (1 ▸ 2 ▸ 3), thereby avoiding pleats and bunching.

Figure 3-2 *The skin tightening sequencing and the vectors for skin flap insetting.*

DEEP PLANE SEQUENCING AND DEEP PLANE VECTORS

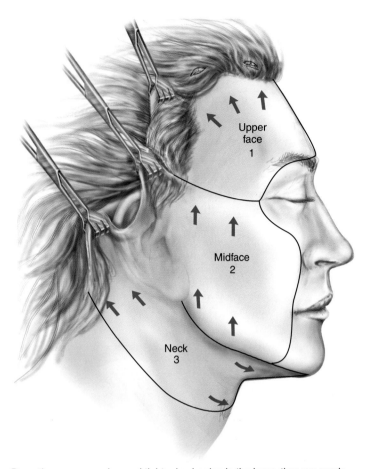

Deep tissue suspension and tightening begins in the brow, then proceeds to the midface, and ends in the neck (1 → 2 → 3). The vectors are radial in the brow, vertical in the midface, and bidirectional oblique in the neck.

Figure 3-3   *The deep subcutaneous tissue sequencing and the vectors for deep subcutaneous tissue insetting.*

INDICATIONS

The introduction of botulinum toxin type A (Botox, Allergan Inc., Irvine, California) has revolutionized the options available for surgical rejuvenation of the upper face, and Botox therapy has become an adjunctive staple in the plastic surgeon's repertoire. There is a common misconception in the public, however, that Botox rejuvenates the upper face without the need for surgery. In fact, some patients who come to the office seeking improvement in the appearance of the upper face seem positively shocked when eyelid and brow surgery is advised rather than serial injections of Botox. In this current nonsurgical cosmetic climate, it behooves the plastic surgeon to be fully cognizant of the risks and benefits of Botox therapy when advising patients about cosmetic improvements in the upper face.

Carefully planned serial injections of Botox have become the standard of care for a large majority of patients who complain about unsightly dynamic forehead and glabellar lines. These patients are usually in their late 20s, 30s, and early 40s and more often than not present with other cosmetic surgery complaints as well (Fig. 3-4A). Once patients with dynamic forehead lines also have the physical signs of blepharochalasis with imminent brow ptosis, however, blepharoplasty or brow lift or both, not serial forehead injections of Botox, should be advised (Fig. 3-4B and C). These patients usually must rely on tonic frontalis muscle activity to elevate the brows to an aesthetically pleasing height and to lessen the heavy appearance of the upper eyelids and brow. Serial glabellar injections of Botox can be helpful if significant depressor overactivity is present; however, forehead injections of Botox in these patients lower the eyebrows, accentuate the already heavy appearance of the upper eyelids, and make applying eye makeup nearly impossible. Although the forehead may be as smooth as glass, the inability to raise the now ptotic eyebrows gives the face an "angry" look the patient simply cannot will away. An unhappy patient invariably results.

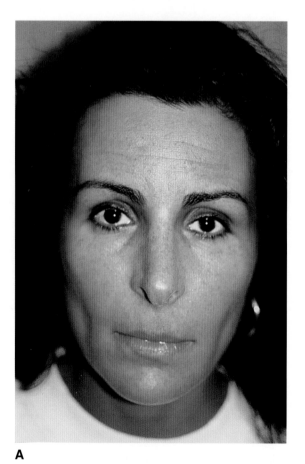

A

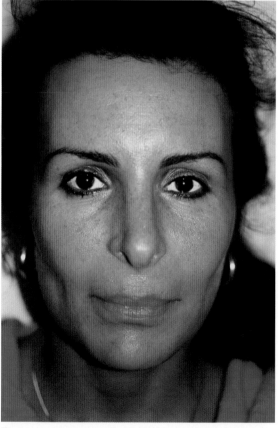

B

Figure 3-4 ***A*** *and* ***B,*** *The ideal candidate for Botox is the 30-something patient with dynamic forehead and glabellar lines.* ***C–F,*** *Once patients with dynamic forehead lines develop the physical stigmata of blepharochalasis and brow ptosis, blepharoplasty and/or brow lift, not serial forehead injections of Botox, is recommended.* ***C*** *and* ***E,*** *These sisters both required near-constant frontalis muscle activity to elevate the brows to an aesthetically pleasing height and to lessen the heavy appearance of the upper eyelids and brow.* ***D*** *and* ***F,*** *Although both were poor candidates for forehead Botox injections, excellent results were achieved with upper blepharoplasty. The older sister* ***(F)*** *also underwent concomitant endoscopic brow lift.*

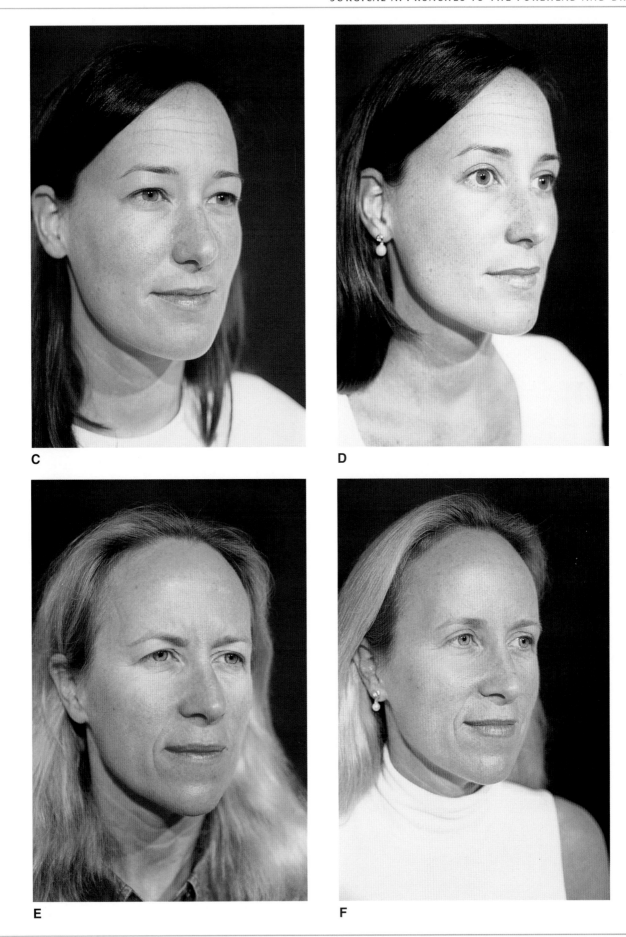

C

D

E

F

When forehead and glabellar lines are static in nature, that is, when they are permanent and appear along with true dermal furrows, then a combination of soft tissue fillers and laser resurfacing should also be offered. These patients have usually entered middle age and have long ago established a vicious loop pattern of depressor and elevator muscle overactivity to counteract gravimetric ptosis of the soft tissues of the forehead and brow.

Although many of these patients come into the office requesting Botox, soft tissue fillers, and resurfacing, they also need to be warned that Botox injections should be limited exclusively to the glabella and central forehead if surgical rejuvenation is declined. Forehead injections of Botox for this type of patient in the absence of blepharoplasty and brow lift will strongly accentuate brow ptosis even if fillers and resurfacing are added (Fig. 3-5).

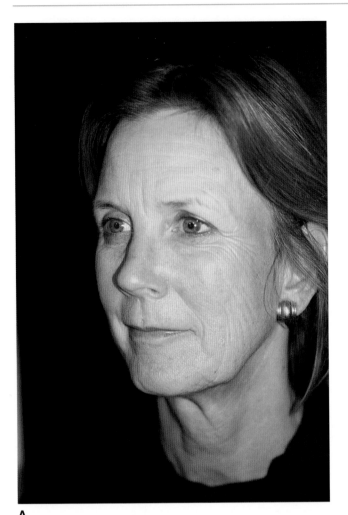
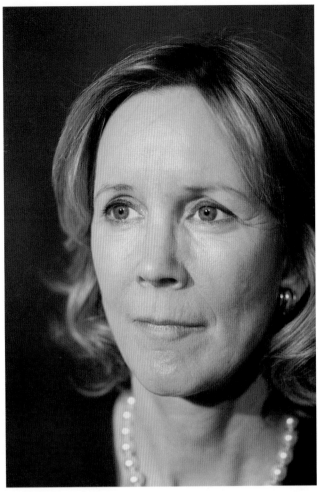

A   **B**

Figure 3-5   *Suboptimal candidates for Botox are middle-aged patients with brow ptosis and static forehead and glabellar lines.* **A,** *This 52-year-old woman underwent full-face laser resurfacing, facelift, and glabella and forehead injections of Botox.* **B,** *The Botox smoothed out her forehead nicely but accentuated her upper eyelid blepharochalasis and lateral brow ptosis.*

The primary indication for surgical rejuvenation of the upper face is gravimetric soft tissue ptosis of the forehead, brow, and temporal regions and static glabellar and forehead lines. Surgical rejuvenation of the upper face is accomplished by three well-known techniques, any of which can be combined with blepharoplasty, laser resurfacing, and soft tissue fillers. These techniques are the temporal lift, the endoscopic brow lift, and the coronal lift (Fig. 3-6). The choice of surgical technique for the upper face depends on the extent and degree of temporal and brow soft tissue ptosis, the depth and degree of glabellar and forehead lines, and the quality and height of the hairline.

The ideal candidate for the temporal lift is the middle-aged or older patient with mild to moderate lateral brow ptosis, temporal soft tissue ptosis, and extensive crow's feet. In many cases, the patient's primary reason for undergoing cosmetic facial surgery is not upper facial complaints but rather the signs of midfacial and neck aging. Accordingly, the primary indication for using a temporal lift is to prevent post-facialplasty temporal and lateral brow bunching. The temporal lift, as classically practiced, has no effect on glabellar or forehead lines, cannot "lift" ptotic medial brow soft tissue, and cannot vertically elevate the eyebrows at their apex points. In addition, because no neurotomies or myotomies are performed with the temporal lift, no permanent alteration of dynamic facial expression is produced. Only slight elevation of the temporal hairline is produced by the temporal lift, unless the pretrichal approach is used.

The ideal candidate for the endoscopic brow lift is the 30- or 40-something patient with glabellar frown lines and brow ptosis. A temporal lift can be added if temporal soft tissue ptosis and extensive crow's feet are present. If the patient is undergoing simultaneous midfacial and neck rejuvenation, a temporal lift is usually necessary. If procerus and corrugator myotomies are performed, then the endoscopic brow lift permanently reduces depressor muscle function. The endoscopic brow lift, in and of itself, does not directly alter elevator muscle function (i.e., frontalis muscle); however, vertical repositioning of the brow and forehead results in a pleasing reduction of forehead lines. This improvement occurs because the frontalis muscle is vertically elevated by the endoscopic lift and no longer requires an extensive resting tone in order to elevate the eyebrows. True vertical elevation of the medial and lateral brows at their apex points is effected by the endoscopic brow lift. Slight elevation of the frontal hairline is produced by the endoscopic forehead lift, unless the pretrichal approach is used.

The ideal candidate for the coronal brow lift is the middle-aged or older patient with deep glabellar and forehead lines, thick oily corrugated forehead skin, and moderate to severe medial brow, lateral brow, and temporal soft tissue ptosis. One of the main advantages of the coronal brow lift is that procerus, corrugator, and frontalis myotomies can be performed, thereby permanently reducing depressor and elevator muscle function. True vertical elevation of the entire brow and temporal region is produced by the coronal technique, making the coronal lift the technique of choice for patients complaining of severe brow and temporal ptosis, as well as for patients complaining of significant eyebrow asymmetry. Elevation of the frontal and temporal hairlines is also produced by the coronal lift, making the coronal lift the technique of choice for patients with short, deeply corrugated foreheads. In addition, with the pretrichal coronal approach, the forehead can be shortened and narrowed, making the coronal approach the technique of choice for patients with extremely high and broad foreheads who desire reduction.

KEY POINTS

1) The primary indication for surgical rejuvenation of the upper face is soft tissue ptosis of the forehead, brow, and temporal regions, forehead height disparities, and permanent static glabellar and forehead lines.

2) The ideal candidate for the temporal lift is the middle-aged or older patient with lateral brow ptosis, temporal soft tissue ptosis, and extensive crow's feet.

3) The ideal candidate for endoscopic brow lift is the youngish to middle-aged patient with glabellar frown lines and moderate brow ptosis.

4) The ideal candidate for the coronal brow lift is the middle-aged or older patient with deep glabellar and forehead lines, thick oily corrugated forehead skin, forehead height disparity, and moderate to severe brow and temporal soft tissue ptosis.

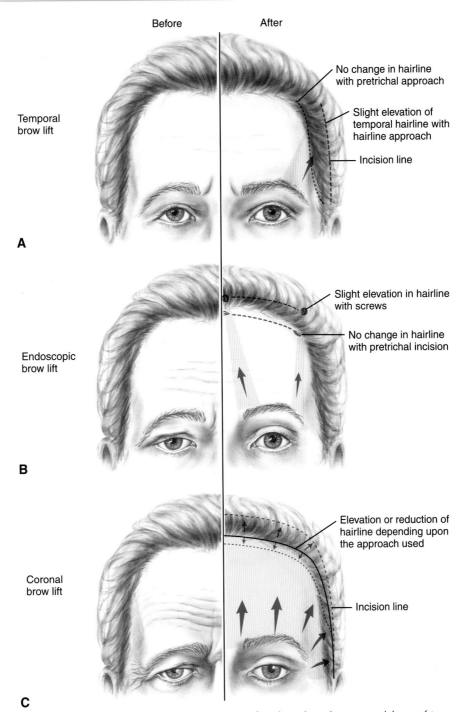

Before   After

Temporal brow lift

No change in hairline with pretrichal approach

Slight elevation of temporal hairline with hairline approach

Incision line

A

Slight elevation in hairline with screws

No change in hairline with pretrichal incision

Endoscopic brow lift

B

Elevation or reduction of hairline depending upon the approach used

Incision line

Coronal brow lift

C

Figure 3-6 *The choice of surgical technique for the upper face depends on the extent and degree of temporal and brow soft tissue ptosis, the depth and degree of glabellar and forehead lines, and the quality and height of the hairline.*

ANATOMICAL CONSIDERATIONS

Anatomical considerations include (1) the position of the incisions chosen for upper facial surgical rejuvenation relative to the location of the motor and sensory nerves and (2) the proper release and relocation of the retaining ligament system of the upper face (Fig. 3-7).

Incisional approaches chosen for brow- and forehead-plasty must respect the course of the motor and sensory nerves in the region. The frontal branch of the facial nerve leaves the parotid gland below the zygomatic arch, penetrates the gland at a right angle, crosses the midportion of the zygomatic arch along the superficial surface, courses within the temporoparietal fascia through the temporal region, and, at approximately halfway along its course, crosses the sentinel vein. The frontal branch then enters the frontalis muscle and deep portion of the orbicularis muscle slightly above the level of the superior orbital rim. The frontal branch of the superficial temporal artery parallels and remains above the nerve along its course. The sentinel vein and the frontal branch of the superficial temporal artery are surface landmarks that serve to indicate the approximate subcutaneous position of the nerve.

The supraorbital nerve exits the supraorbital foramen and quickly splits into a medial superficial and a lateral deep division. The deep division is deep to the galeal fat pad and passes along the floor of the glide plane space. The deep division also lies deep to the corrugator muscle. The deep division acutely angles out deep to the frontalis muscle and galea and arcs superiorly parallel to and within 2 cm of the temporal fusion line. The deep division provides sensation to the frontoparietal scalp. The medial superficial division resides within the galeal fat pad and is superficial to the corrugator muscle. This nerve pierces the frontalis muscle along with the supratrochlear nerve to innervate the forehead and anterior scalp.

The orbital ligaments and the periosteal zones of adhesion represent the true and false retaining systems of the upper face, respectively. These are the structures that require release if elevation of the brow and forehead is to be successful on a long-term basis. The orbital retaining ligaments are true dermal to periosteal retaining ligaments, 6 to 8 mm in length, and centered over the zygomaticofrontal suture. These firm, taut white fibers are contiguous with the temporal crest and the temporal fusion line. A small artery, a sensory nerve, and several large veins are evident within the area. In the event of injury to any of these, endoscopically assisted ligation may be necessary if packing the area is unsuccessful. The periosteal zone of adhesion is a wing-shaped band 1.5 to 2.5 cm in width. This zone of adhesion begins at the nasofrontal junction, runs laterally across the forehead above the supraorbital rims, and meets the orbital ligaments at the zygomaticofrontal junction. The periosteal zone of adherence is an adherence of the deep galea to periosteum. The deep galea serves as both the roof and the floor of the glide plane space, the areolar tissue–lined space that allows for near-frictionless movement of the forehead and glabella musculature over the frontal bone. The glide plane space also serves as the plane through which the soft tissues of the forehead and brow descend—the more frowning we do, the lower the brow goes over time; the more eyebrow elevation we feel we need to do, the more forehead and glabellar lines we develop; the more brow ptosis we develop; and so on. Subperiosteal release of the orbital ligaments and the periosteal zone of adhesion elevates the galea fusion band, the glide plane space, and ptotic forehead and brow soft tissue. Cephalic fixation must be within the deep galea in order for elevation to be effective.

KEY POINTS

1) Incisional approaches for brow- and foreheadplasty must respect the course of the motor and sensory nerves in the region. These include the frontal branch of the facial nerve, the superficial and deep divisions of the supraorbital nerve, and the supratrochlear nerve.

2) The orbital ligaments and the periosteal zones of adhesion represent the true and false retaining systems of the upper face. They must be released and fixed at a higher level if vertical elevation of the brow and forehead soft tissue is desired.

3) The orbital retaining ligaments are true dermal to periosteal retaining ligaments, 6 to 8 mm in length, and are centered over the zygomaticofrontal suture.

4) The periosteal zone of adhesion is a wing-shaped 1.5 to 2.5 cm band of adherence of the deep galea to the periosteum. This begins at the nasofrontal junction, runs across the forehead above the supraorbital rims, and coalesces with the orbital ligaments at the zygomaticofrontal junction.

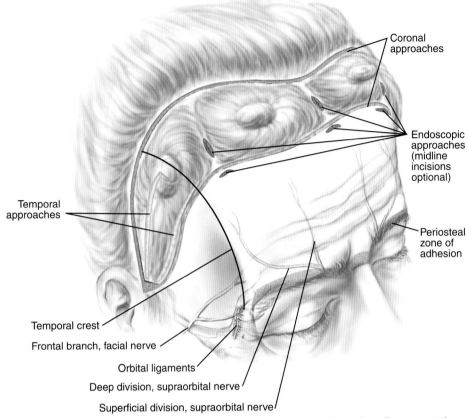

Coronal approaches

Endoscopic approaches (midline incisions optional)

Temporal approaches

Periosteal zone of adhesion

Temporal crest

Frontal branch, facial nerve

Orbital ligaments

Deep division, supraorbital nerve

Superficial division, supraorbital nerve

Figure 3-7 *Anatomical considerations in brow- and foreheadplasty: incision options, ligaments and nerves, and zones of adhesion.*

AESTHETIC CONSIDERATIONS

Aesthetic considerations include (1) placement of incisions above or below the hairline, (2) the configuration and height of the eyebrow, (3) the height of the hairline and the thickness and quality of the hair, and (4) patient concerns with minor hair loss (Fig. 3-8).

Whatever the choice of approach, incisions can be placed either within the hairline or in a pretrichal location. This decision depends on several factors: the configuration of the eyebrows, the height of the hairline, and hair loss concerns. If the patient is pleased with the configuration of her eyebrows, if the patient's hairline is low, or if the patient's primary concern is the aesthetic outcome, then a hairline approach is appropriate and indicated. However, if the patient desires a major alteration of eyebrow configuration, if the patient's hairline is high or borderline acceptable, or if the patient is exceedingly concerned with even a minor amount of hair loss, then a pretrichal approach is appropriate and indicated.

When an approach within the hairline is chosen, the incisions should respect the fashion of the patient's hairstyle. The incision should not be placed on or crossing natural "parts" in the scalp, and the incision should be beveled in order to avoid injuring the hair follicles. When a pretrichal approach is chosen, the incisions should be placed as close as possible to the hairline, should be "stair-stepped" slightly to avoid deforming the natural hairline, and should be closed with fine sutures in multiple layers to avoid unsightly depressions.

The configuration and height of the eyebrows should be discussed with the patient prior to surgery. In general, aesthetically pleasing eyebrows are symmetrical and obliquely peaked laterally, and apex points are positioned at or slightly higher than the supraorbital rims when observed with the patient in the upright position. If significant alteration to the configuration of the eyebrows is desired, then a pretrichal endoscopic approach is preferable because of the short distance between the incision site and the eyebrow. The endoscopic approach also allows for subcutaneous browpexy with minimal scar burden to the patient. If the configuration of the eyebrows is acceptable, then a hairline approach, which can be either endoscopic or coronal, is indicated. If brow ptosis is isolated to the lateral brow and the eyebrow configuration is acceptable, then a temporal approach is preferable.

KEY POINTS

1) If the patient is pleased with the configuration of her eyebrows, if the hairline is low, or if the patient's concern is primarily the aesthetic outcome, then an approach with incisions placed within the hairline is indicated for upper facial rejuvenation.

2) If the patient desires a change in the configuration of her eyebrow, if the hairline is high or borderline acceptable, or if the patient is exceedingly concerned with even a minor amount of hair loss, then a pretrichal approach is indicated for upper facial rejuvenation.

3) Hairline incisions should respect the fashion of the patient's hairstyle, should not be placed on or cross natural parts in the scalp, and should be beveled at an angle that avoids hair follicle injury.

4) Pretrichal incisions should be placed as close as possible to the hairline, should be stair-stepped slightly to avoid deforming the natural hairline, and should be closed with fine sutures in multiple layers to avoid unsightly depressions.

5) When significant alteration to the configuration of the ptotic eyebrows is desired, then a pretrichal endoscopic approach is preferable.

6) When the configuration of the eyebrows is acceptable, then hairline approaches, whether endoscopic or coronal, are preferable.

7) When brow ptosis is isolated to the lateral brow and the eyebrow configuration is acceptable, the temporal approach is preferable.

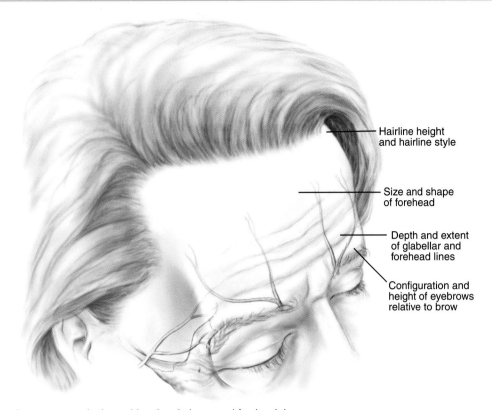

Hairline height
and hairline style

Size and shape
of forehead

Depth and extent
of glabellar and
forehead lines

Configuration and
height of eyebrows
relative to brow

Figure 3-8 *Aesthetic considerations in brow- and foreheadplasty.*

TECHNIQUES

Temporal Lift

Temporal lifts are ideal for two types of patients: (1) middle-aged patients with brow ptosis isolated to the lateral brow whose primary reason for undergoing cosmetic surgery is signs of midfacial and neck aging (Figs. 3-9*A* and *B* and 3-10) and (2) older patients who complain of lateral brow ptosis, temporal soft tissue ptosis, and extensive crow's feet in addition to signs of midfacial and neck aging (Figs. 3-11 and 3-12). Conservative upper blepharoplasty is usually indicated in the vast majority of patients desiring a temporal lift. Markings for the upper eyelids should be performed with the patient in the upright position prior to surgery. Modifications to the markings can then be made after the patient assumes the supine position on the operating room table and the temporal lift has been completed. The temporal lift has no effect on glabellar or forehead lines and cannot "lift" ptotic medial brow soft tissue. In addition, because no neurotomies or myotomies are performed with this technique, no permanent alteration of dynamic facial expression is effected. Slight elevation of the temporal hairline is produced by the temporal lift unless the pretrichal approach is chosen.

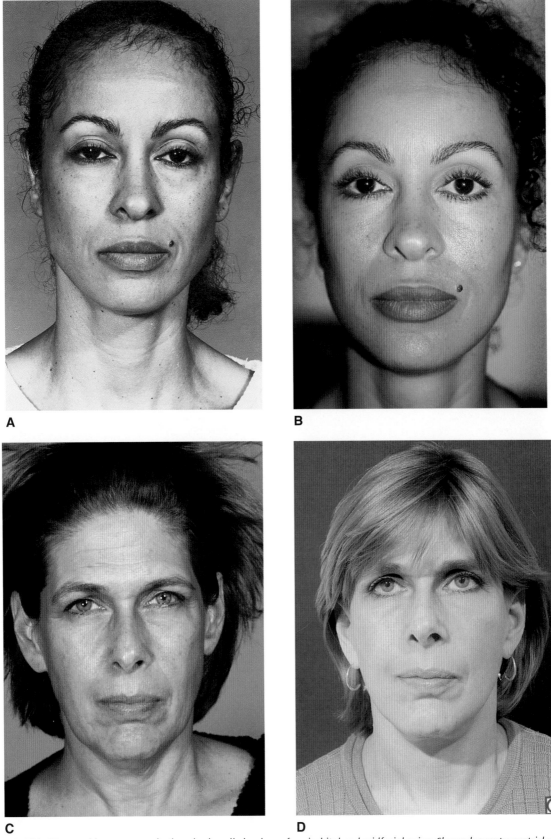

A

B

C

D

Figure 3-9   ***A,*** *This 42-year-old woman was bothered primarily by signs of periorbital and midfacial aging. She underwent a pretrichal temporal and minimal-incision midfacial lift, transconjunctival lower blepharoplasty, and conservative upper blepharoplasty.* ***B,*** *Her postoperative appearance.* ***C,*** *This 50-year-old woman was bothered primarily by lateral brow, midfacial, and neck soft tissue ptosis. She underwent a classic temporal lift and two-flap rhytidectomy. No upper blepharoplasty was performed.* ***D,*** *Her postoperative appearance.*

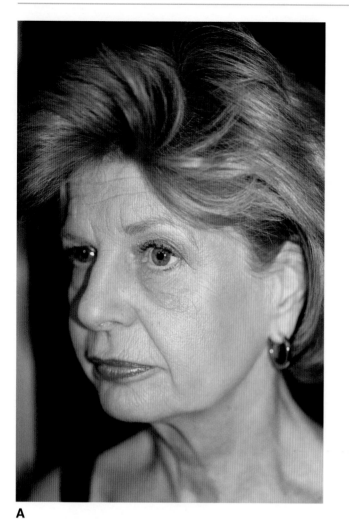

A

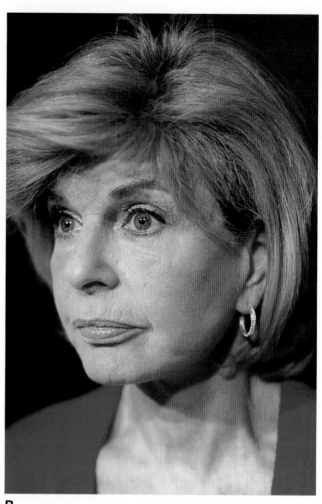

B

Figure 3-10 **A,** *This 54-year-old woman complained of signs of lateral brow, midfacial, and neck aging. A slight modification of the lateral eyebrow configuration was desired. The patient was exceedingly concerned with the potential for hair loss. A pretrichal approach for temporal lift was chosen to complement two-flap rhytidectomy and upper blepharoplasty.* **B,** *Her postoperative appearance.*

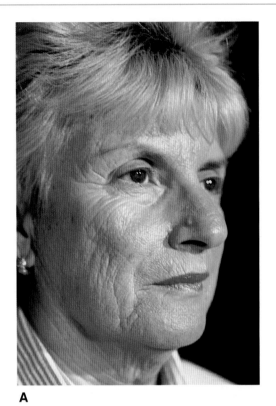
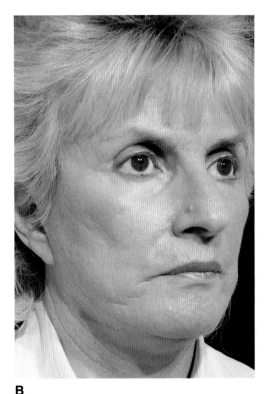

A
B

Figure 3-11 **A,** *This 65-year-old woman complained of extensive crow's feet as well as temporal and lateral brow ptosis and signs of midfacial and neck aging. A slight modification of lateral eyebrow configuration was desired. The patient was concerned about any hair loss related to the surgery.* **B,** *Extensive laser resurfacing, a pretrichal approach for temporal lift, and a conservative upper blepharoplasty complemented the facelift.*

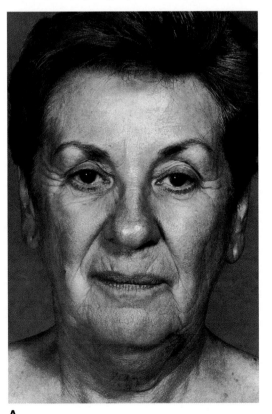
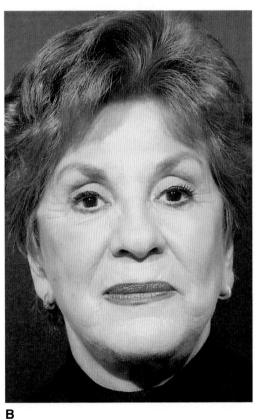

A
B

Figure 3-12 **A,** *This 67-year-old woman complained of lateral brow ptosis as well as signs of midfacial and neck aging. The configuration of the eyebrows was acceptable, and the patient was not overly concerned with a minor amount of hair loss. A temporal lift using a hairline approach was performed with her facelift, as well as a conservative blepharoplasty.* **B,** *Her postoperative appearance.*

The classic approach for the temporal lift is a gently curved incision which mirrors and is 5 to 6 cm behind the temporal hairline (Fig. 3-13). This incision must reach the temporal fusion line. A transverse sideburn incision can and should be added. A temporal dart near the temporal fusion line should also be added, which assists vertical elevation of the temporal flap. If a facelift is to be performed, this incision can easily be joined with the preauricular incision. As noted previously, the incision must respect the pathways of the motor and sensory nerves in the region.

The pretrichal approach for the temporal lift is optional and used only if a minimal incision rhytidectomy is to be used simultaneously. This incision is stair-stepped 1 to 2 mm anterior to the temporal hairline and connected to the preauricular incision through the transverse sideburn incision. Again, the pretrichal incision must reach the temporal fusion line. No superior dart is required when the pretrichal temporal lift is performed.

After the incisions have been fashioned and the hair has been rearranged, anesthetic solution consisting of 0.5% lidocaine and 1:200,000 epinephrine is infiltrated into the region. The incisions are beveled in the direction of the hair follicles. The incisions are carried through the temporoparietal fascia to expose the temporalis fascia. Hemostasis is obtained.

The first portion of the dissection is carried out in the subgaleal plane (Fig. 3-14). This is performed in the areolar layer using a curved Gorney scissors. This portion of the dissection is assisted by Lahey clamp retraction of the temporal flap. Subgaleal dissection proceeds to the anterior hairline only. The frontal branch of the facial nerve resides along the deep surface of the temporoparietal fascia in the temporal region and is subject to injury if subgaleal dissection proceeds any further anterior than the temporal hairline.

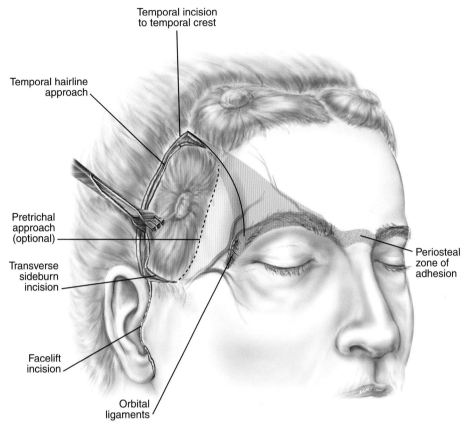

Figure 3-13   *The classic approach for the temporal lift is a gently curved incision that mirrors and is 5 to 6 cm behind the temporal hairline. This incision must reach the temporal fusion line. Additional incisions include a transverse sideburn incision and a temporal dart near the temporal fusion line. The optional pretrichal approach can be stair-stepped 1 to 2 mm anterior to the hairline.*

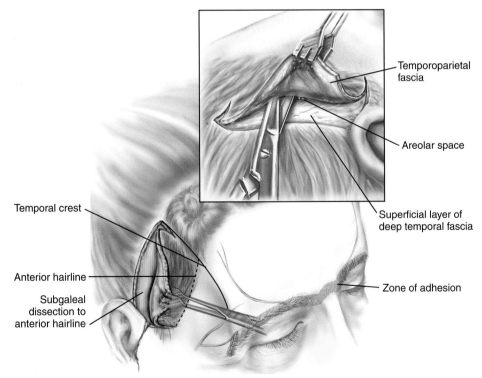

Figure 3-14   *The first portion of the dissection for the temporal lift is carried out in the subgaleal plane, using a curved Gorney scissors in the areolar layer (inset).*

The second portion of the dissection is carried out in the subperiosteal plane (Fig. 3-15). This is performed using a curved flat sharp periosteal elevator. Subperiosteal dissection is begun superiorly at the temporal fusion line. Resistance to dissection is felt where the soft tissues are densely adherent to the periosteum, but once dissection is medial to the temporal fusion line, dissection without resistance is appreciated until the periosteal zone of adherence and orbital ligaments are reached along the bony orbital ridge. Subperiosteal release of the periosteal zone of adherence proceeds lateral to the supraorbital notch, and subperiosteal release of the orbital ligaments proceeds along the zygomaticofrontal suture by using a Daniel endoforehead elevator. The frontal branch of the facial nerve and the deep division of the supraorbital nerve are safely within the temporal flap at this point of the dissection. A small vein and arteriole are often noted during dissection of the orbital ligaments. Endoscopically assisted cauterization of these vessels greatly reduces the need for more rigorous hemostasis. Traction on the temporal flap results in mobility of the lateral brow at this juncture. If mobility is restricted, subperiosteal dissection of the lateral orbit and anterior zygoma is necessary. Before flap transposition is performed, however, excision of a small 2.0 × 3.0 cm area of temporalis fascia should be performed, which promotes long-term cicatricial adhesion of the temporal flap.

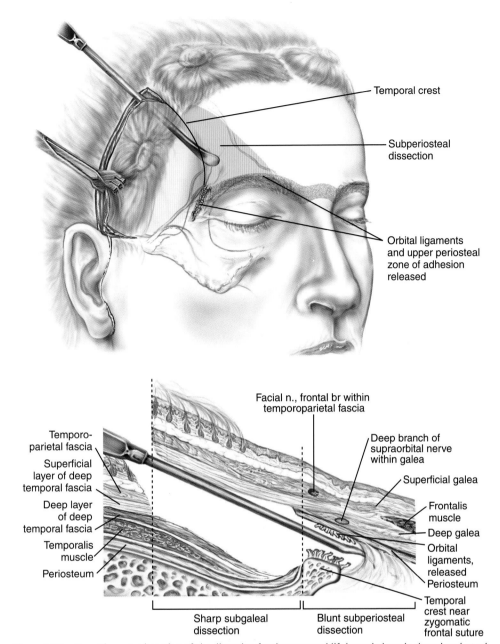

Temporal crest

Subperiosteal dissection

Orbital ligaments and upper periosteal zone of adhesion released

Facial n., frontal br within temporoparietal fascia

Temporo-parietal fascia

Superficial layer of deep temporal fascia

Deep layer of deep temporal fascia

Temporalis muscle

Periosteum

Deep branch of supraorbital nerve within galea

Superficial galea

Frontalis muscle

Deep galea

Orbital ligaments, released

Periosteum

Temporal crest near zygomatic frontal suture

Sharp subgaleal dissection

Blunt subperiosteal dissection

Figure 3-15 **Top,** *The second portion of the dissection for the temporal lift is carried out in the subperiosteal plane, using a curved flat sharp periosteal elevator to release the periosteal zone of adhesion and the orbital ligaments.* **Bottom,** *Cross-sectional anatomy. The deep branch of the supraorbital nerve and the frontal branch of the facial nerve are well protected within the flap.*

Fixation of the temporal flap is performed along a radial-based superolateral vector by a series of horizontal mattress stitches placed between the temporoparietal fascia and superficial temporal fascia on the temporal flap and the temporalis muscle and temporal fascia layers of the patient's scalp (Fig. 3-16). These stitches should be evenly placed and tied sequentially from below upward. Permanent sutures of 2-0 Mersilene are best for fixation. Transposition of the flap is aided by excision of a superior dart of scalp at the temporal fusion line.

Redundant scalp after the temporal lift has been set can be relieved by posterior subgaleal dissection for 2 to 3 cm (Fig. 3-17). This maneuver allows the posterior scalp to retract enough that the scalp can be closed without significant redundancy and bunching. Several deep 3-0 Vicryl sutures can be placed and the scalp closed with staples. Residual minor scalp redundancy will resolve within 6 weeks. Resection of hair-bearing scalp should be avoided at all costs.

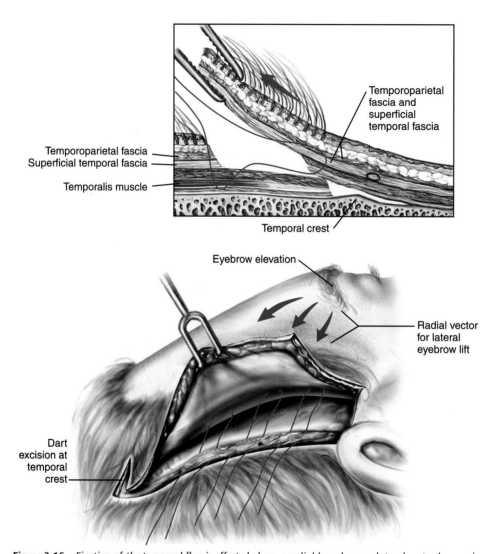

Figure 3-16 *Fixation of the temporal flap is effected along a radial-based superolateral vector by a series of horizontal mattress stitches placed between the temporoparietal fascia and superficial temporal fascia on the temporal flap and the temporalis muscle and temporal fascia layers of the patient's scalp.* **Top,** *Cross-sectional anatomy.* **Bottom,** *Drawing—intraoperative view.*

SETTING THE TEMPORAL LIFT AND RELIEVING SCALP AND TEMPORAL BUNCHING

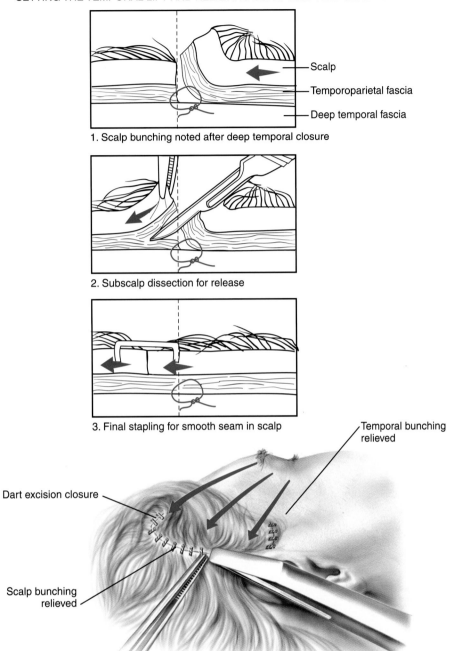

1. Scalp bunching noted after deep temporal closure

2. Subscalp dissection for release

3. Final stapling for smooth seam in scalp

Figure 3-17 *Redundancy of scalp after the temporal lift has been set can be relieved by posterior subgaleal dissection for 2 to 3 cm.* **Top,** *1–3: Cross-sectional anatomy and surgical maneuvers.* **Bottom,** *Drawing—postoperative appearance.*

CLINICAL PEARLS

- The incision within the hairline for temporal lift must reach the temporal fusion line for optimal translocation of the flap. A temporal dart near the temporal fusion line assists vertical elevation of the flap.
- The initial dissection within the hairline is performed in the subgaleal plane, followed by subperiosteal plane dissection to the eyebrows. This bilevel plane of dissection prevents injury to the frontal branch of the facial nerve and the deep division of the supraorbital nerve.
- For optimal temporal flap mobilization, subperiosteal release of the periosteal zone of adherence and the orbital ligaments is necessary.
- If mobility of the temporal flap is restricted, subperiosteal dissection of the lateral orbit and anterior zygoma is necessary.
- Before the temporal flap is transposed, excision of a small 2.0 × 3.0 cm area of temporalis fascia will aid long-term cicatricial adhesion of the temporal flap.
- Fixation of the temporal flap is performed along a radial-based superolateral vector with a series of horizontal mattress stitches placed between the temporoparietal fascia and superficial temporal fascia on the temporal flap and the temporalis muscle and temporal fascia layers of the patient's scalp.
- Scalp redundancy and bunching are relieved by posterior subgaleal dissection for 2 to 3 cm. Residual minor scalp redundancy resolves within 6 weeks. Resection of hair-bearing scalp should be avoided at all costs.

Endoscopic Lift

Endoscopic lifts are ideal for two types of patients: (1) younger to middle-aged patients with early brow ptosis and upper eyelid blepharochalasis (Figs. 3-18*A* and 3-19) and (2) middle-aged or older patients with brow ptosis, glabellar and transverse forehead lines, and signs of mid-facial and neck aging (Figs. 3-20 and 3-21). Conservative upper blepharoplasty is indicated in the vast majority of patients undergoing an endoscopic lift. Markings for upper blepharoplasty are performed with the patient in the upright position prior to surgery. Modifications to the markings can then be made after the patient has assumed the supine operating position and the endoscopic lift has been completed. A temporal lift can also be added if temporal soft tissue ptosis and extensive crow's feet are present. The endoscopic brow lift permanently reduces depressor muscle function when procerus and corrugator myotomies are performed. The endoscopic brow lift, in and of itself, does not directly alter the frontalis muscle; however, if depressor myotomies are performed and vertical repositioning of the brow and forehead soft tissues is effectively achieved, a more pleasing appearance of the upper face results that is comparable with results achieved by coronal lifts (Fig. 3-22). True vertical elevation of the medial and lateral brows at their apex points is effected by the endoscopic brow lift. Elevation of the frontal hairline can result when the endoscopic lift is performed through an approach within the hairline.

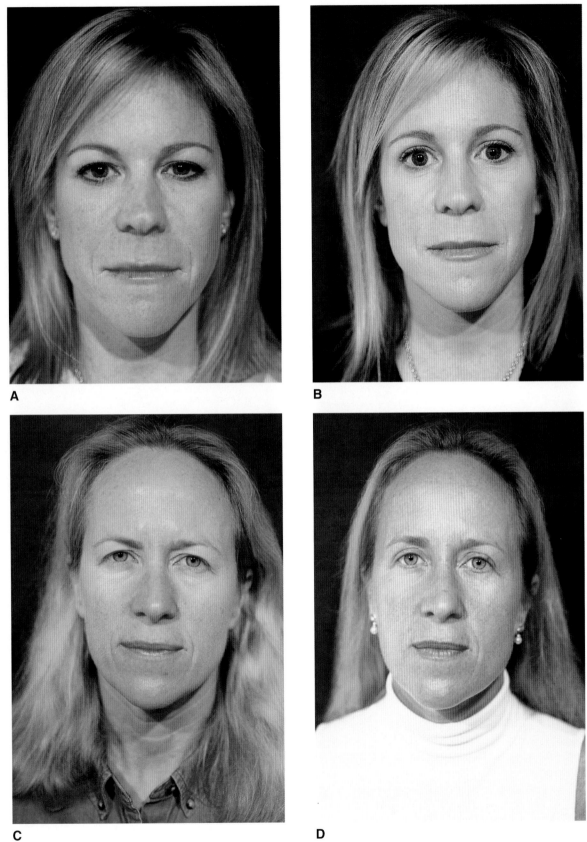

A

B

C

D

Figure 3-18 **A** and **C,** *These two patients, both in their early 40s, already had high foreheads and did not want the hairline elevated further despite complaining about heavy brows and hooded upper eyelids.* **B** and **D,** *Conservative upper blepharoplasty along with an endoscopic brow lift via the pretrichal approach improved brow and eyelid aesthetics yet did not significantly alter the hairline. Lower blepharoplasty was performed as well.*

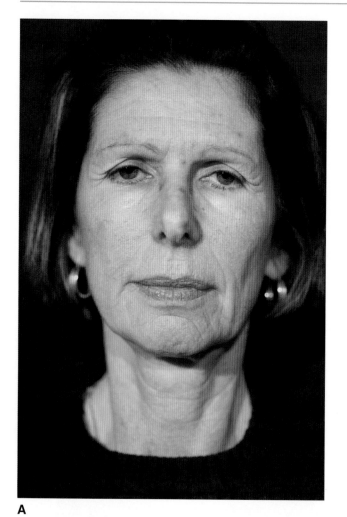

A

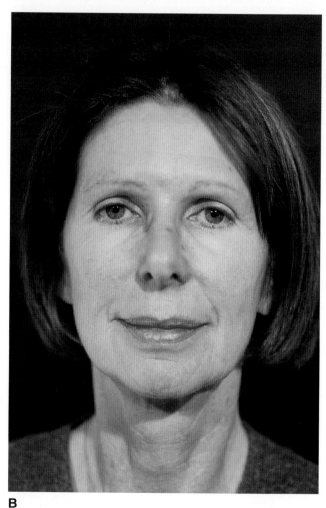

B

Figure 3-19   **A,** *This 52-year-old woman complained of a heavy lateral brow, "sad eyes," and transverse forehead and frown lines. She did not want a facelift.* **B,** *Conservative upper blepharoplasty, an endoscopic brow lift with incisions placed behind the hairline, and laser resurfacing of the forehead, lower eyelids, and mouth improved her facial aesthetics without a facelift.*

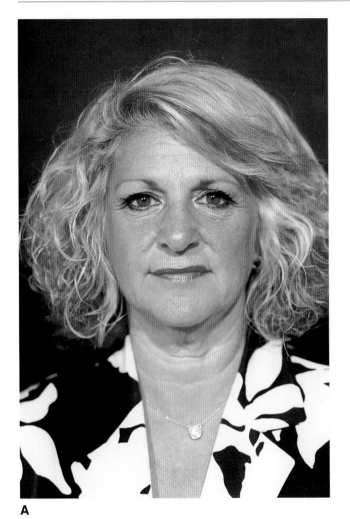

A

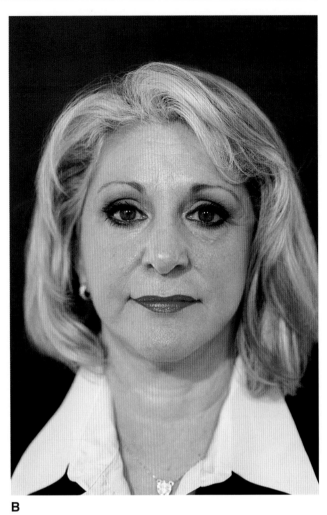

B

Figure 3-20   **A,** *This 53-year-old woman wanted "everything done." She had a short forehead, brow ptosis, and glabellar and transverse forehead lines, in addition to blepharochalasis and signs of facial and neck aging. Upper and lower blepharoplasty, an endoscopic browlift, and a face and neck lift with forehead and perioral laser resurfacing were performed.* **B,** *Her postoperative appearance.*

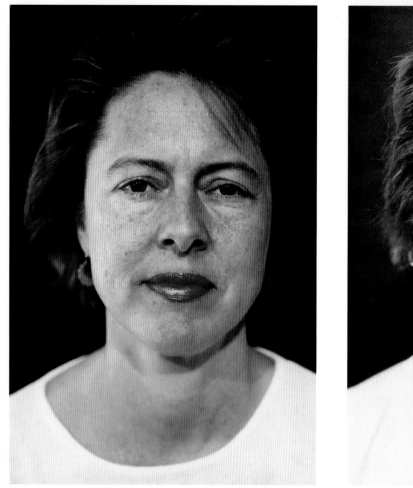

A

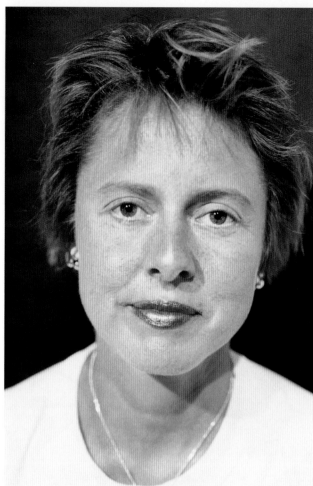

B

Figure 3-21   *This 50-year-old woman complained of a ptotic brow and baggy and hooded eyelids. She was an excellent candidate for an endoscopic brow lift along with blepharoplasty, which greatly contributed to her end result.*

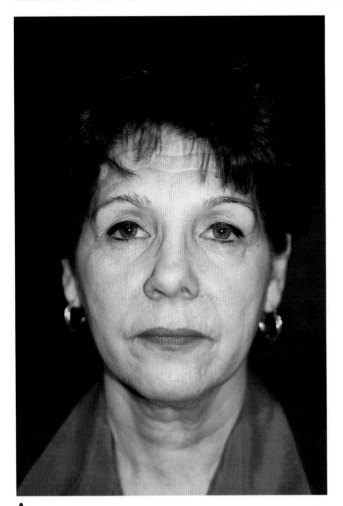

A

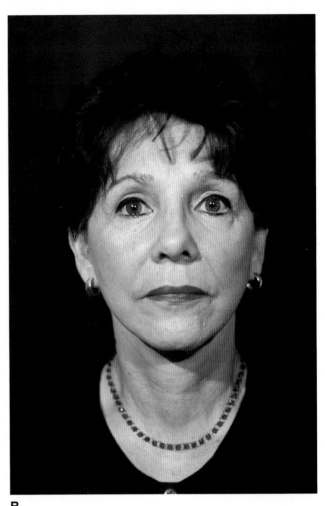

B

Figure 3-22 Although an endoscopic brow lift, in and of itself, does not directly alter the frontalis muscle, if depressor myotomies are performed and vertical repositioning of the brow and forehead soft tissues is achieved with the endoscopic lift, a more pleasing appearance of the forehead lines results. **A,** This 57-year-old woman complained about brow ptosis, a lined forehead, and signs of perioral, midfacial and neck aging. An endoscopic lift, extensive laser resurfacing, and a two-flap rhytidectomy were performed. **B,** The improvement in her upper facial appearance achieved by the endoscopic lift was comparable with that expected with a coronal lift.

Incisions for the endoscopic lift can be either within the hairline or pretrichal, depending on the patient's and the surgeon's preferences (Fig. 3-23). The incisions must respect the pathways of the motor and sensory nerves in the region. In general, three incisions are mandatory for endoscopic procedures: one for the scope and the other two for instruments. The paramedian incisions should parallel the temporal crest and be situated directly above the apex of the eyebrows, and the third, optional incision is central in location. If an approach within the hairline is chosen, the incisions are best oriented vertically and placed several centimeters behind the frontal hairline. If a pretrichal approach is chosen, the incisions are best oriented horizontally and placed very close to the frontal hairline. Both types of incisions should be no greater than 1 to 2 cm in length and should be beveled in the direction of the hair follicles. A third, central incision is optional; whether it is used depends on the surgeon's adeptness with the endoscope and the patient's aesthetic requirements. If medial brow ptosis is significant, with crowding of the brows, then a central incision is mandatory for fixation and elevation.

After the incisions have been fashioned and the hair has been rearranged, anesthetic solution consisting of 0.5% lidocaine and 1:200,000 epinephrine is infiltrated into the region. The incisions are carried down to the frontal bone. Once the periosteum is visualized, a round flat subperiosteal elevator is inserted and subperiosteal dissection of the forehead, glabella, and eyebrows is performed (Fig. 3-24). The periosteal zone of adherence and orbital ligaments are released with the aid of Daniel curved endoforehead elevators. The endoplastic scope should be inserted when subperiosteal dissection proceeds around the supraorbital foramen, such that the supraorbital nerves are preserved. A small vein and arteriole are often noted during dissection of the orbital ligaments. Endoscopically assisted cauterization of these vessels greatly reduces the need for more rigorous hemostasis.

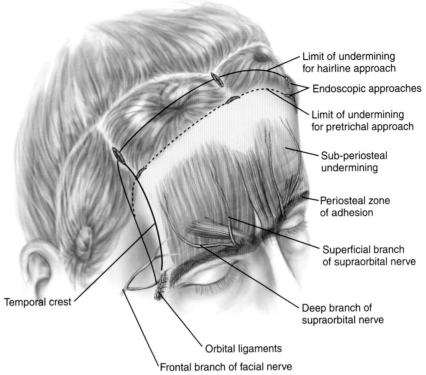

Figure 3-23 *Incisions for the endoscopic lift can be either within the hairline or pretrichal, depending on the patient's and the surgeon's preferences.*

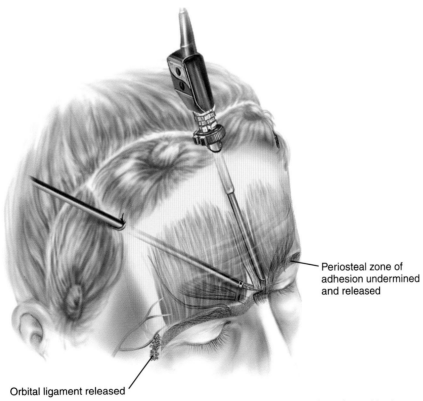

Figure 3-24 *Subperiosteal dissection of the forehead, glabella, and eyebrows is performed in the designated areas with full release of the periosteal zone of adherence and the orbital ligaments.*

Use of an endoforehead canula greatly assists retraction and visualization for the myotomy segment of the procedure (Fig. 3-25). Myotomies can be performed in either blunt or sharp fashion. A Hester square-ended reverse elevator is preferred for blunt myotomies of the corrugator and procerus musculature. The reverse elevator is used to avulse the muscle bundles apart. Blunt myotomies are complete when the galeal fat pad is visualized. Great care must be exercised in performing the procerus myotomies to avoid injury to the supratrochlear nerve, because the nerve is immediately superficial and lateral to the muscle. Occasionally, a slip of the deep head of the orbicularis muscle also needs to be divided for complete lysis of brow depressor function. This strip of deep orbicularis muscle is lateral to the corrugator muscle and supraorbital nerve. If sharp myotomies are chosen, a Ramirez curved sharp endoscopic scissors is preferred. The author has found that blunt myotomies are intrinsically more hemostatic and safer than sharp myotomies, especially with regard to the potential for sensory nerve injuries.

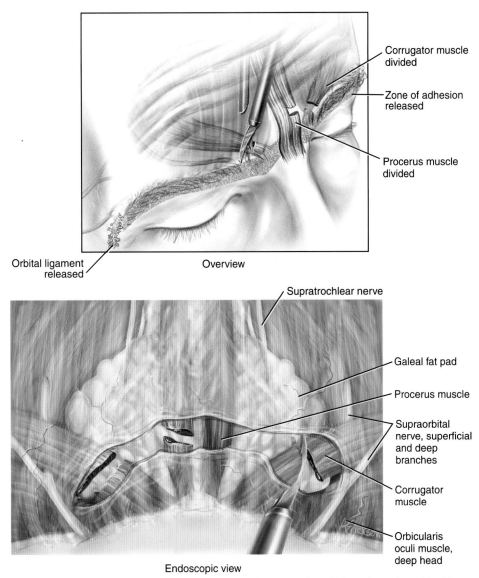

Corrugator muscle divided

Zone of adhesion released

Procerus muscle divided

Orbital ligament released

Overview

Supratrochlear nerve

Galeal fat pad

Procerus muscle

Supraorbital nerve, superficial and deep branches

Corrugator muscle

Orbicularis oculi muscle, deep head

Endoscopic view

Figure 3-25 *Use of an endoforehead cannula greatly assists myotomies, which can be performed in either blunt or sharp fashion. Myotomies are complete when the galeal fat pad is completely visualized. Great care must be exercised to avoid injury to the supraorbital and supratrochlear nerves.* **Top,** *Surgical overview.* **Bottom,** *Endoscopic view.*

Fixation for the endobrow lift ranges from the simple to complex. Some surgeons perform no fixation at all. They simply insert a closed suction drain, close the incisions, and place a compression dressing, depending on periosteal readhesion for fixation. The assumption is that if depressor muscle function has been effectively arrested by corrugator and procerus myotomies, the eyebrows and forehead will naturally reset at a higher level within several hours, when frontalis muscle function returns. Other surgeons place several external suspension sutures of 3-0 nylon into the eyebrows, tie them under slight tension to the staples that were used to close the hairline incisions, and incorporate this entire "suspension system" into a light gauze dressing. The dressing and the suspension sutures are removed along with the staples on the third to the fifth postoperative day.

When more reliable means for fixation are judged to be necessary, several other fixation techniques are available. Of utmost importance, cephalic fixation must be performed within the deep galea for vertical elevation of the eyebrows to be effective. One must remember that the glide plane space, which allows for descent of forehead and eyebrow soft tissues, is located between the leaflets of the galea.

If an approach within the hairline has been chosen, fixation is performed using endoscopic brow fixation screws (Stryker-Leibinger, Kalamazoo, Michigan) (Fig. 3-26). Subperiosteal undermining is performed in an arc 1 to 2 cm above the vertical hairline incisions. A 1.5 mm × 42 mm twist drill bit with a Stryker shaft end and a working length of 3.1 mm is used to cut a hole in the outer cortical table of the frontal bone within the upper half of the incision (Leibinger, Freiburg, Germany). This bit allows for a drill hole to be cut in the outer table without undue concern for injury to the diploic space or the inner cortical table. If excessive bleeding is encountered after the drill hole has been cut, hemostasis will immediately be obtained if the screw is rapidly inserted. Depending on the thickness of the patient's scalp, 12, 14, or 16 mm long self-tapping 2.0 mm diameter endoscopic brow fixation screws are inserted. Two-finger tightness is optimal for screw insertion and prevents screw stripping or bone fractures. The heads of the screws should sit several millimeters above the scalp to facilitate removal. A mattress stitch of 2-0 Polysorb suture on a GU-46 tapered needle (Ethicon Co., Somerville, New Jersey) is placed with good purchase into the proximal deep galea. Skin hooks are placed to elevate the forehead and eyebrows to the desired height and configuration, and the sutures are simultaneously tied above the screws. A horizontal mattress stitch of 3-0 Vicryl suture is used to close the dermis, and staples are placed to close the scalp incision. If the procedure has been unusually "wet," a 7 mm round Jackson-Pratt drain can be placed through one of the hairline incisions, to be removed on the following day. The screws, along with the staples, are removed after 7 to 10 days.

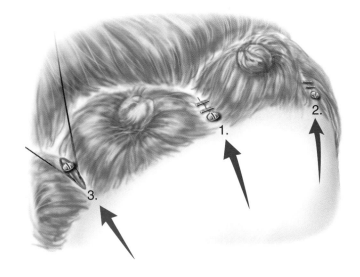

A

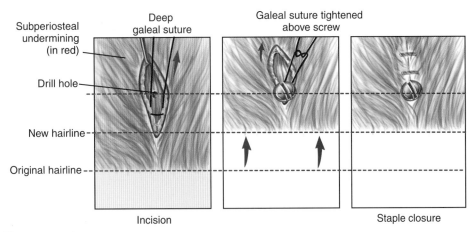

Subperiosteal undermining (in red)

Deep galeal suture

Galeal suture tightened above screw

Drill hole

New hairline

Original hairline

Incision

Staple closure

B

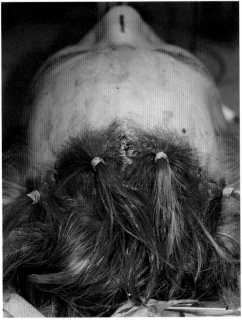

C

Figure 3-26 **A–C,** *For approaches within the hairline, miniscrew fixation to the outer cortical table of the frontal bone optimizes vertical elevation of the brow. A drill hole is cut within the upper half of the stab incision, and depending upon the thickness of the patient's scalp, 12, 14, or 16 mm self-tapping miniscrews are inserted. The head of the miniscrew should sit several millimeters above the scalp to facilitate removal. A mattress stitch of 2-0 Vicryl suture is placed into the deep galea adjacent to the frontal hairline. While skin hooks vertically elevate the scalp, forehead, and eyebrows to their desired height, the Vicryl sutures are simultaneously tied above the screw. Staples are used for scalp closure.*

If a pretrichal approach has been chosen, fixation is performed with "T to V" galeal advancement (Fig. 3-27). Subperiosteal undermining is not performed above the horizontal pretrichal incisions. Once the necessary amount of brow elevation is determined, a small vertical incision is carried onto the forehead at the center of the horizontal incision. A mattress stitch of 2-0 Vicryl suture (Ethicon Co.) on a GU-46 tapered needle is placed with good purchase into the deep galea. Skin hooks are placed to elevate and separate the forehead and eyebrows to their desired height and configuration, and the sutures are tied simultaneously. A horizontal mattress stitch of 3-0 Vicryl suture closes the dermis, and fine vertical mattress stitches of 6-0 nylon are then used to close the incisions. If the procedure has been unusually "wet," a 7 mm round Jackson-Pratt suction drain is placed through a stab incision within the hairline and removed on the following day. The nylon sutures are removed in 5 days and replaced with Steri-Strips.

CLINICAL PEARLS

- Incisions for the endoscopic lift can be either within the hairline or pretrichal, depending on the patient's complaints and the surgeon's preferences.
- If an approach within the hairline is chosen, the incisions are best oriented vertically and placed several centimeters behind the frontal hairline. If a pretrichal approach is chosen, the incisions are best oriented horizontally and placed along the frontal hairline.
- Paramedian incisions are mandatory, and if medial brow ptosis is significant, then a central incision is necessary to vertically elevate the eyebrows and forehead for fixation at a higher location.
- The dissection plane is subperiosteal, and the dissection must release the periosteal zone of adherence and orbital ligaments. This is greatly aided by use of a Daniel curved endoforehead elevator.
- Procerus and corrugator myotomies are performed either bluntly or sharply and are complete when the galeal fat pad is completely visualized. Blunt myotomies are intrinsically more hemostatic and slightly safer in preventing sensory nerve injuries than sharp myotomies.
- Cephalic fixation must be performed at the deep galeal level for vertical elevation of the eyebrows to be effective. If an approach within the hairline has been chosen, fixation is performed using screws. If a pretrichal approach has been chosen, fixation is performed with T to V galeal advancement.

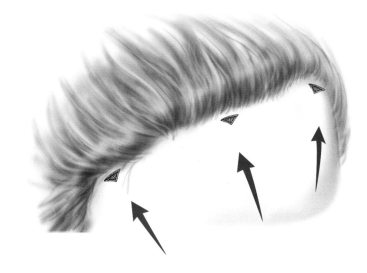

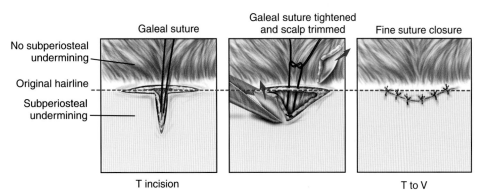

Figure 3-27 *For pretrichal approaches, fixation is performed with "T to V" galeal advancement. Once the necessary amount of brow elevation is determined, a small vertical incision is carried onto the forehead at the center of the horizontal incision. A mattress stitch of 2-0 Polysorb suture on a GU-46 tapered needle is placed with good purchase into the deep galea. Skin hooks are placed to elevate the forehead and eyebrows to their desired height and configuration, and the sutures are simultaneously tied. Fine sutures are used for closure.*

Coronal Lift

Coronal lifts are ideal for three types of patient: (1) the middle-aged or older patient with a short, thick, corrugated forehead and brow or temporal soft tissue ptosis (Fig. 3-28), (2) the patient with a high, broad forehead who desires reduction (Fig. 3-29), and (3) the patient with significant forehead and brow asymmetries (Fig. 3-30*A* and *B*). For the patient with a short, constricted forehead, true vertical elevation and widening of the entire forehead and eyebrows, along with elevation of the frontal and temporal hairlines, are produced when the classic gull-wing approach is used (see Fig. 3-28). Conversely, for the patient with a high, broad forehead, true shortening and narrowing of the forehead and temple, as well as elevation of ptotic eyebrows, are produced when the pretrichal approach is used. This approach significantly lowers the frontal and temporal hairlines (see Fig. 3-29). A conservative upper blepharoplasty is indicated in the vast majority of patients undergoing coronal brow lift. Markings for upper blepharoplasty are performed with the patient in the upright position prior to surgery. Modifications to the markings can then be made after the patient assumes the supine position on the operating room table and the coronal lift has been completed. One of the main advantages of the coronal brow lift is that procerus, corrugator, and frontalis myotomies are performed, thereby permanently reducing depressor and elevator muscle function. For patients with significant forehead and brow asymmetries, myotomies can be performed in asymmetrical fashion and brow ptosis corrected asymmetrically to optimize the aesthetic result.

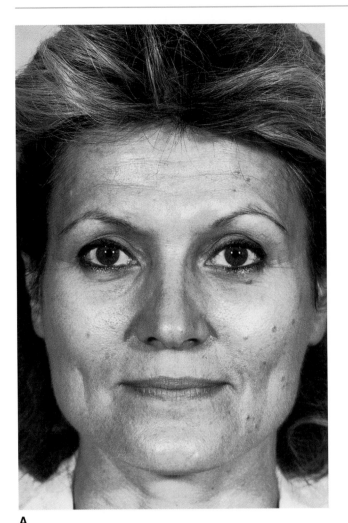

A

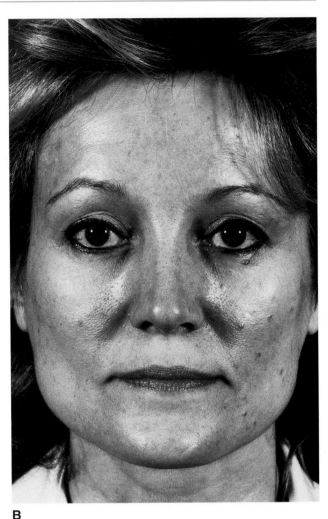

B

Figure 3-28 *Coronal lifts are ideal for the middle-aged and older patient who complains of a short, thick, corrugated forehead and brow or temporal soft tissue ptosis.* ***A,*** *This 48-year-old woman's short, constricted forehead was lengthened and broadened and her frontal and temporal hairlines were elevated by coronal lift performed through the classic gull-wing approach. She also underwent facelift. No blepharoplasty was performed.* ***B,*** *Her forehead lines were permanently softened, the forehead skin was thinned, and her brow was maintained at a pleasing height by this technique.*

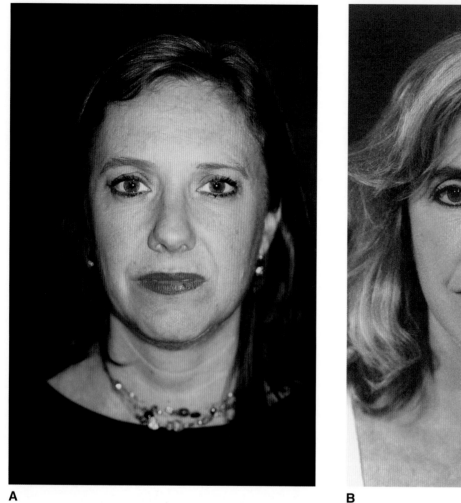

A

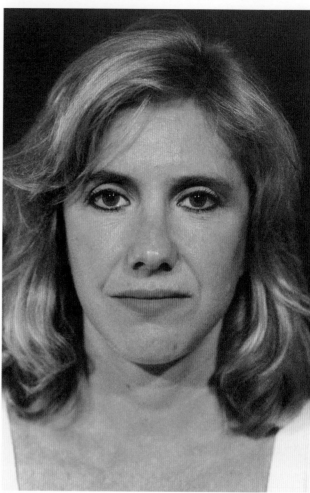

B

Figure 3-29 *Coronal lifts are also ideal for patients with high, broad foreheads who desire reduction.* **A,** *This 47-year-old woman was always bothered by a high, crowned forehead.* **B,** *Her forehead was shortened and narrowed by a coronal lift performed through a pretrichal approach. She also had a facelift and a conservative upper blepharoplasty.*

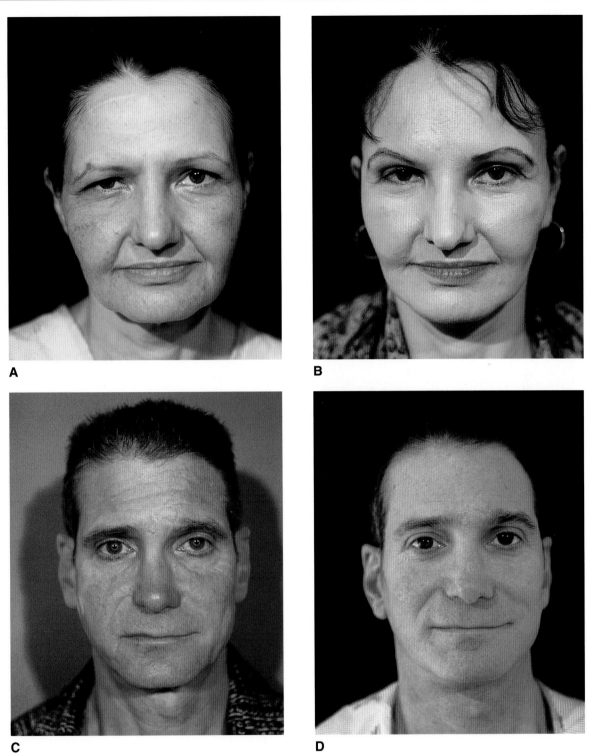

A

B

C

D

Figure 3-30 *Significant post-traumatic forehead and brow asymmetries are best corrected by coronal lifts. Brow ptosis can be corrected in asymmetrical fashion to optimize the aesthetic result. **A,** This 52-year-old woman was extremely distressed by asymmetrical post-traumatic brow ptosis. She was also bothered by signs of premature midfacial and neck aging. **B,** Asymmetrical coronal lift performed through the classic gull-wing approach, facelift, and blepharoplasty resulted in improvement of her facial features. **C,** This 50-year-old man complained about asymmetrical forehead lines and brow ptosis as a result of a car accident over 30 years ago. He was also bothered by signs of facial and neck aging. **D,** Asymmetrical coronal lift with resection and temporal fascia grafting of the left frontalis, cross-hatch scoring of the right frontalis, and facelift resulted in a more symmetrical upper facial appearance as well as a more youthful look.*

Once a coronal lift has been chosen, either a classic gull-wing scalp incision or a pretrichal incision is designed (see Fig. 3-7). Both incisions transect the deep division of the supraorbital nerve; however, the gull-wing incision transects the nerve at a much higher level, thereby minimizing frontoparietal scalp sensory loss. The pretrichal incision should be stair-stepped within 1 to 2 mm of the temporal and frontal hairlines. Both incisions should be beveled along the direction of the hair follicles and combined with transverse sideburn incisions to aid access.

After the incisions have been fashioned and the hair has been rearranged, anesthetic solution consisting of 0.5% lidocaine and 1:200,000 epinephrine is infiltrated into the region. The incisions are beveled along the direction of the hair follicles and carried directly down to the loose areolar plane. Below the temporal crest the incision is carried through the temporoparietal fascia and the superficial layer of the deep temporal fascia to expose the temporalis fascia. Hemostasis is obtained, and subgaleal dissection of the upper half of the forehead is performed with a flat wide periosteal elevator (Fig. 3-31). Subperiosteal dissection of the lower forehead and brow is best performed with a sharp round periosteal elevator, because the skin in this region is densely adherent to bone. Release of the subperiosteal zone of adhesion and the orbital ligaments must be thoroughly performed for effective release of the soft tissues. Dissection below the temporal crest is performed deep to the superficial layer of deep temporal fascia in order to elevate the temporal fat pad and to prevent injury to the frontal branch of the facial nerve.

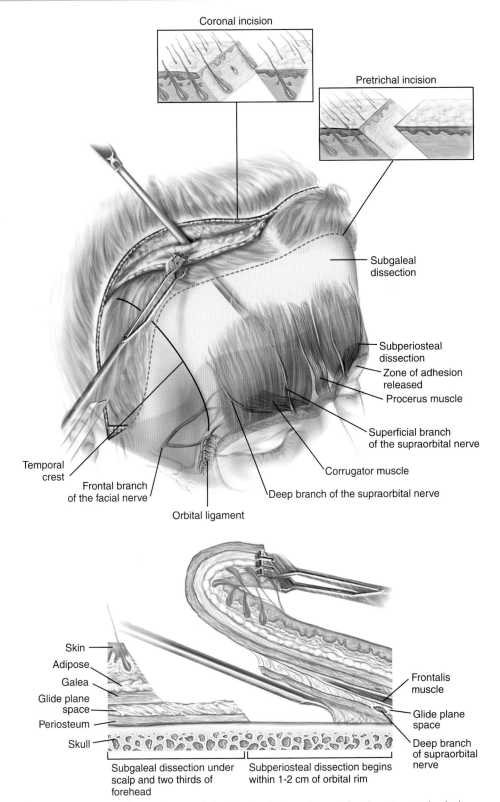

Coronal incision

Pretrichal incision

Subgaleal dissection

Subperiosteal dissection

Zone of adhesion released

Procerus muscle

Superficial branch of the supraorbital nerve

Corrugator muscle

Deep branch of the supraorbital nerve

Orbital ligament

Frontal branch of the facial nerve

Temporal crest

Skin

Adipose

Galea

Glide plane space

Periosteum

Skull

Frontalis muscle

Glide plane space

Deep branch of supraorbital nerve

Subgaleal dissection under scalp and two thirds of forehead

Subperiosteal dissection begins within 1-2 cm of orbital rim

Figure 3-31 **Top,** *Incisions and anatomic landmarks.* **Bottom,** *Cross-sectional anatomy. Subgaleal dissection proceeds to the midforehead followed by subperiosteal dissection to release the supraorbital zone of adherence and the orbital ligaments. The supraorbital nerve and the frontal branch of the facial nerve are well protected within the flap.*

Once the dissection has fully released the forehead and brow soft tissue, with care taken to preserve the supraorbital and supratrochlear nerves, myotomies of the frontalis, corrugator, and procerus musculature are sharply performed (Fig. 3-32). The frontalis myotomy can be performed by either resection or scoring. When the frontalis muscle is stout and short, resection is best; however, when the frontalis is thin and wide, full-thickness scoring with a scalpel or electrocautery blade in a crosshatch pattern is best. If resection is performed, a graft of temporal fascia or AlloDerm (LifeCell Co., Branchburg, New Jersey) should be inset to avoid a secondary contour defect. Care must be exercised in dissecting and preserving the supraorbital and supra-trochlear nerves during performance of the frontalis myotomy. The procerus and corrugator myotomies require only dissection and transection, unless unusually stout muscles are encountered. In such cases, resection of a small segment of the muscles is necessary, and a small fat graft should be interposed to prevent contour irregularity.

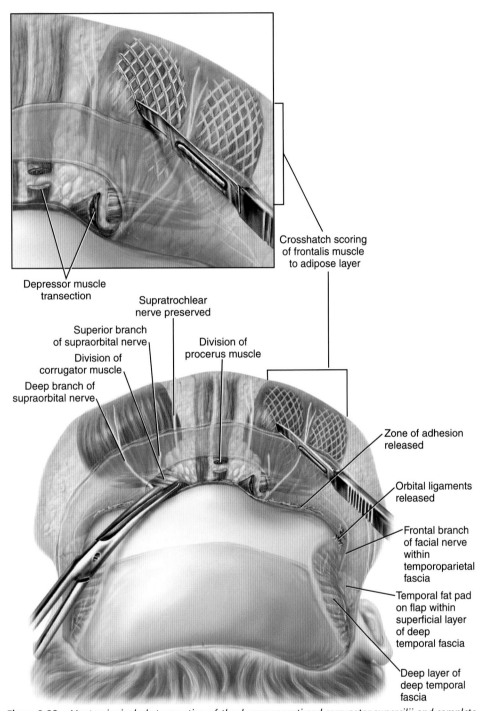

Crosshatch scoring
of frontalis muscle
to adipose layer

Depressor muscle
transection

Supratrochlear
nerve preserved

Superior branch
of supraorbital nerve

Division of
procerus muscle

Division of
corrugator muscle

Deep branch of
supraorbital nerve

Zone of adhesion
released

Orbital ligaments
released

Frontal branch
of facial nerve
within
temporoparietal
fascia

Temporal fat pad
on flap within
superficial layer
of deep
temporal fascia

Deep layer of
deep temporal
fascia

Figure 3-32   *Myotomies include transection of the depressor septi and corrugator supercilii and complete crosshatch scoring of the frontalis muscle. The superficial and deep branches of the supraorbital nerve and the supratrochlear nerve should be preserved, and the superficial layer of the deep temporal fascia should be preserved on the flap to protect the frontal branch of the facial nerve.*

After hemostasis is obtained, fixation of the coronal flap is performed (Fig. 3-33). Key stitches are placed for vertical elevation of the flap in three locations: the medial eyebrow, the peak eyebrow, and the lateral eyebrow. Lahey clamps are placed on the coronal flap to aid retraction, and vertical cuts are made in the flap to customize vertical elevation at these locations. This is performed with buried galeal stitches of 2-0 Vicryl suture. The vectors for vertical brow displacement are radial to the midline, thereby "opening" a crowded medial brow as well as elevating the ptotic soft tissue component. In order to achieve this radial and vertical displacement of the eyebrows, it is best to place these key stitches alternating between sides—right medial, then left medial; right peak, then left peak; right lateral, then left lateral. Each stitch should be placed and each suture tied before the next stitch is placed. Once the key sutures have been properly placed, resection of excess scalp can be performed along the direction of the hair follicles. This resection should be performed in a tension-free manner, because tension for the closure has been placed at the three key stitch sites. The coronal flap should literally fall into place.

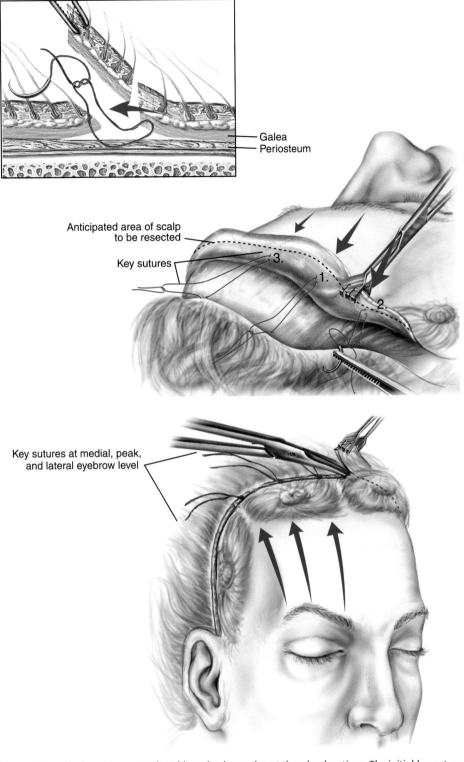

Galea
Periosteum

Anticipated area of scalp
to be resected

Key sutures

Key sutures at medial, peak,
and lateral eyebrow level

Figure 3-33 *The key sutures are placed into the deep galea at three key locations. The initial key suture is placed to fixate the apex of the brow, followed by the lateral brow and then the medial brow, making certain to lift and slightly separate the medial eyebrows and glabella. Excess scalp is then conservatively resected.*

Several deep alignment stitches of 3-0 Vicryl suture are placed for deep closure. Staples are used for scalp closure (Fig. 3-34). A closed suction drain is placed exiting in the temporal scalp, and finally, dressings are placed.

CLINICAL PEARLS

- Once a coronal lift has been chosen, either a classic gull-wing scalp incision or a pretrichal incision is designed, in combination with a transverse sideburn incision to aid access.
- Subperiosteal dissection of the lower forehead and brow is best performed with a sharp round periosteal elevator, because the skin in this region is densely adherent to bone.
- Release of the subperiosteal zone of adhesion and the orbital ligaments must be thoroughly performed for effective release of the soft tissues.
- Dissection below the temporal crest is performed deep to the superficial layer of deep temporal fascia to elevate the temporal fat pad and to prevent injury to the frontal branch of the facial nerve.
- The frontalis muscle can be either resected, if it is stout and short, or scored full-thickness, if it is thin and wide. If frontalis resection is performed, a graft of temporal fascia should be inset to avoid a secondary contour defect.
- Great care must be exercised in dissection to preserve the supraorbital and supratrochlear nerves during the frontalis myotomy portion of the procedure.
- The procerus and corrugator myotomies require only dissection and transection, unless a short, stout muscle is encountered. In such cases, then resection of a small segment of the muscle is necessary, and a small fat graft should be interposed to prevent contour irregularity.
- The vectors for vertical brow displacement are radial to the midline, thereby "opening" a crowded medial brow as well as elevating the ptotic soft tissue component.
- Three key buried galeal stitches of 2-0 Vicryl suture are used for vertical elevation of the medial eyebrow, peak eyebrow, and lateral eyebrow.
- Scalp resection should be performed in a tension-free manner, with tension placed at the three key stitch sites—the coronal flap should literally fall into place.

Key References

Connell B, Lambros V, Neurohr G: The forehead lift: Techniques to avoid complications and produce optimum results. Aesth Plast Surg 13:217, 1989.

Daniel R, Tirkanits B: Endoscopic forehead lift: An operative technique. Plast Reconstr Surg 98:1148, 1996.

Dayan S, Perkins S, Vartanian A, Wiesman I: The forehead lift: Endoscopic versus coronal approaches. Aesth Plast Surg 25:35, 2001.

De la Fuente A, Santamaria A: Endoscopic forehead lift: Is it effective? Aesth Surg J 22:113, 2002.

Isse N: Endoscopic facial rejuvenation: Endoforehead, the functional lift. Case Reports. Aesth Plast Surg 18:21, 1994.

Knize D: Limited incision foreheadplasty. Plast Reconstr Surg. 103:271, 1999.

Matarasso A, Hutchinson O: Evaluating rejuvenation of the forehead and brow: An algorithm for selecting the appropriate technique. Plast Reconstr Surg 106:687, 2000.

Ramirez O: Endoscopic techniques in facial rejuvenation. Aesth Plast Surg 18:141, 1994.

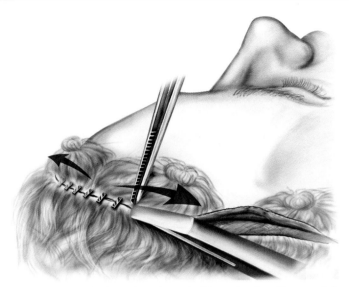

Figure 3-34 *Scalp closure is performed with staples placed from medial to lateral, making certain to evert the wound edges slightly.*

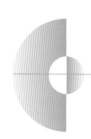

CHAPTER FOUR

One-Layer Approaches to the Face and Neck

The subcutaneous one-layer approach for facelift incorporates the traditional skin flap approach with small-cannula liposculpture and fat grafting lipostructure. For the purposes of this text, the subcutaneous layer in the face and neck is defined as the epidermis, dermis, and hypodermis, or superficial fat layer. This superficial fat layer is uniform throughout the face and neck and held into a tight lattice-like arrangement by fibrous tissue extensions between the reticular dermis and the superficial layer of the investing fascia, or superficial musculoaponeurotic system (SMAS). The SMAS also has a deep component with roots that weave through the deep fat layer and around the mimetic musculature. Because of this intricate investiture, the SMAS, along with the broad platysma muscle, can be raised as a separate and independent surgical flap for facial and neck recontouring. The two-layer approach for facelift, which includes independent SMAS, SMAS-platysma, and deeper fascial techniques, is discussed in the next chapter ("Two-Layer Approaches to the Face and Neck").

When I trained in the 1980s, the one-layer subcutaneous approach for facelift meant raising skin flaps comprising very little superficial fat. The one-layer subcutaneous technique went by many names, depending on the author primarily responsible for popularizing a specific version of the technique. From a conceptual standpoint, however, the surgeon primarily achieved *skin tightening* when using this technique. Then, in the 1990s, the thickness of superficial fat included within the skin flaps of the subcutaneous technique increased. Many plastic surgeons began including as much superficial fat as possible on facial and neck skin flaps. The one-layer subcutaneous technique evolved, and surgeons began to achieve a second goal: *superficial fat repositioning.* The new millennium brought a variety of dependable techniques for facial and neck liposculpture and primary structural fat grafting. This added wood to the plastic

surgeon's fire, so that a third, very important goal was achieved with the one-layer subcutaneous techniques, a goal previously attainable only by independent two-layer techniques: *facial and neck reshaping.* The one-layer subcutaneous technique had gone from a technical exercise in skin tightening to a sculptural art form. There still, however, are three very important principles separating one-layer subcutaneous techniques from two-layer techniques: (1) one-layer subcutaneous techniques involve only one layer, no matter how thick nor how sculpted the fat; (2) the flaps can be fashioned along only one vector of skin tension, which makes them dependent on a single wound for healing; and (3) no surgical manipulation of the underlying SMAS and platysma muscle is performed.

As discussed in Chapters One and Two, the face, which is composed of concentric layers of lamellar tissue, most closely resembles an onion in structure. Aging in the face begins superficially and proceeds with unremitting intensity inward—like a rotting onion, the skin of which peels and dies before the core goes soft. The superficial subcutaneous tissues of the face and neck are exposed at all times, subject to the trauma that the elements pose, as well as the shearing forces created by the demands of everyday life. Once the forces of facial aging have eroded through the subcutaneous tissues and into the mimetic muscular, fascial, and ligamentous system that suspends the face and neck from the underlying craniofacial skeleton, techniques designed to manipulate these deeper structures are necessary if serious rejuvenation is desired. This injunction is not meant to minimize how important one-layer subcutaneous technique is to the plastic surgeon. Mastery and proper performance of the subcutaneous technique are a sine qua non for optimal facelifting. For even with today's powerful deep fascial and muscle techniques, by which the surgeon can sculpt a virtual Venus de Milo under the skin, if he or she covers that with a crumpled, asymmetrical, or wasted skin envelope, beauty will most certainly not be served. Subcutaneous sculpting techniques and deeper plane fascial and muscle engineering techniques are like the right and left hands of the plastic surgeon—both hands need to work together in a coordinated and balanced effort in order to achieve optimal aesthetic results.

One-layer subcutaneous technique is examined in great detail in this chapter, with both illustrations and operative photographs of each and every step provided. Although at today's state-of-the-art plastic surgery meetings the emphasis always seems to be on baking the more complexly flavorful and intricately arranged "deep plane cake," it is the velvety-smooth "subcutaneous frosting" that gets the attention of patients and their friends the quickest.

KEY POINTS

1) One-layer thin-flap subcutaneous facelift technique achieves skin tightening.

2) One-layer thick-flap subcutaneous facelift technique achieves skin tightening and superficial fat repositioning.

3) One-layer thick-flap subcutaneous facelift technique, when combined with liposculpture and lipostructure, can also achieve facial and neck reshaping, comparable to that attainable with two-layer techniques, as long as significant ligamentous and musculofascial laxity is not present.

4) If significant ligamentous and musculofascial laxity is present, two-layer techniques are advisable.

INDICATIONS

Thin-flap subcutaneous techniques are most commonly used for the outer layer in performing two-layer surgery. The subcutaneous flap for the two-layer technique does need to be thin because a significant portion of the superficial fat must remain on the SMAS layer. The SMAS layer must have enough substance to allow the surgeon to develop an independent flap that repositions the superficial fat effectively along different vector lines and reshapes the face and neck artistically.

Thick-flap one-layer subcutaneous techniques incorporate as much superficial fat as possible in the skin flap. This technique is indicated primarily for patients without deeper tissue ptosis—youthful patients with skin folds and minimal ligamentous or musculofascial laxity. Thick-flap one-layer subcutaneous techniques are especially useful when combined with the minimal-incision approach for facelift. Liposculpture and lipostructure are added depending on the patient's needs.

Variable-thickness-flap one-layer subcutaneous techniques include a predetermined amount of superficial fat on the skin flaps. This technique is indicated for the secondary face- and neck lift patient, in whom the first procedure has determined the thickness of the subcutaneous flap. Variable-thickness techniques must, by necessity, include liposculpture and lipostructure to achieve facial and neck reshaping.

Thin-flap, variable-thickness-flap, and thick-flap techniques achieve their best results when combined with superficial liposculpture and fat grafting using the fat scaffolding technique of Coleman. It seems illogical to discuss surgical procedures indicated for the youthful patient and for the secondary facelift patient before reviewing the surgical options available for the middle-aged prospective "novice," the most common patient desiring rhytidectomy. But as my wry plastic surgery mentor Dr. Thomas Rees once observed, there is usually a good reason traditional surgical techniques are called traditional!

Other rare indications for one-layer subcutaneous techniques include cosmetic procedures in patients who have undergone previous head and neck surgery, especially superficial parotidectomy. In these patients, the facial nerve has been transposed to a very superficial and extremely vulnerable position within a scarred subcutaneous bed. In addition, in patients who have received silicone injections for vague cosmetic reasons, unfortunately a concrete-like scar that encases the subcutaneous layers of the face and neck is typically seen. Rather than embark on a futile search for traditional surgical planes of dissection and risk injury to deeper vital structures, a traditional subcutaneous facelift is a far better option.

KEY POINTS

1) Thin-flap one-layer subcutaneous facelift technique forms the outer layer for two-flap techniques and is indicated primarily for patients with significant ligamentous and musculofascial laxity.

2) Thick-flap one-layer subcutaneous facelift technique is indicated primarily for the youthful patient with significant skin folds and minimal ligamentous or musculofascial laxity. Liposculpture and lipostructure are used depending on the patient's needs.

3) Variable-thickness-flap one-layer subcutaneous facelift technique is indicated primarily for secondary facelift patients, and liposculpture and lipostructure are mandatory.

OPERATIVE STRATEGIES

The Youthful Patient

Selection of the ideal surgical approach for youthful patients with skin folding and minimal ligamentous ptosis poses several problems. These patients are in a dilemma: They see themselves aging in the mirror, but do they really need a facelift? The plastic surgeon is also in a dilemma: Will *superficial liposculpture and primary fat grafting* be enough to treat a few skin folds and creases, or should the subcutaneous fat be repositioned and the skin tightened with a *thick-flap one-layer subcutaneous facelift* performed through minimal incisions? Many youthful patients make this decision for the surgeon by refusing a facelift for personal reasons. They simply will not accept the stigma of a facelift—after all, their mother didn't "need" a facelift until she was in her 60s. Then the plastic surgeon begins to wonder: Will superficial liposculpture and fat grafting meet the expectations of such a patient?

The answer to this dilemma lies in the degree and amount of skin folding in the patient's face. If the woman, no matter what her age, has supple skin with minimal skin folding and little, if any, ligamentous laxity, then superficial liposculpture with or without lipostructure will yield good recontouring results (Fig. 4-1). If the patient has microgenia, then a chin implant can improve the results even further (Fig. 4-2). Some of the apparent cervical skin excess will be used to recontour the neck after the liposculpture, and whatever remains can be literally drawn forward and "lifted" by the chin augmentation (Fig. 4-3). In some youthful patients, the only thing that bothers them is a deep nasolabial fold. If ligamentous laxity is minimal and the patient has no other cheek folds, then fat grafting alone can yield good results. The patient does not need a subcutaneous one-layer facelift as long as the deep nasolabial fold is the only feature perceived as requiring correction. If the face is thin, then fat grafting of the crease using the fat scaffolding technique and small, precise amounts of fat is all that is necessary (Fig. 4-4). If the face is full, liposculpture of the heavy fold with fat grafting of the deep crease using fat scaffolding technique keeps the face in balance (Fig. 4-5). Facial and neck liposculpture and lipostructure, once considered ancillary techniques for facial rejuvenation, have become frontline treatments for the youthful patient, as well as for the patient who has undergone facelift but desires a minor revision (Fig. 4-6).

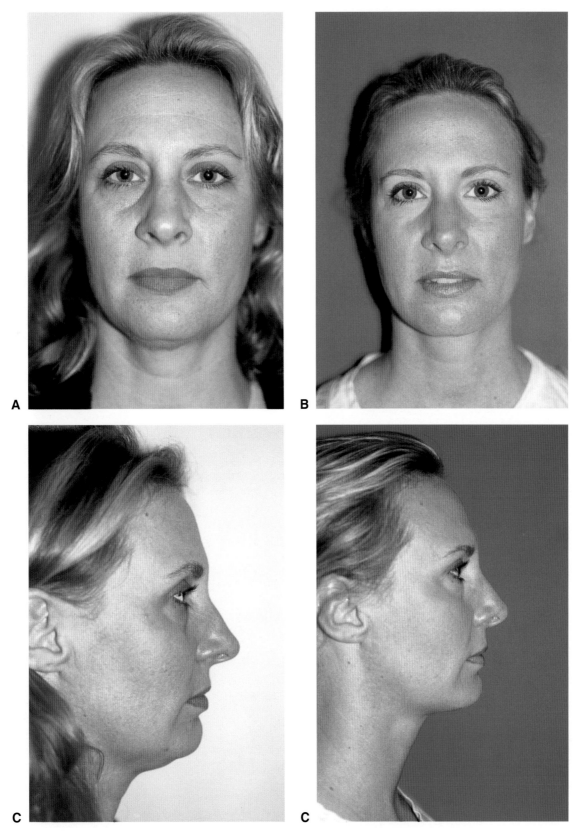

Figure 4-1 *The Youthful Patient: Cervical and Jowl Liposculpture.* ***A*** *and* ***C,*** *This 42-year-old woman had heavy subcutaneous fat collections in the jowl and anterior neck regions. She has supple skin, a minimal nasolabial fold, and minor ligamentous laxity.* ***B*** *and* ***D,*** *Superficial liposculpture of the anterior neck and jowls yielded good recontouring results at 1 year. Note: A rhinoplasty and lower blepharoplasty were added.*

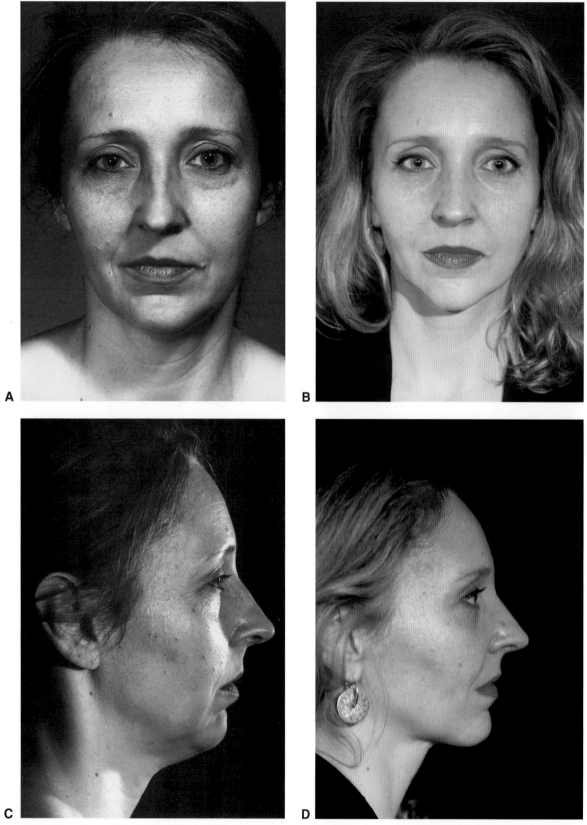

Figure 4-2 *The Youthful Patient: Chin Implant with Cervical and Jowl Liposculpture/Lipostructure.* **A** *and* **C,** *This 41-year-old woman complained of jowls and lack of jawline and neck definition. She has a thin face, a weak jaw, and minimal ligamentous laxity despite her plump jowls and anterior neck.* **B** *and* **D,** *A chin implant, along with superficial liposculpture and fat grafting over the lateral chin, yielded good recontouring results at 1 year. Note that some of the apparent cervical skin excess was drawn forward and up by the chin augmentation. The patient also had four-lid blepharoplasty.*

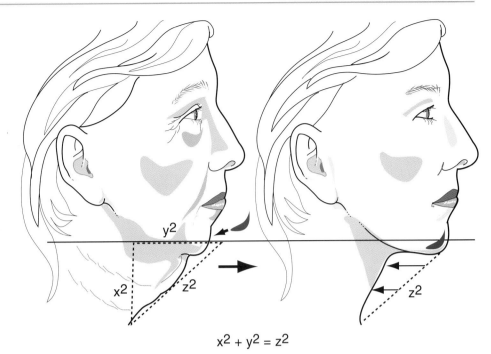

Figure 4-3 *Liposculpture. After anterior neck liposculpture, the apparent cervical skin excess is used to recontour the neck. Beware: In the patient with significant skin folds, skin tightening will not result from superficial liposculpture, even if lipostructure is added!*

$$x^2 + y^2 = z^2$$

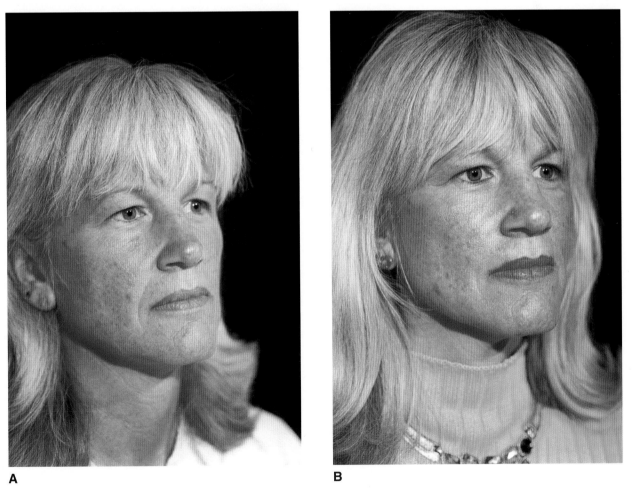

A   **B**

Figure 4-4 *The Youthful Patient: Lipostructure of the Nasolabial Crease. **A,** This 39-year-old woman has a thin face, minimal ligamentous ptosis, and a simple deep nasolabial crease. **B,** Fat grafting of the crease (with 5 mL of fat per side) using the fat scaffolding technique yielded good results at 2 years.*

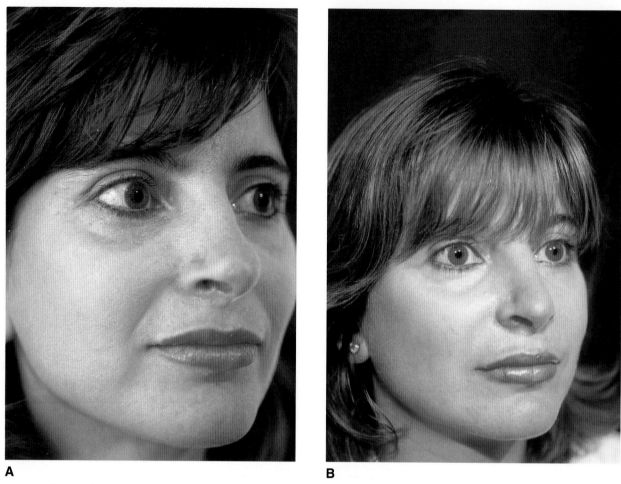

A   **B**

Figure 4-5 *The Youthful Patient: Liposculpture of Nasolabial Fold and Lipostructure of the Nasolabial Crease. **A,** This 43-year-old woman has a full face, minimal ligamentous laxity, and a simple deep nasolabial fold. **B,** Liposculpture of the folds and fat grafting of the crease (with 5.0 mL of fat per side) using the fat scaffolding technique yielded a good result that preserved facial balance at 1 year.*

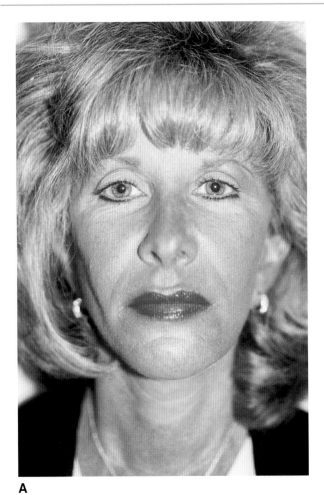

A

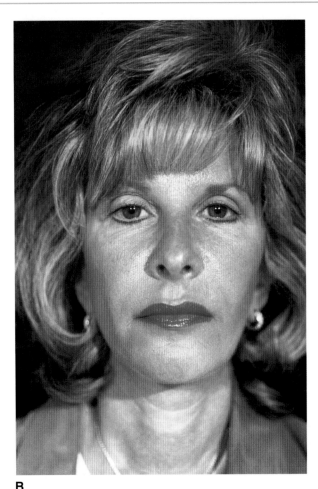

B

Figure 4-6 *Liposculpture of Nasolabial Fold and Lipostructure of the Nasolabial Crease after Facelift.* **A,** *This 52-year-old woman, at 2 years after two-layer facelift using the extended SMAS/platysma technique, was bothered by a persistent nasolabial fold.* **B,** *Liposculpture of the fold and fat grafting of the crease (with 6.0 mL of fat per side) using the fat scaffolding technique yielded improvement at 1 year.*

When the degree of skin folding becomes significant, especially in the youthful patient with a thin face, a deep nasolabial crease, and lateral cheek folds, then superficial liposculpture and lipostructure are not enough. *Liposculpture and lipostructure do not tighten lax, excessive skin.* Once skin folding is significant, especially in the cheek, then thick-flap one-layer subcutaneous facelift is necessary if substantial improvement is desired (Figs. 4-7 to 4-9). On close examination, these patients usually present with rhytides beyond those expected for their youthful number of years. If platysma banding is evident in the neck at rest, anterior neck corset-like platysmaplasty performed through the submental approach with or without suspension sutures should be added (Figs. 4-10 to 4-12). If musculofascial and ligamentous laxity is present and the patient desires optimal results, then two-layer techniques are advisable despite the patient's age (Figs. 4-13 and 4-14). A simple test for ligamentous and musculofascial laxity in the face and neck is to have the patient bring the chin down to the chest while leaning forward; if the facial and neck soft tissues sag off the face rather than simply bunching up, then ligamentous and musculofascial laxity is significant, and the plastic surgeon should seriously consider a two-layer technique (Fig. 4-15).

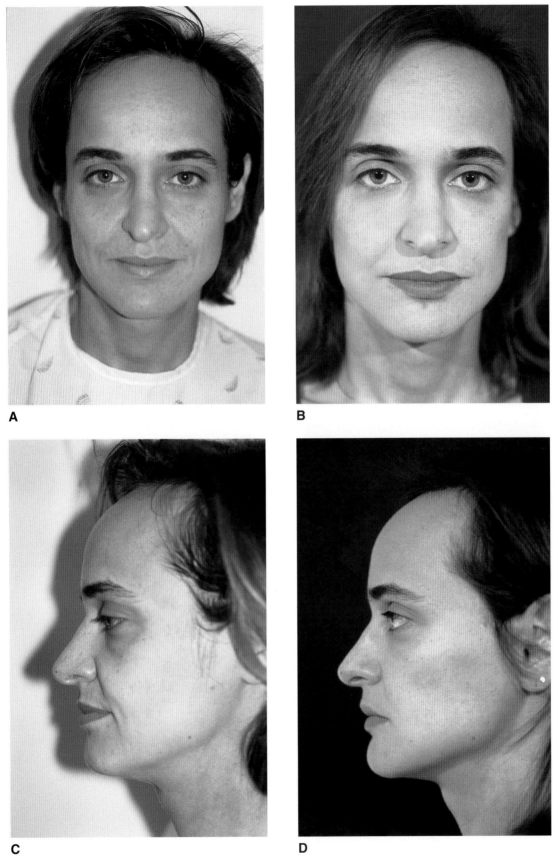

A

B

C

D

Figure 4-7 *The Youthful Patient: Thick-Flap One-Layer Subcutaneous Facelift. **A** and **B,** This 39-year-old woman has a thin face, minimal ligamentous laxity, deep nasolabial creases, and deep cheek folds. **C** and **D,** Thick-flap one-layer subcutaneous facelift performed through a minimal incision approach resulted in correction after 1 year.*

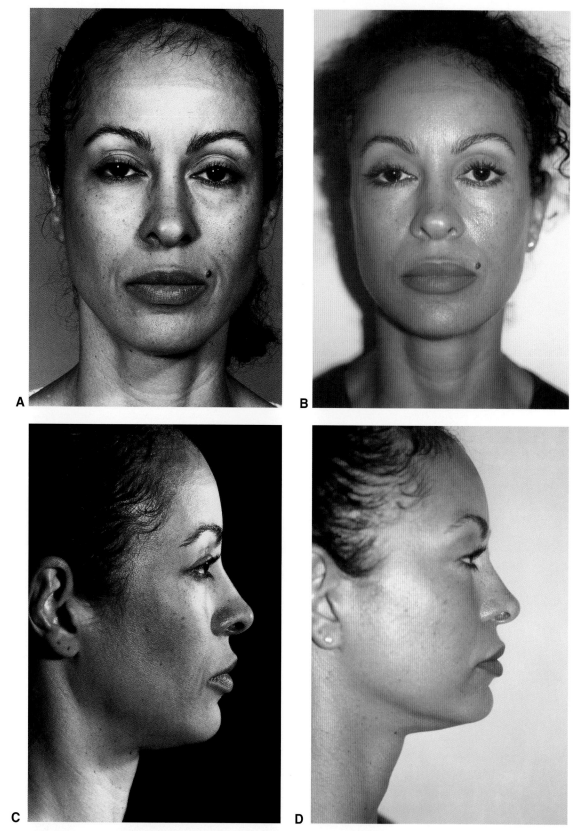

Figure 4-8 *The Youthful Patient: Thick-Flap One-Layer Subcutaneous Facelift and Liposculpture.* ***A*** *and* ***C,*** *This 40-year-old woman has a thin face, minimal ligamentous laxity, fine nasolabial creases, and fine cheek folds.* ***B*** *and* ***D,*** *Thick-flap one-layer subcutaneous facelift performed through a minimal-incision approach and cervical liposculpture softened these features. Note: Four-lid blepharoplasty was also performed. The patient would have benefited from fat grafting but refused this procedure.*

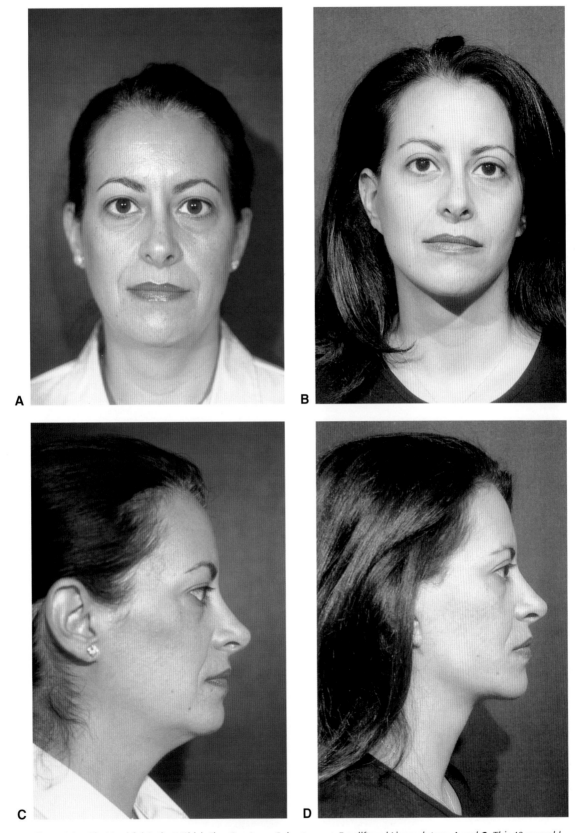

Figure 4-9 *The Youthful Patient: Thick-Flap One-Layer Subcutaneous Facelift and Liposculpture.* ***A*** *and* ***C,*** *This 40-year-old woman has a thin face, early jowls and nasolabial creases, and musculoligamentous neck laxity.* ***B*** *and* ***D,*** *Thick-flap one-layer subcutaneous facelift with lateral platysmaplasty performed through a minimal-incision approach and cervical liposculpture resulted in improvement at 1 year. Note: Lower blepharoplasty was also performed. Fat grafting of the nasolabial creases would have benefited the patient.*

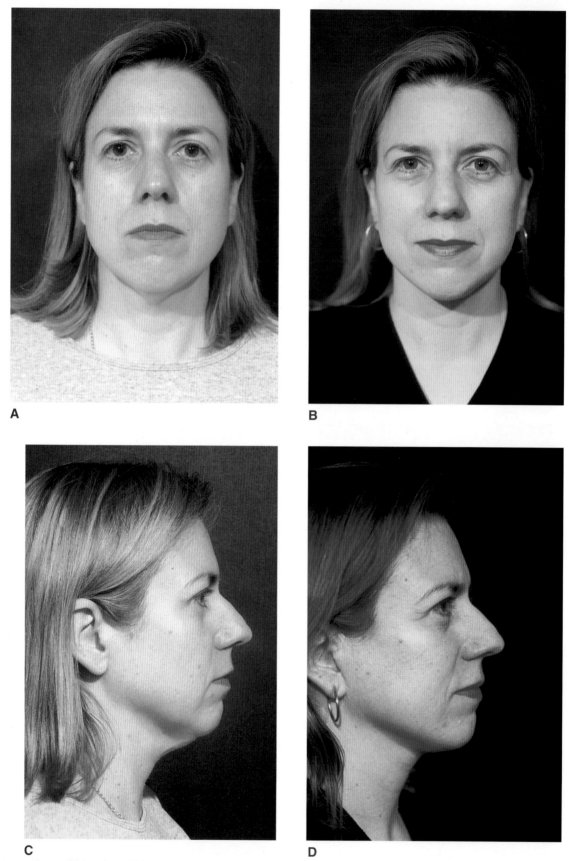

Figure 4-10   *The Youthful Patient: Thick-Flap One-Layer Subcutaneous Facelift and Liposculpture/Lipostructure.* ***A*** *and* ***C,*** *This 40-year-old woman has a thin face and musculoligamentous neck laxity.* ***B*** *and* ***D,*** *One-layer thick-flap subcutaneous facelift with anterior corset-like platysmaplasty, cervical liposculpture, and nasolabial crease fat grafting (with 6.0 mL of fat per side) yielded correction at 2 years.*

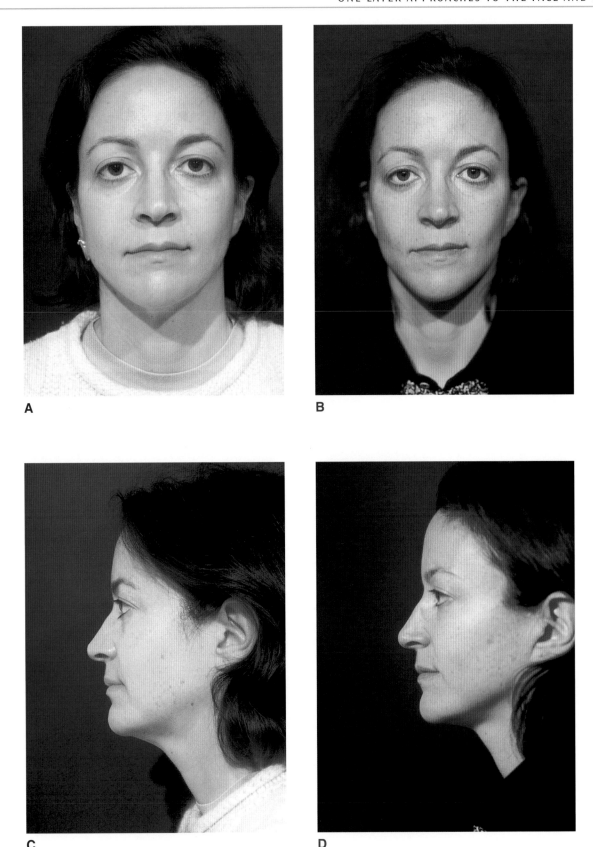

A

B

C

D

Figure 4-11   *The Youthful Patient: Thick-Flap One-Layer Subcutaneous Facelift and Liposculpture/Lipostructure.* ***A*** *and* ***C,*** *This 40-year-old woman has a thin face and musculoligamentous neck laxity.* ***B*** *and* ***D,*** *Thick-flap one-layer subcutaneous facelift with anterior corset-like platysmaplasty, cervical liposculpture, and nasolabial crease fat grafting (with 6.0 mL of fat per side) yielded correction at 1 year.*

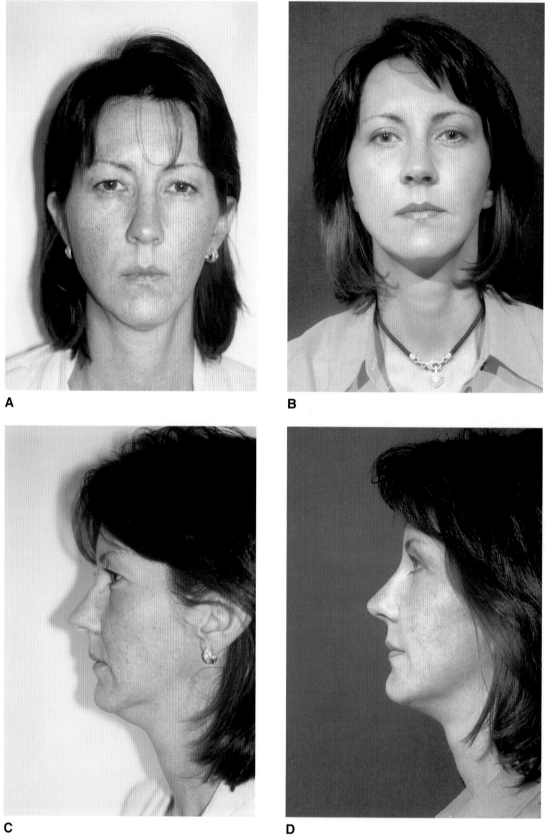

A

B

C

D

Figure 4-12   *The Youthful Patient: Thick-Flap One-Layer Subcutaneous Facelift and Liposculpture/Lipostructure.* **A** *and* **C,** *This 40-year-old woman has a thin face and musculoligamentous neck laxity.* **B** *and* **D,** *Thick-flap one-layer subcutaneous facelift with anterior corset-like platysmaplasty, cervical liposculpture, and nasolabial/marionette crease fat grafting (with 5.0 mL of fat per side) yielded correction at 1 year. Upper blepharoplasty was added. Note: The patient has a low hyoid bone.*

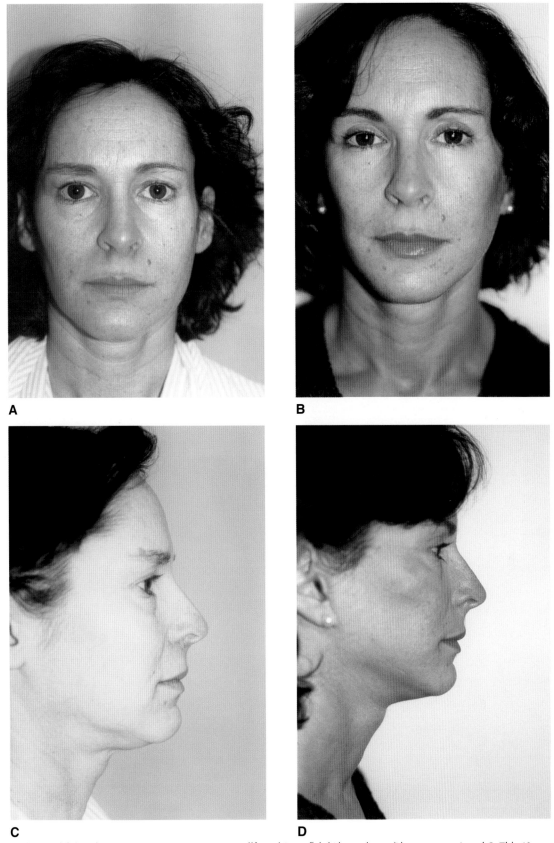

A

B

C

D

Figure 4-13 *The Youthful Patient: Two-Layer SMAS-ectomy Facelift and Superficial Liposculpture/Lipostructure. **A** and **C**, This 40-year-old woman has significant facial and neck ligamentous laxity despite her age. **B** and **D**, Lateral SMAS/platysma-ectomy facelift, cervical liposculpture, and nasolabial/marionette crease and lateral chin fat grafting (with 8.0 mL of fat per side) was performed through the minimal-incision approach and yielded correction at 1 year. Note: Four-lid blepharoplasty was also performed.*

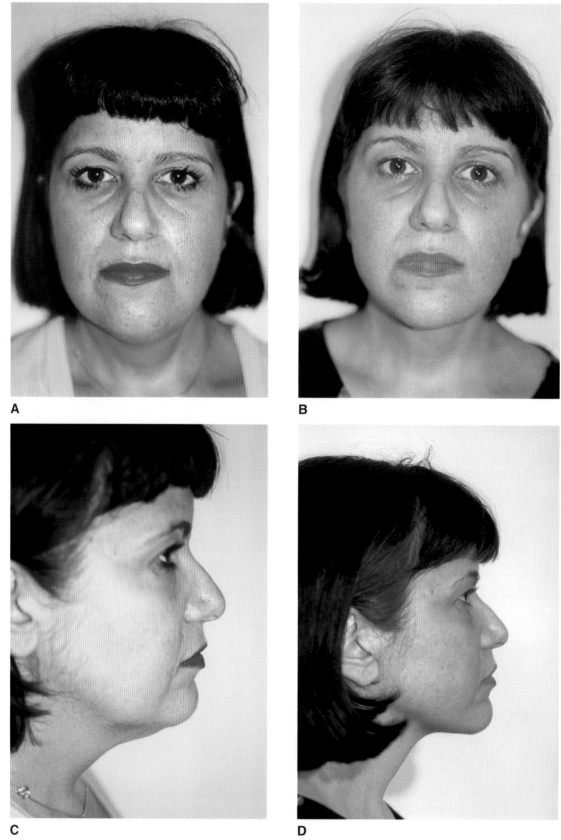

Figure 4-14 *The Youthful Patient: Two-Layer Extended SMAS/Platysma Facelift and Superficial Liposculpture/Lipostructure.* **A** *and* **C,** *This 40-year-old woman has significant facial and neck ligamentous laxity despite her age.* **B** *and* **D,** *Two-layer extended SMAS/platysma facelift and cervical, jowl, and nasolabial fold liposculpture with fat grafting (with 5.0 mL of fat per side) yielded correction at 1 year. Contrast this result with the results obtained using liposculpture/fat grafting alone (see Figs. 4-16 and 4-17).*

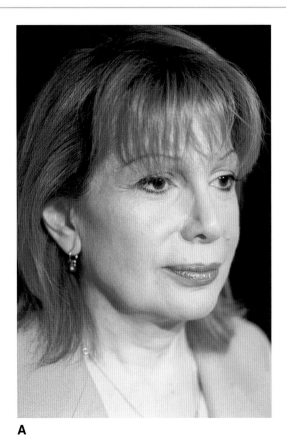
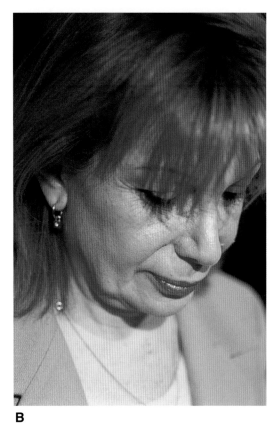

A   **B**

Figure 4-15   ***A*** *and* ***B,*** *A simple test for ligamentous laxity in the face and neck is to have the patient bring the chin down to the chest while leaning forward. If the facial and neck soft tissues sag off the face rather than simply bunching up, then ligamentous and musculofascial laxity is significant. In such cases, the deep layer needs to be addressed, and two-layer techniques are advisable.*

Another problem encountered in youthful patients who are heavy is that underlying musculofascial laxity often coexists within the neck despite its firmness and fullness. The fat literally blankets the underlying platysma muscle, which really is excessive and lax. Such patients often refuse a facelift, feeling that this procedure is for those with saggy skin. They believe that the main problem is excess fat, so that liposuction must be the solution. In many cases, significant improvement can be obtained with superficial liposculpture of the face and neck alone (Fig. 4-16). Removing the fat, however, will also unmask the platysma excess, and platysma banding at rest will become evident several months postoperatively (see Fig. 4-16). These patients need to be counseled about the potential pitfalls of liposculpture before surgery and be forewarned that platysma muscle laxity, as well as skin laxity, may persist, even if chin implants and lipostructure are added (Fig. 4-17). They also need to understand that

despite what they may have read or seen, liposuction and fat grafting are not going to tighten skin and muscle and give them the well-sculpted jawline they envision. A facelift will be necessary if that is truly what they desire.

One solution that has been proposed by several surgeons to address this potential pitfall of liposculpture is the limited anterior platysmaplasty. The author has found that limited anterior platysmaplasty is best used as a secondary procedure for correcting residual platysma bands after a facelift has been performed, and not for the youthful patient with a bad neckline who refuses a facelift. When the limited anterior platysmaplasty is used with liposculpture and lipostructure to treat the youthful patient with a heavy neck or platysma excess, persistent neck seromas and small localized neck infections can result. These problems will negate any potential benefits the procedure provides, even if that procedure has been combined with suspension sutures.

KEY POINTS

1) Superficial liposculpture with lipostructure alone yields good recontouring results in youthful patients with supple skin, minimal skin folding, and minimal ligamentous laxity.

2) A chin implant improves neck recontouring results initially achieved by liposculpture and lipostructure.

3) Even in youthful patients, liposculpture and lipostructure do not tighten lax, excessive skin.

4) Once significant skin folding exists in the youthful patient, especially in the cheeks, then thick-flap one-layer subcutaneous facelift is advisable if substantial improvement is desired.

5) If platysma excess and banding are evident in the neck, anterior neck corset-like platysmaplasty with or without suspension sutures should be added to the subcutaneous facelift.

The Secondary Facelift Patient

Surgery in the secondary face- and neck lift patient poses several problems. First, in many secondary and tertiary procedure patients, a well-developed bed of fibrous scar tissue exists in the subcutaneous tissues—a remnant from the previous facelift. This plane is technically easy to undermine and less bloody than it is at first procedures. The thickness of the subcutaneous flap, however, has already been determined at the original procedure. How thick to make the skin flap cannot be decided until the dissection is begun. Hence, the technique used for

secondary patients is called *variable-thickness*. In a majority of secondary patients this scar tissue plane is composed of so much fibrous tissue that it actually obscures the anatomical details of the underlying SMAS and platysma muscle. In such cases, a deeper plane two-layer technique is fraught with unnecessary difficulty, bleeding, and danger. Fortunately, for most secondary patients we can capitalize on the presence of this scar tissue plane. After all, it has much of the strength and substance of the SMAS anyway. The scar tissue plane can actually become the carrier in skin tightening and superficial fat repositioning (Fig. 4-18).

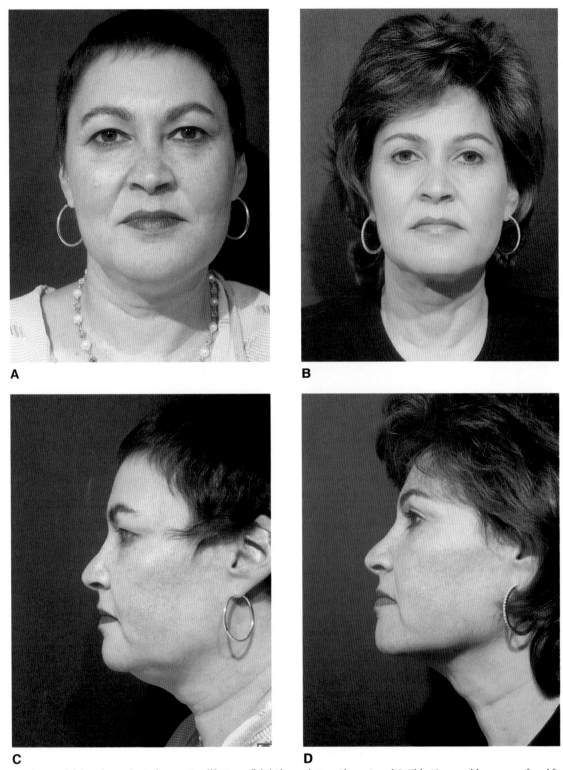

A

B

C

D

Figure 4-16   *The Youthful Patient Who Refuses a Facelift: Superficial Liposculpture Alone.* **A** *and* **C,** *This 40-year-old woman refused facelift and desired liposuction only. In youthful patients who are heavy, underlying platysma muscle laxity can be obscured by the fat.* **B** *and* **D,** *Although significant improvement can be noted after superficial liposculpture of the face and neck, removing the fat will unmask this platysma excess, and platysma banding will become evident several months postoperatively.*

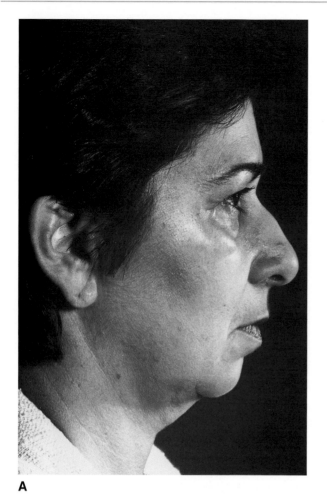

A

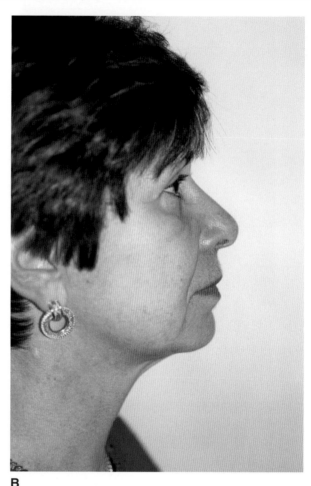

B

Figure 4-17   *The Middle-Aged Patient Who Refuses a Facelift: Superficial Liposculpture/Lipostructure and Chin Implant.* **A,** *This 50-year-old woman obviously needed a facelift for significant cosmetic improvement, but refused. She was counseled preoperatively about the potential pitfalls of liposculpture only, and forewarned that skin and platysma muscle laxity may persist after liposculpture* **(B),** *despite adding a chin implant and large-volume fat grafting to the lateral chin, nasolabial fold, and marionette line areas. Patients need to be counseled that despite what they may have read or seen, liposuction and fat grafting are not going to tighten skin or reposition muscle and cannot give them the sculpted look that a facelift can.*

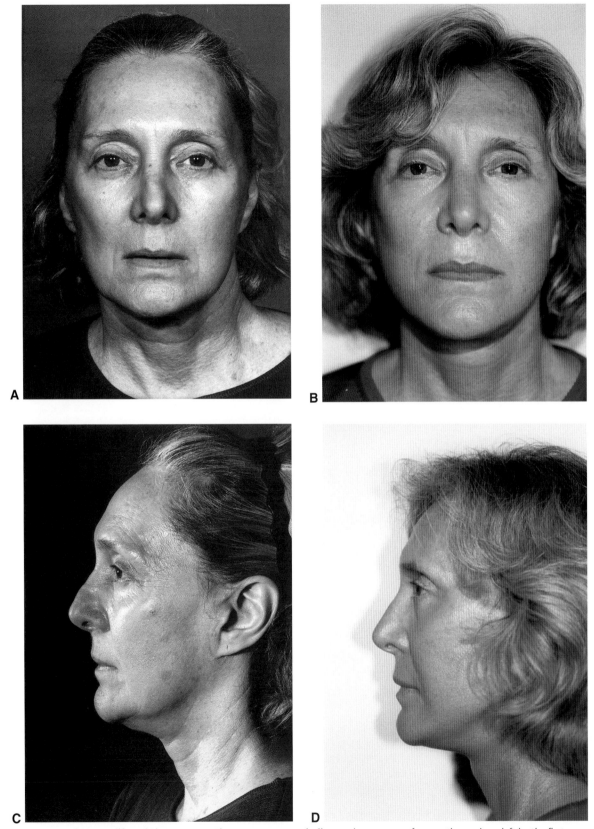

Figure 4-18   *Secondary Facelift and Lipostructure. The surgeon can capitalize on the presence of a scar tissue plane left by the first procedure by using it as the carrier for a one-layer subcutaneous "lift." This scar tissue has much of the strength and substance of the SMAS anyway.* **A** *and* **C,** *This 58-year-old secondary facelift patient had a subcutaneous scar tissue plane of such good quality that SMAS and platysma muscle surgery was judged to be unnecessary. Fat grafting of the nasolabial crease and marionette crease (with 6.0 mL of fat per side) was also performed.* **B** *and* **D,** *Her postoperative appearance.*

Second, in patients who have had their first procedure well over a decade ago, this scar tissue plane may not be plentiful enough for the present surgical purposes. After the skin flap has been undermined, if laxity of the SMAS and platysma is noted and the deeper layer anatomy is straightforward, then the surgeon can choose a two-layer procedure. More often than not, however, the SMAS and platysma are found to be thinned and stretched from the previous surgery and woefully inadequate to serve the present surgical needs. Old suture material is found, along with rents between the fibers of the platysma muscle through which small pseudoherniations of deep fat and fascia can be noted. Minor facial and anterior neck asymmetries suddenly make sense when the patient's preoperative photographs are reviewed. When this happens, the plastic surgeon must rely on the one-layer subcutaneous flap technique for the "lift" (Fig. 4-19). If that lift is well performed, long-term results comparable to those obtained with the two-layer deeper plane techniques can be achieved with the one-layer subcutaneous technique (Fig. 4-20).

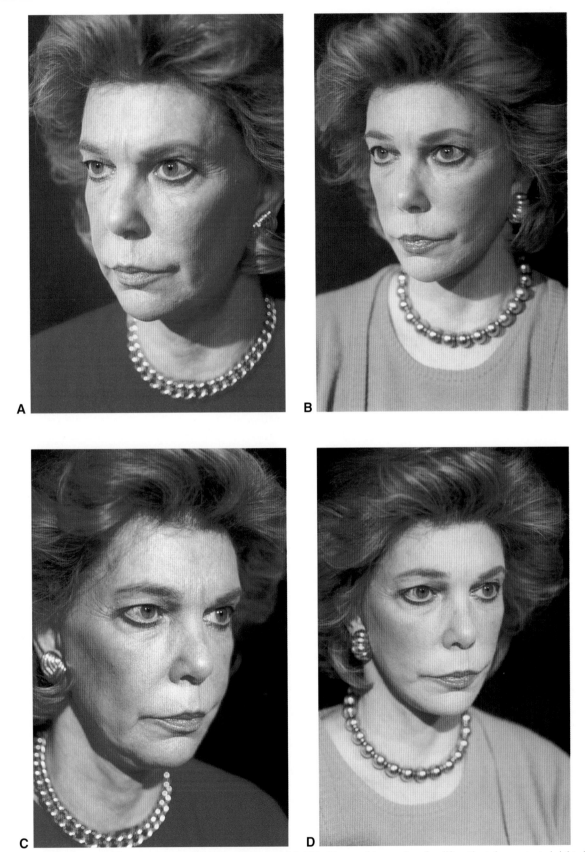

Figure 4-19 *Secondary Facelift Asymmetry and Lipostructure.* **A** *and* **C,** *This 62-year-old secondary facelift patient demonstrated right-sided excessive tissue redundancy in the jowl and anterior neck regions. The previously raised SMAS/platysma flaps were found to be severely thinned and stretched at surgery.* **B** *and* **D,** *Secondary subcutaneous rhytidectomy with asymmetrical vectors and asymmetrical tissue resection, and lipostructure of the left lateral chin, oral commissures, and marionette creases (with 8 mL of fat per side) yielded near-symmetrical secondary correction at 1 year.*

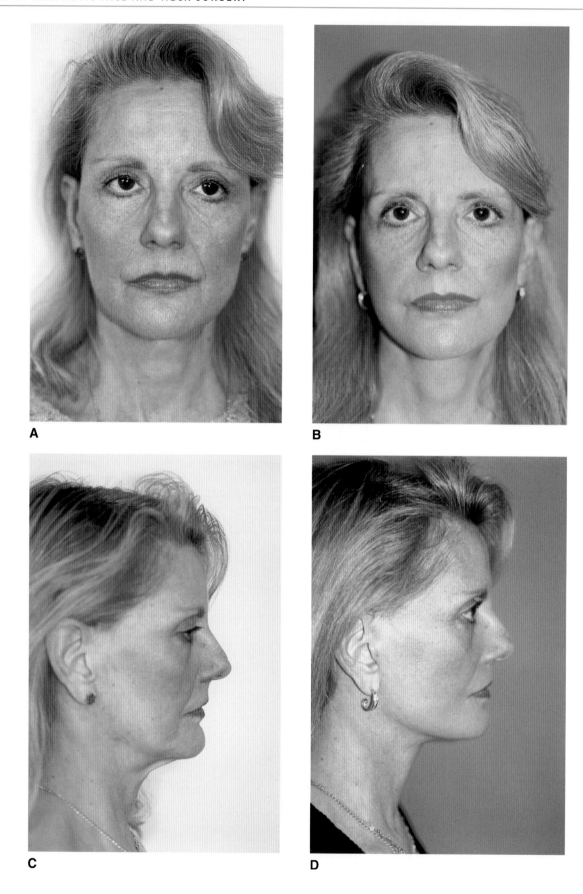

A

B

C

D

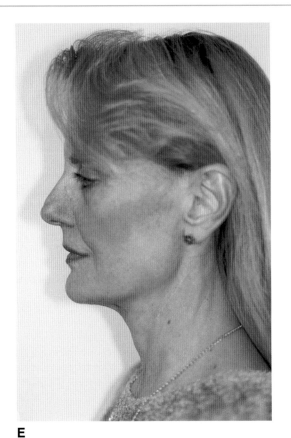

E

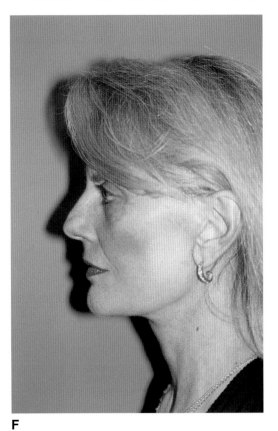

F

Figure 4-20   *Secondary Facelift Asymmetry and Lipostructure.* **A, C,** *and* **E,** *This 52-year-old woman demonstrated right jowl and platysma excess and banding.* **B, D,** *and* **F,** *Left-sided thick-flap one-layer subcutaneous facelift and right-sided two-layer lateral SMAS/platysma-ectomy and lipostructure of the nasolabial, marionette, and oral commissural creases (with 7 mL of fat on the left and 5 mL on the right) yielded a pleasing and symmetrical result more than a year later.*

Third, in many secondary facelift patients, the facial nerve may not lie at its usual anatomical depth. If a resective or two-layer technique was employed for the previous procedure, especially if absorbable sutures were used and tied under great tension, separation of the deeper plane plication may eventuate. The net result for the patient is that the facial nerve and its branches literally float up to a more vulnerable subcutaneous plane. If a significant scar tissue reaction is present that obscures anatomical detail, the stage is then set for motor nerve injury—the most dreaded of all facelift complications. Rather than risk injury to branches of the facial nerve, especially the more superficially located frontal and marginal mandibular branches, it is far safer to perform a thick one-layer subcutaneous lift for skin tightening and superficial fat suspension, and to supplement areas of contour deficiency with fat grafting. SMAS and lateral platysma plication sutures can be added, if safely indicated. And, of course, anterior neck corset-like platysmaplasty with or without suspension sutures can also be performed, if indicated, which will optimize the patient's surgical result (Figs. 4-21 and 4-22).

KEY POINTS

1) A well-developed bed of fibrous scar tissue exists in the subcutaneous tissues of most secondary facelift patients, a remnant from the previous surgery.

2) This scar tissue plane is easy to undermine and bleeds the least; however, the fibrous component can also obscure some of the anatomical details of the underlying SMAS and platysma muscle, making deeper plane two-layer techniques difficult, bloody, and dangerous.

3) The subcutaneous scar tissue bed in many secondary patients has much of the strength and substance of the SMAS anyway, obviating the need for deeper two-layer lifts and allowing a safer procedure.

4) If a previous resective or two-layer technique has been employed using absorbable sutures tied under tension, separation of the deeper plane plication can result, and the facial nerve and its branches can float up to a more vulnerable location.

5) Rather than risk injury to branches of the facial nerve, especially the more superficially located frontal and marginal mandibular branches, it is far safer in secondary procedures to perform a thick one-layer subcutaneous lift with fat grafting, using the fat scaffolding technique, to supplement areas of contour deficiency.

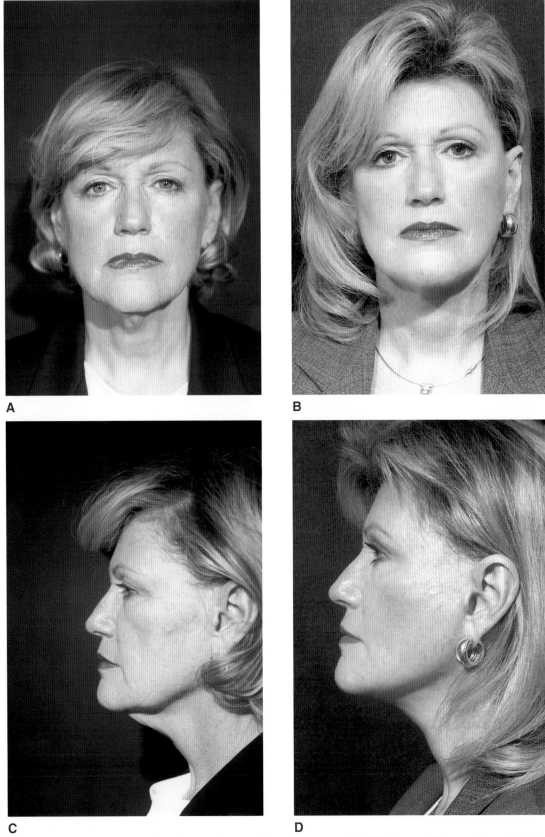

A

B

C

D

Figure 4-21   *Secondary Facelift with Corset-like Platysmaplasty and Lipostructure.* **A** and **C,** This 54-year-old woman demonstrated ligamentous and musculofascial face and neck laxity. Scarring obscured anatomical detail. Rather than risk injury to branches of the facial nerve, a thick-flap one-layer subcutaneous lift was performed. Fat grafting of the nasolabial, marionette, and oral commissural creases (with 7 mL of fat per side) was performed. **B** and **D,** Anterior corset-like platysmaplasty complemented her result at 1 year. Note: The patient declined a brow lift.

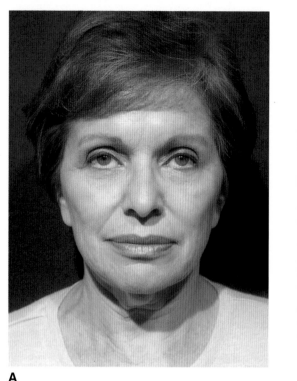
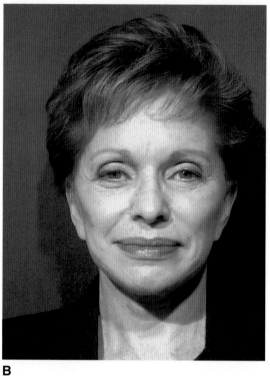

A   B

Figure 4-22   *Secondary Facelift with Corset-like Platysmaplasty and Suspension Sutures.* **A** *and* **C,** *This 61-year-old woman demonstrated ligamentous and musculofascial face and neck laxity.*

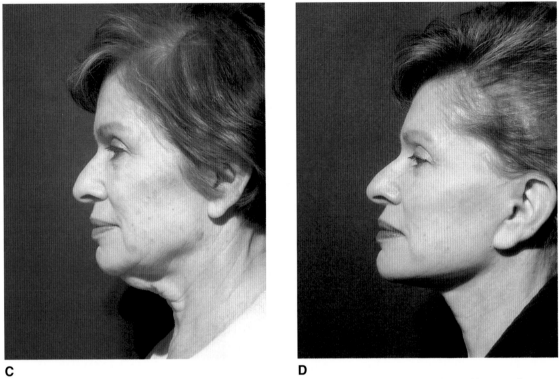

C

D

Figure 4-22, cont'd   ***B*** *and* ***D,*** *A thick-flap one-layer subcutaneous lift and anterior neck corset-like platysmaplasty with suspension sutures were performed. The combination significantly improved the patient's appearance at 1 year.*

TECHNIQUE

Subcutaneous facelift surgery involves several sequentially planned steps. These steps, which constitute the basic building blocks of the technique, are marking of incisions, anesthetization, undermining and defatting of subcutaneous flaps using both sharp and blunt (suction-assisted lipectomy [SAL]) techniques, hemostasis, and fashioning of the flaps along a cephaloposterior-directed vector along with fat grafting using the fat scaffolding technique. Fashioning the flaps is the most elaborate of the steps and includes placement of the deep key anchor sutures; rotation, advancement, and closure of the flaps; excess skin and soft tissue trimming; and placement of drains.

Step 1: Marking the Incisions

The basic incisions are illustrated in Figure 4-23. These incisions are used in combination and should always be placed in inconspicuous locations. Incisions in hair-bearing tissues should be beveled to avoid injury to the hair follicles with resultant bald scars. Pretrichal incisions, used more often in men, should be beveled at a more acute angle to spare pretrichal follicles, which sprout at more of an acute angle to the skin.

The markings include some combination of the following: (1) a gently curving temporal incision of variable length well behind the anterior hairline, (2) a transverse sideburn incision, which can be extended upward along the anterior hairline as a substitute for the temporal incision (used mainly in men), (3) a preauricular incision extending along the entire length of the ear with either pretragal (used in men only) or post-tragal (suitable for both women and men) modifications, and (4) a postauricular incision of variable length. The postauricular incision can be either the classic high incision, carried out above the sulcus on the ear cartilage and then diverging perpendicular to the ear and angling into the posterior hairline for a variable distance, or a low, curved incision in the sulcus that follows the posterior hairline for the vascular-compromised patient (i.e., a smoker); for the youthful patient, the minimal-incision approach can be used. Stab incisions in furrows and skin folds are used for liposculpture and lipostructure. The "workhorse" incision used in the vast majority of the author's middle-aged female patients is illustrated in Figure 4-24.

CLINICAL PEARLS

- Beveling of incisions in hair-bearing areas prevents bald scars.
- Incisions must be in inconspicuous locations.
- Pretrichal incisions are best for men.
- Post-tragal incisions are used in women as well as in men, but pretragal incisions should be used only in men.
- The classic postauricular incision is carried out above the sulcus on the ear cartilage and then diverges high and perpendicular to the ear and angles into the posterior hairline for a variable distance.
- The minimal-incision approach, combining transverse sideburn, post-tragal preauricular, and very limited postauricular incisions, is best for the youthful patient.

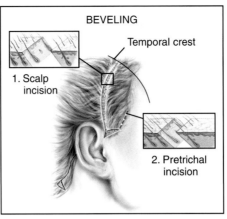

Figure 4-23 *Basic Incisions.
Preauricular incisions: 1, temporal
incision parallel and posterior to the
anterior hairline; 2, transverse sideburn
incision, which can be extended along
the anterior hairline as a substitute for
the temporal incision (i.e., in men); and
3, an incision along the entire length of
the ear in either a pretragal position (A,
used in men) or a post-tragal position
(B, for use in women). Postauricular
incisions may be either (1) the classic
high incision carried out on the ear
cartilage above the sulcus angling into
the posterior hairline or (2) a low,
curved incision in the sulcus for the
vascular-compromised patient (i.e., a
smoker); (3) the minimal-incision
approach can be used for younger
patients.*

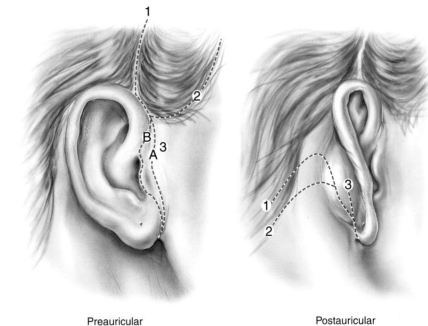

Preauricular   Postauricular

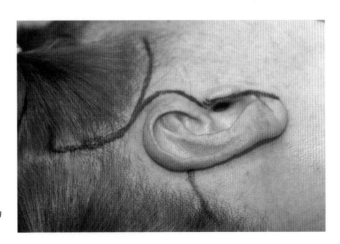

Figure 4-24 *The "workhorse" incision
used for the vast majority of patients.*

Step 2: Anesthetization

The preferred solution for anesthetization is 0.3% lidocaine with 1:200,000 epinephrine in Ringer's lactate. This is easily mixed by ancillary staff preoperatively by adding 50 mL of 2% and 50 mL of 1% lidocaine to 2.5 mL of 1:1000 epinephrine and diluting the solution with 400 mL of Ringer's lactate. The total volume of the solution is usually divided between the facial (75%) and the forehead and brow (25%) portions of the procedure.

After induction of the patient with intravenous sedation by the anesthesiologist, a 20-gauge spinal needle is used with the Klein Infiltration System (Wells Johnson Co., Tucson, Arizona) for anesthetization of the upper face, midface, and lower face and neck subunits. The setting for the Klein Infiltration System varies between 3 and 10. Forehead and brow portions of the procedure are performed initially as reviewed in the previous chapter. For the facial procedure, the anterior neck is anesthetized first, because this is the first subunit to undergo surgery. The spinal needle is introduced along the anticipated line of the submental incision with the neck extended (Fig. 4-25A). The anesthetic solution is infiltrated as the spinal needle is advanced over the neck in the subcutaneous plane, the fluid pushing aside tissue planes as the needle is advanced (Fig. 4-25B). This technique of anesthetization avoids direct injury to neurovascular and deeper vital structures. The injection does not need to be exactly placed in the plane to be lifted—that is, subcutaneous, SMAS, or sub-SMAS—because diffusion of the anesthetic solution is quite rapid throughout the face and neck fascial planes. The angle of introduction of the spinal needle is altered after the first pass (Fig. 4-25C) to cover adjacent areas. The entire anterior neck is completely anesthetized after a few passes (Fig. 4-25D). The spinal needle is reintroduced along the anticipated posterior hairline incision and advanced over the posterior neck using the same technique (Fig. 4-25E). Complete anesthetization of the neck is accomplished after several passes (Fig 4-25F).

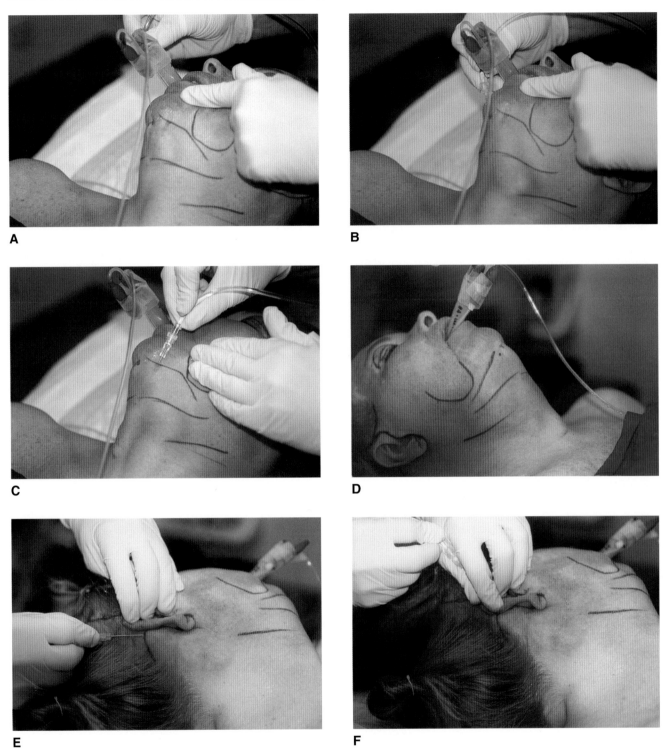

A

B

C

D

E

F

Figure 4-25 *Anesthetization: The Neck.* **A,** *For anterior neck anesthetization, the spinal needle is introduced with neck extended and infiltration of anesthetic solution begun.* **B,** *Infiltration of anesthetic solution proceeds as the spinal needle is advanced over the neck, gently pushing aside tissue planes as the needle is advanced, with care taken to avoid direct injury of vital structures.* **C,** *The angle of introduction of the spinal needle is altered in order to anesthetize the entire anterior neck.* **D,** *The anterior neck anesthetization is completed.* **E,** *The spinal needle is reintroduced and advanced over the posterior neck using the technique illustrated in* **A** *and* **B.** **F,** *The posterior hairline is also infiltrated with this technique, completing neck anesthetization.*

The face is similarly anesthetized. The spinal needle is introduced through the anticipated temporal incision and anesthetic solution infiltrated into the subfollicular plane. The needle is advanced into the preauricular region while infiltration is performed (Fig. 4-26*A*). Slight alteration of the angle of introduction of the needle is performed without withdrawing the needle, and the needle is "popped" deep to the temporoparietal fascia (Fig. 4-26*B*). Anesthetization of the remainder of the temporal region is performed to the anterior hairline. The needle is reintroduced along the anticipated sideburn incision and advanced while infiltrating over the face (Fig. 4-26*C*). The operator should attempt to keep the needle in the deep subcutaneous plane superficial to the SMAS for infiltration of the face. Staying within the anticipated region of preauricular skin resection, the spinal needle is advanced and infiltration performed over the rest of the face (Fig. 4-26*D*).

CLINICAL PEARLS

- The preferred solution is 50 mL of 2% and 50 mL of 1% lidocaine, 2.5 mL of 1:1000 epinephrine, and 400 mL of Ringer's lactate split between the facial (75%) and forehead and brow portions of the procedure (25%).
- The anesthetic solution is infiltrated using a 20-gauge spinal needle advanced over the face and neck in the subcutaneous plane, the fluid pushing aside tissue planes as the needle is advanced, with care taken to avoid direct injury to neurovascular and deeper vital structures.
- The injection does not need to be exactly placed in the plane to be lifted (i.e., subcutaneous, SMAS, or sub-SMAS) because diffusion of the anesthetic solution is quite rapid throughout the face and neck fascial planes.

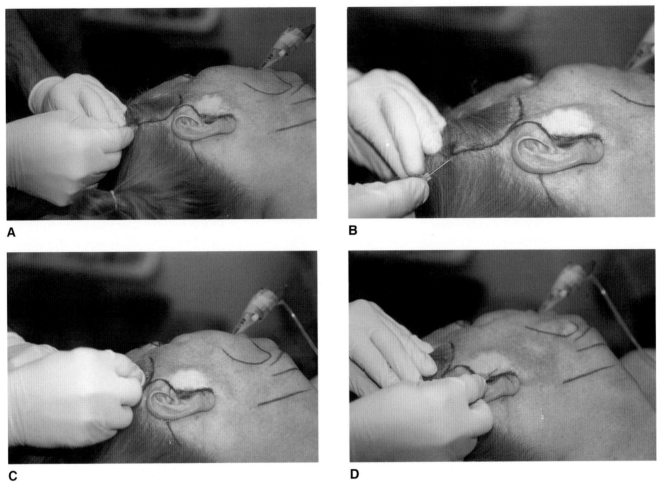

A

B

C

D

Figure 4-26 *Anesthetization: The Face.* **A,** *The spinal needle is introduced under the planned temporal incision, and the temporoparietal fascia and preauricular region are infiltrated.* **B,** *The angle of introduction of the spinal needle is altered, and the temporal region deep to the temporoparietal fascia is anesthetized to the level of the anterior hairline.* **C,** *At the level of the sideburn, the spinal needle is reintroduced, and the entire preauricular region of the face is infiltrated in a plane superficial to the SMAS.* **D,** *Staying within the anticipated region of preauricular skin resection, the spinal needle is advanced and infiltration performed over the rest of the face.*

Step 3: Liposculpture and Undermining

The surgical portion of the subcutaneous facelift procedure begins in every patient with conservative superficial liposculpture. The objectives of liposculpture are (1) defatting of heavy subcutaneous fat collections and (2) blunt undermining and creation of broad-based flaps preserving neurovascular structures. Liposculpture is especially helpful in the neck, where a broad-based subcutaneous flap extending from the clavicles to within several centimeters of the trapezius muscle is created. This broad-based subcutaneous flap, after it is sharply lifted through the periauricular incisions, heals much more securely to the underlying platysma and deep fascia than if only SAL were used to remove a small collection of fat in the submental region.

The liposculpture technique used is similar to the one used for body contouring, except in the neck. Liposculpture in the face and neck should always be *conservative,* because fat adds suppleness to the skin. The anterior neck is approached first. Pretunneling is unnecessary. A single submental stab incision is performed, and with gentle piston-like action, a 2 or 3 mm flat-tipped cannula is passed, more frequently in the center of the topographical "bull's eye" and less frequently along the periphery (Fig. 4-27). Vacuum action predominates in the area with greatest fat content (Fig. 4-28*A*), and tapering is performed at the periphery. (Fig. 4-28*B*). Cross-tunneling through a preauricular stab incision is added to defat and undermine the lateral neck (Fig. 4-28*C*). Superficial liposculpture for patients with heavy jowls is also performed through either the preauricular or the nasal alar approach (Fig. 4-28*D*). SAL of the jowls as well as heavy nasolabial folds is *extremely conservative,* thereby avoiding difficult-to-correct secondary deformities. The amount of liposuctioned fat in the jowls should be no greater than a couple of cubic centimeters per side (Fig. 4-28*E*).

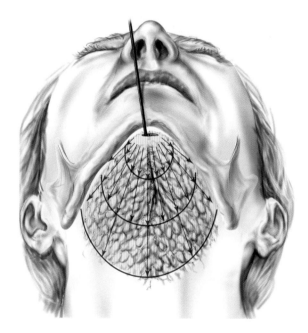

Figure 4-27 *Liposculpture. In the submental region, a single stab incision is performed. With gentle piston-like action, a 2 or 3 mm flat-tipped cannula is passed, more frequently in the center of the topographical "bull's eye" and less frequently along the periphery. Vacuum suction predominates in the area with greatest fat content, and tapering is performed at the periphery.*

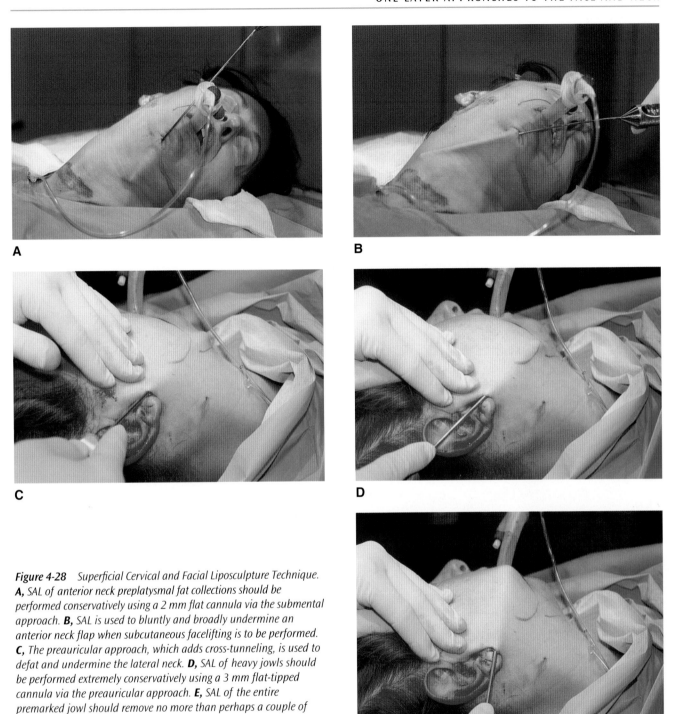

Figure 4-28 *Superficial Cervical and Facial Liposculpture Technique.* ***A,*** *SAL of anterior neck preplatysmal fat collections should be performed conservatively using a 2 mm flat cannula via the submental approach.* ***B,*** *SAL is used to bluntly and broadly undermine an anterior neck flap when subcutaneous facelifting is to be performed.* ***C,*** *The preauricular approach, which adds cross-tunneling, is used to defat and undermine the lateral neck.* ***D,*** *SAL of heavy jowls should be performed extremely conservatively using a 3 mm flat-tipped cannula via the preauricular approach.* ***E,*** *SAL of the entire premarked jowl should remove no more than perhaps a couple of cubic centimeters of fat per side.*

The next segment of the procedure involves sharp undermining. This begins with *lateral temporal dissection.* The scalpel is used to create a beveled incision through the scalp in the temporal hair-bearing region. This incision is connected with the transverse sideburn incision. The temporoparietal fascia and the temporal branch of the superficial temporal artery and vein are exposed (Fig. 4-29A). Electrocautery is used to incise the temporoparietal fascia (Fig. 4-29B). If the temporal branches of the superficial temporal artery and vein

impede further dissection, they can be ligated; otherwise, they are preserved. Gentle blunt dissection reveals the areolar plane below the temporoparietal fascia (Fig. 4-29C). Undermining to the anterior hairline is performed with Rees or Gorney scissors utilizing countertraction (Fig. 4-29D). The frontal branches of the superficial temporal artery and vein are dissected, which are also ligated if found to impede dissection (Fig. 4-29E). The superficial layer of the deep temporal fascia is fully exposed (Fig. 4-29F).

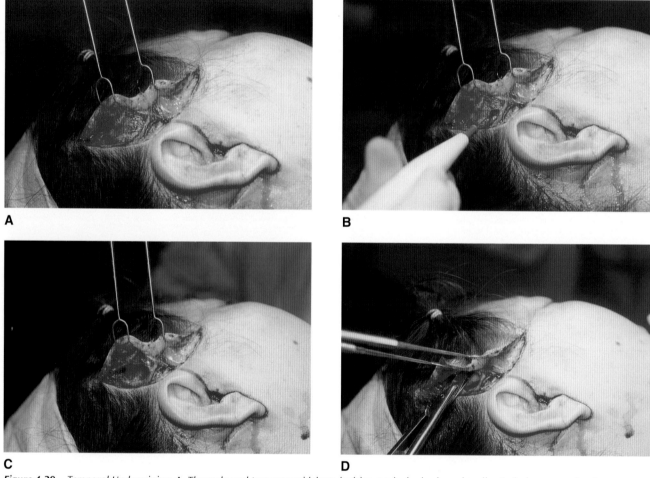

A **B** **C** **D**

Figure 4-29 *Temporal Undermining.* **A,** *The scalp and transverse sideburn incision are incised using a beveling technique, exposing the temporoparietal fascia and the temporal branches of the superficial temporal vessels. If found to impede further dissection, these vessels can be divided; otherwise, they are preserved.* **B,** *With skin hook retraction, electrocautery is used to incise the temporoparietal fascia.* **C,** *The areolar plane between the temporoparietal fascia and the deep temporal fascia is exposed with blunt finger dissection.* **D,** *With skin hook countertraction, Rees or Gorney scissors are used to dissect anteriorly to the anterior hairline and superiorly over the lateral temporal region.* **E,** *The frontal branches of the superficial temporal vessels are exposed, which if found to impede further dissection can also be ligated.* **F,** *The glistening white layer of the deep temporal fascia is evident over the temporalis muscle.*

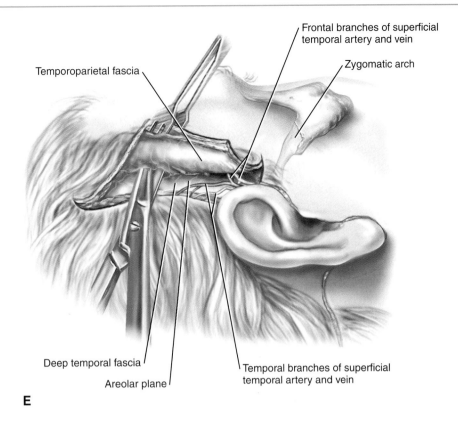

Temporoparietal fascia

Frontal branches of superficial temporal artery and vein

Zygomatic arch

Deep temporal fascia

Areolar plane

Temporal branches of superficial temporal artery and vein

E

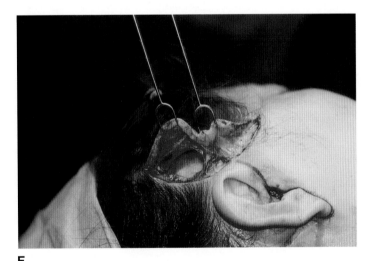

F

The scalpel is used to incise and perform *preauricular dissection* (Fig. 4-30*A*). Using countertraction, as much fat as possible should be preserved on the midfacial flap, especially because maximal tension will later be placed on this flap. SMAS and platysma remain on the patient during the one-layer subcutaneous approach. It is vital to make certain that the subcutaneous dissection does not violate the temporoparietal fascia near the zygomatic arch. This creates the "meso-temporalis," which protects the superficially located frontal branch

of the facial nerve from injury (Fig. 4-30*B*). Traction is placed on the ear, and the scalpel is used to incise and perform *postauricular dissection* (Fig. 4-30*C*). Again, all fat is left on the skin flap, while cervical investing fascia and platysma are left on the patient (Fig. 4-30*D*). This incision is given clearance from the lobule to preserve space for ear piercing. The vestigial muscles of the ear are exposed, as well as the mastoid fascia. The scalpel dissection portion of the procedure is now complete (Fig. 4-30*E*).

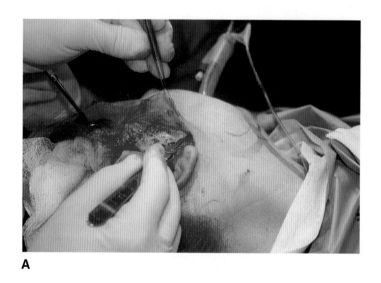

A

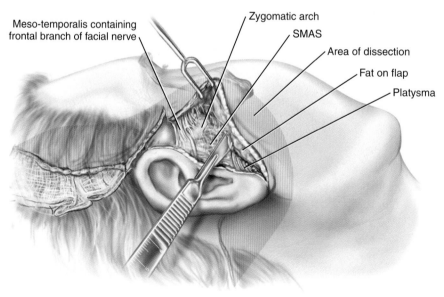

B

Figure 4-30 *Scalpel Undermining.* **A,** *Preauricular sharp supra-SMAS and supra-platysma dissection is carried out with a scalpel, preserving as much superficial fat of the skin flap as possible, especially in the midface, and leaving the SMAS and platysma on the patient.* **B,** *The "meso-temporalis" is created over the zygomatic arch, composed of temporoparietal fascia, protecting the superficially located frontal branch of the facial nerve.*

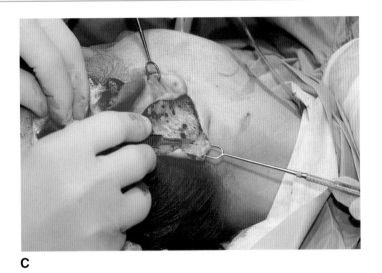

C

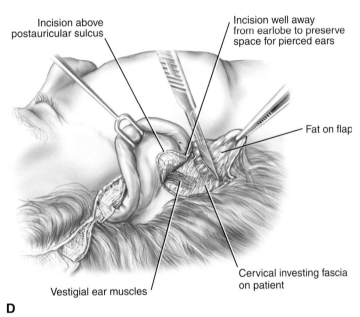

Incision above
postauricular sulcus

Incision well away
from earlobe to preserve
space for pierced ears

Fat on flap

Vestigial ear muscles

Cervical investing fascia
on patient

D

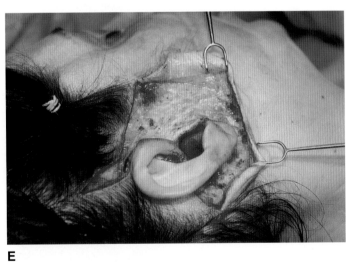

E

Figure 4-30, cont'd **C,** *Postauricular sharp suprafascial dissection is carried out with a scalpel raising the flap on the fascia and preserving all fat on the flap.* **D,** *The postauricular incision should be far enough away from the earlobe to preserve space for ear piercing.* **E,** *The scalpel dissection is completed with a posterior hairline incision high and angled into the posterior hairline.*

Scissors undermining using a curved Rees or Gorney scissors against skin hook countertraction is performed over the face and neck. The dissection is begun in the lateral neck. If blunt undermining with the liposuction cannula has been performed, little resistance is met (Fig. 4-31*A*). Scissors undermining then proceeds over the anterior neck (Fig. 4-31*B*) and upward over the jowl (Fig. 4-31*C*). SMAS and platysma are preserved on the patient, and as much superficial fat as possible is left on the skin flap (Fig. 4-31*D*). The scissors is flipped with points upward during dissection over McGregor's patch in the preauricular region, to avoid injury to branches of the zygomatic branches of the facial nerve, which become quite superficial over this region (Fig. 4-31*E*). Once past McGregor's patch, the scissors is replaced with points downward, and undermining is performed over the premalar region. The premalar region is where two-layer SMAS techniques deviate from thick subcutaneous techniques. In thick-flap one-layer subcutaneous techniques, undermining with elevation of as much superficial fat as possible is performed over the premalar region to well within 1 or 2 centimeters of the nasolabial fold (Fig. 4-31*F*). In two-layer techniques, the superficial fat is preserved on the SMAS in the premalar region such that the SMAS becomes the carrier for superficial

fat repositioning and facial reshaping. The only exception is the deep-plane technique of Hamra, which is discussed separately in the next chapter.

CLINICAL PEARLS

- The subcutaneous facelift procedure begins in every patient with superficial liposculpture, which achieves *conservative* superficial defatting and aggressive wide and blunt undermining, especially in the anterior neck.
- Superficial liposculpture for heavy nasolabial folds and jowls is performed *extremely conservatively*, with removal of no greater than perhaps a couple of cubic centimeters of fat per side.
- Undermining is performed with elevation of superficial fat of variable thickness on the skin flaps, depending on the surgeon's objectives.
- SMAS and platysma muscle are not included at all with the skin flaps in the one-layer subcutaneous facelift technique.
- During dissection over McGregor's patch in the preauricular region, it is best to flip the curved scissors points upward to avoid injury to the zygomatic branches of the facial nerve, which can become quite superficial over this region.
- In thick-flap one-layer subcutaneous techniques, undermining with elevation of as much superficial fat as possible is performed over the premalar region, whereas in two-layer techniques, the superficial fat is preserved on the SMAS in the premalar region such that the SMAS becomes the carrier for superficial fat repositioning and facial reshaping.

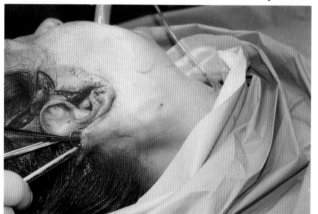

A

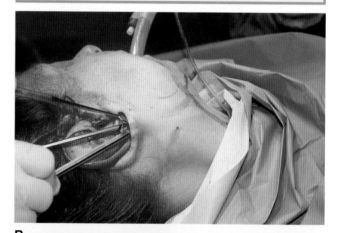

B

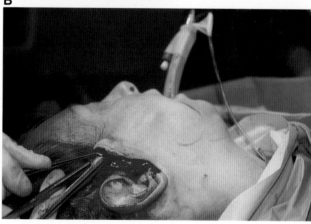

C

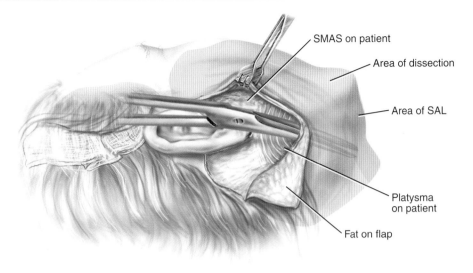

SMAS on patient

Area of dissection

Area of SAL

Platysma
on patient

Fat on flap

D

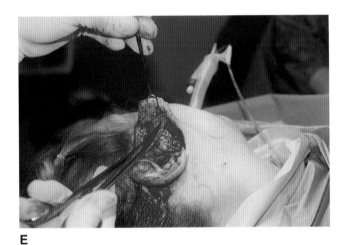

E

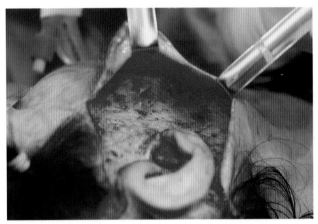

F

Figure 4-31   *Scissors Undermining.* **A,** *Scissors undermining begins in the deep posterior neck over the cervical fascia, with countertraction aided by skin hooks.* **B,** *Scissors undermining over the platysma is performed to abut the region of the anterior neck undermined using SAL technique.* **C,** *Scissors dissection is performed over the jowls and lower face is performed above the platysma. Note: Undermining in this region is greatly aided when SAL of the jowls has been previously performed.* **D,** *In the traditional subcutaneous technique, great effort is made to preserve all superficial fat on the skin flap and all SMAS and platysma on the patient.* **E,** *Midfacial dissection of the zygomatic ligaments (McGregor's patch) is greatly aided by flipping the curved scissors such that the points are directed upward, thereby avoiding facial nerve injury.* **F,** *Dissection of the difficult premalar region in the traditional subcutaneous technique is in the superficial fat plane, which greatly varies from SMAS and platysma techniques, covered in the next chapter.*

Step 4: Hemostasis

Hemostasis may be the most tedious and boring portion of the procedure, but it is often vital in preventing the most common and annoying complication—hematoma. Using the anesthetization technique illustrated and continually packing the wound with gauze soaked in 0.5% lidocaine with 1:200,000 epinephrine diminish the time spent on hemostasis. That does not mean that time spent on hemostasis is not time well spent. Hemostasis is aided by using a fiberoptic retractor with a good light source and insulated forceps with fine teeth, both integral parts of the surgical armamentarium (Fig. 4-32). Hemostasis on the skin flap should be performed with gentle retraction of the tissues off the skin flap such that cautery burns and subsequent pox-like areas of full-thickness flap slough are avoided. This nasty complication can spoil an otherwise pleasing result.

CLINICAL PEARLS

- Continually packing the wound with gauze soaked with 0.5% lidocaine with 1:200,000 epinephrine and using tumescent anesthetization technique diminish the time spent on hemostasis.
- Hemostasis on the skin flap should be performed with gentle retraction of the tissues off the flap such that cautery burns are avoided.

Step 5: Fashioning the Flaps, Closure, and Lipostructure

Overview

Fashioning the skin flaps and closure constitute the most complex and confusing aspect of the subcutaneous facelift. This "crescendo" part of the procedure can be best understood by first reviewing the major components before tackling the details—and this portion of the procedure involves quite a few details. As the great architect Mies van der Rohe said, "God is in the details!"

Setting the *skin tension vectors* and the *sequencing of closure* are paramount for achieving symmetrical and pleasing results (Fig. 4-33). The neck is set first, with closure along a skin tension vector that roughly follows the jawline. The midface is set next, with closure along a skin tension vector that follows the axis of the ear—a more vertical vector than the neckline vector. The upper face is set last, with closure along skin tension vectors set radial to the curve of the temporal incision. Proper setting of skin tension vectors and proper sequencing of closure avoid secondary residual skin folds, so-called lateral sweep, in the face.

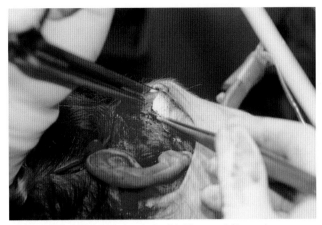

Figure 4-32 *Hemostasis is greatly aided by use of fiberoptic retractors and insulated forceps, which are integral parts of the surgical armamentarium.*

SKIN TENSION VECTORS AND CLOSURE SEQUENCING
1 ➔ 2 ➔ 3

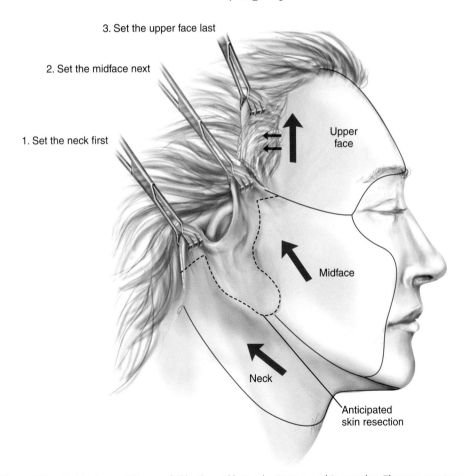

3. Set the upper face last

2. Set the midface next

1. Set the neck first

Upper face

Midface

Neck

Anticipated skin resection

Figure 4-33 *Fashioning and Closure of Skin Flaps: Skin Tension Vectors and Sequencing. The proper vectors for skin tension and correct sequencing of closure of the subcutaneous flaps are paramount for achieving optimal results.*

163

Key anchor sutures should be placed before excess skin is trimmed (Fig. 4-34). These stitches are in three major locations and should be placed in the deep dermis to avoid migrating scars. The first deep dermal anchor suture is placed into the mastoid fascia behind the ear, setting the neck. The second deep dermal suture is placed into the deep temporal fascia and temporalis muscle above the ear, setting the midface. The upper face is set last with a series of sutures that are terraced into the temporoparietal fascia and fixed to the deep temporal fascia and temporalis muscle along the temporal incision. The setting of earlobe and sideburn height, as well as all the trimming of skin excess, should not be performed until these key sutures have been placed.

The only exception to the use of three sets of key anchor sutures is in the *minimal-incision technique* for the youthful patient. In most such cases, the patient complains of midfacial laxity and does not have skin excess in the neck. With this approach, only two key anchor sutures are required to set the midfacial and upper facial flaps. If neck laxity is minor, then a modified third key anchor suture can be placed into the conchal cartilage at the most superior extent of the postauricular incision to set the neck skin flap. The small pleat of excess neck skin behind the ear usually resolves in several months' time. If it does not, then a minor revision can be performed. Revision usually is not necessary. If the neck laxity is significant in the youthful patient, then either a traditional high postauricular incision can be carried out, or a minimal-incision approach with two-flap technique incorporating lateral and anterior platysmaplasty can be used. The apparent cervical skin excess is then used to drape the recontoured neckline.

The *lipostructure* portion of the procedure is performed last. The objective of lipostructure when combined with one-layer subcutaneous facelift is *not* to recontour the entire face and neck with fat grafts, as has been promoted by some surgeons who have spearheaded the use of lipostructure. Rather, once skin tightening and superficial fat repositioning have been achieved with the subcutaneous facelift, lipostructure is used to correct residual furrows and folds in conjunction with laser resurfacing. The technique employed for lipostructure uses the Coleman fat scaffolding technique with centrifuged fat and Coleman needles of various sizes for fat deposition. The amount of fat deposition per region varies greatly, depending on the degree and number of residual facial folds, creases, and furrows. Primary lipostructure is most effective in regions of the face and neck that have not directly been undermined or liposuctioned—the perioral and periorbital regions.

KEY ANCHOR SUTURES WITH ANTICIPATED EXCESS SKIN TRIM

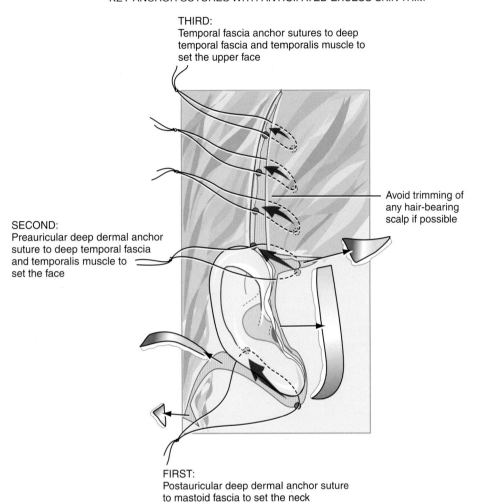

THIRD:
Temporal fascia anchor sutures to deep temporal fascia and temporalis muscle to set the upper face

Avoid trimming of any hair-bearing scalp if possible

SECOND:
Preauricular deep dermal anchor suture to deep temporal fascia and temporalis muscle to set the face

FIRST:
Postauricular deep dermal anchor suture to mastoid fascia to set the neck

Figure 4-34   *Fashioning and Closure of Skin Flaps: Key Anchor Sutures. The key anchor sutures are placed deeply into the dermal and subdermal tissues, followed by the setting of earlobe and sideburn height and the trimming of excess skin. Note: Resection of hair-bearing scalp should be avoided at all cost!*

Technique

Lahey clamps are placed on the neck and midface skin flaps within the area of skin resection, and maximal tension is placed for the *neck skin tension vector* using these clamps (Fig. 4-35*A*). The subdermal postauricular *first key stitch* is placed in buried fashion deep into the mastoid fascia using a 3-0 Vicryl suture (Fig. 4-35*B*). This suture is tied under maximal tension along the neck flap vector (Fig. 4-35*C*). Gentle massaging of the neck flap and prestretching of the neck flap greatly aid receptive relaxation of the skin and allow an easier insetting of the flaps.

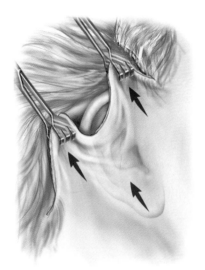

Vectors of tension around the ear

A

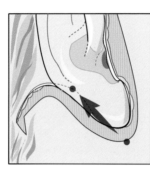

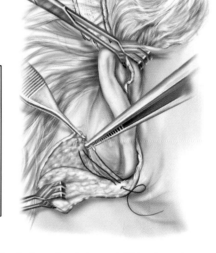

Placement of subdermal postauricular suture into mastoid fascia under maximal tension

B

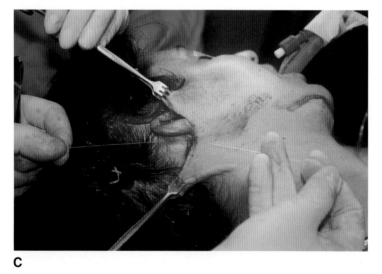

C

Figure 4-35 Setting the Neck Flap. **A,** *The vector of skin tension for neck flap closure is parallel to the jawline.* **B,** *The subdermal postauricular first key anchor stitch is placed deeply into the mastoid fascia behind the ear.* **C,** *This buried key anchor suture is tied with the neck flap placed under maximal tension, and a 3-0 Vicryl suture is used.*

After the first key anchor suture has been placed, *postauricular trim* is performed with a curved or straight Rees or Gorney scissors (Fig. 4-36*A*). Skin trim in this area should allow for good overlap so that closure is in tension-free skin, thereby preventing postauricular scar migration outside the sulcus (Fig. 4-36*B*). The Lahey clamp should distract the neck flap toward the ear while the posterior hairline skin excess is marked (Fig. 4-36*C*). Excess skin trim should allow for good realignment of the posterior hairline and prevention of "dog ears," which in this region often have the annoying tendency to become conspicuous below the hairline (Fig. 4-36*D*).

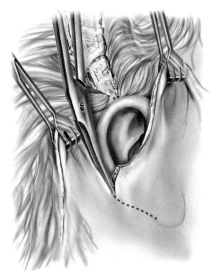

Postauricular trim hugging the postauricular sulcus to the anticipated new earlobe position

A

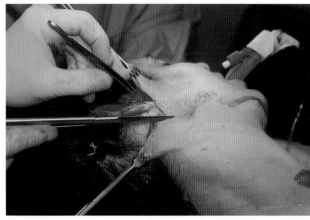

B

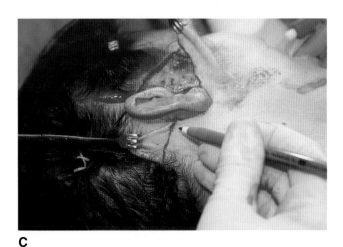

C

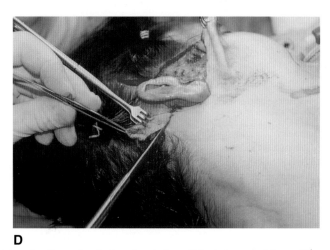

D

Figure 4-36 Setting the Neck. **A,** *The postauricular skin excess is trimmed, hugging the postauricular sulcus to the anticipated new earlobe position.* **B,** *Gentle anterior retraction of the ear greatly aids visualization for trimming of postauricular skin excess, which should allow for good overlap so that inferior migration of scar is prevented.* **C,** *The Lahey clamp is angled toward the ear while the posterior hairline skin excess is marked, to prevent the creation of annoying dog ears.* **D,** *It is essential to realign the posterior hairline while trimming posterior hairline excess.*

Posterior hairline closure is performed in two layers: the first, with deep dermal buried stitches of 4-0 Vicryl suture emphasizing reapproximation of the posterior hairline (Fig. 4-37*A*); the second, with a subcuticular running stitch of 3-0 plain suture for skin closure (Fig. 4-37*B*). Before the suture line is closed completely, a 1 inch Penrose drain trimmed at an angle and opened along one border is placed through the scalp incision (Fig. 4-37*C*). The Penrose drain is positioned flat side down under the skin flap below the jawline, extending for approximately 6 to 8 inches. The surgeon must make certain not to drag hair or particulate debris beneath the flap (Fig. 4-37*D*). The drain is secured with a 3-0 nylon suture.

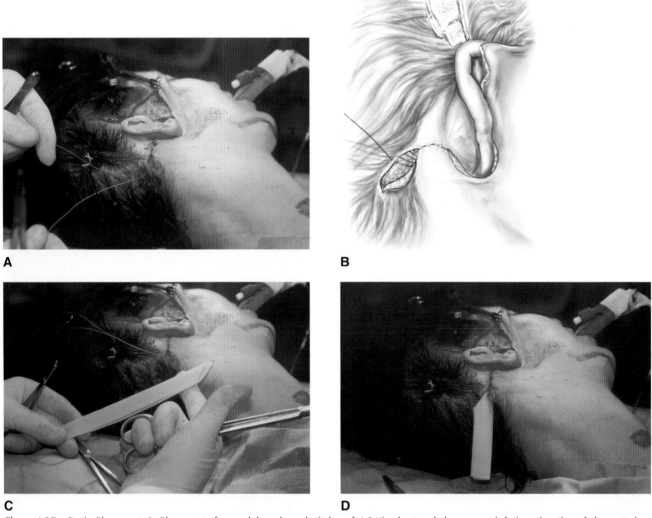

A

B

C

D

*Figure 4-37   Drain Placement. **A,** Placement of several deep dermal stitches of 4-0 Vicryl suture helps prevent inferior migration of the posterior hairline scar. **B,** The second layer of closure should be a subcuticular stitch of 3-0 plain suture. **C,** A Penrose drain, or closed suction drain, can be placed through a small lateral opening within the posterior hairline incision. **D,** The surgeon should be careful not to drag hair beneath the flap, and to secure the drain with a nylon suture.*

The *midface skin tension vector* is set with a Lahey clamp along the axis of the ear or in a slightly more vertical position (Fig. 4-38*A*). It is helpful to also place a Lahey clamp on the upper scalp flap and simultaneously retract the upper scalp flap while marking the anticipated midfacial skin excess (Fig. 4-38*B*). *Vertical skin trim* of the sideburn skin dart is performed with Rees or Gorney scissors (Fig. 4-38*C*), followed by *horizontal skin trim* corresponding to the preauricular skin excess (Fig. 4-38*D*). The remaining midfacial skin flap should be thick and robust, incorporating as much subcutaneous tissue as possible, because tension on this flap will be maximal.

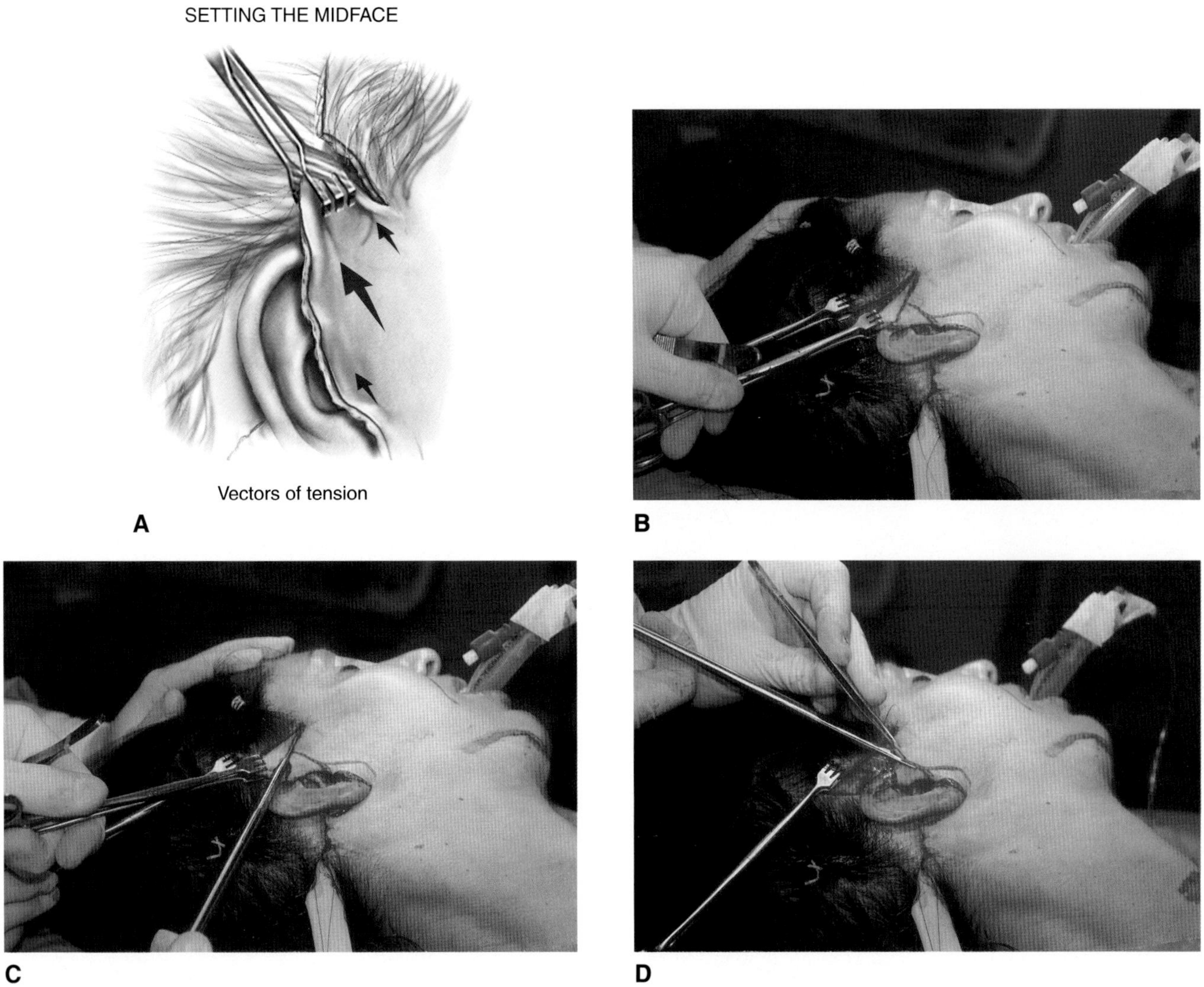

SETTING THE MIDFACE

Vectors of tension

A

B

C

D

Figure 4-38 *Midfacial Flap Trimming.* ***A,*** *The vector of skin tension for setting the midface is along or slightly steeper than the axis of the ear.* ***B,*** *Placement of Lahey clamps on the midface and upper face flaps and retraction along the appropriate vector greatly aid in marking the anticipated skin excess.* ***C,*** *Trim of the vertical skin excess corresponds to the sideburn skin dart.* ***D,*** *Trim of the horizontal skin excess corresponds to the preauricular skin excess.*

The *second key anchor suture* is placed into the deep temporal fascia and temporalis muscle above the ear (Fig. 4-39*A*). This suture is placed deeply into the tissues for strong fixation (Fig. 4-39*B*). If necessary, a second bite is taken of the subcutaneous tissue above the ear for proper alignment of the tissues (Fig. 4-39*C*). A deep dermal pass of the suture on the reciprocal part of the midfacial skin flap is performed with 3-0 Vicryl suture (Fig. 4-39*D*). This buried stitch is tied under maximal tension and supplemented, if necessary (Fig. 4-39*E*). Attention should be given to making certain that the midfacial flap aligns with the ear and does not distort the ear (Fig. 4-39*F*). If misalignment or distortion is noted, this suture should be removed and replaced.

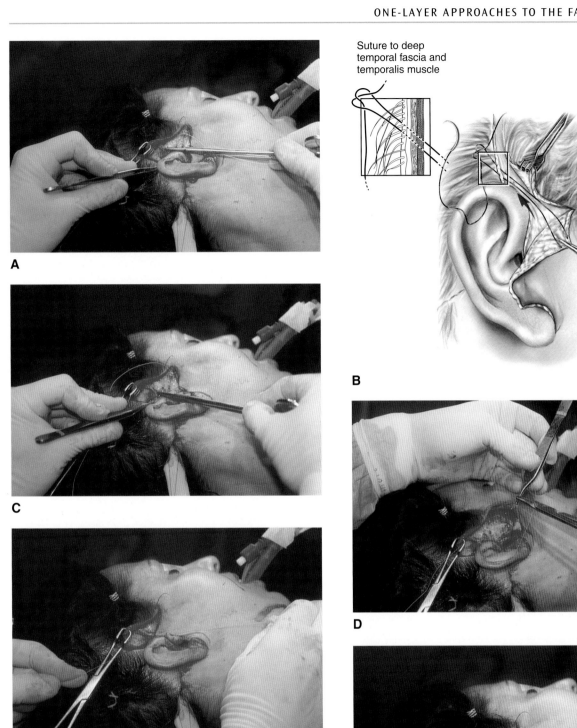

A

B

Suture to deep
temporal fascia and
temporalis muscle

C

D

E

F

Figure 4-39 *Setting the Midfacial Flap.* ***A,*** *The second key anchor suture is placed into the deep tissues above the ear.* ***B,*** *The second suture of 3-0 Vicryl is placed in buried fashion into the deep temporal fascia and temporalis muscle fibers above the ear.* ***C,*** *If necessary, a second pass of the suture is placed through the subcutaneous suture above the ear so that the tissues are properly aligned.* ***D,*** *A deep dermal pass of the buried suture is placed into the appropriate place on the midface flap.* ***E,*** *The buried suture is tied under maximal tension and supplemented.* ***F,*** *If misalignment of the flap or ear distortion is noted, the suture should be removed and replaced.*

Sideburn restoration to its proper height is performed *after* the second key anchor suture has been placed. This maneuver is performed with several deep dermal buried stitches of 4-0 Vicryl suture (Fig. 4-40*A* and *B*). Using this technique, the sideburn should not be elevated more than a few millimeters. If the sideburn is elevated more than this amount and the surgeon believes that this position would be unacceptable to the patient, the position of the second key anchor suture should be altered. Staples can then be applied for scalp closure, or a fine running stitch of 5-0 nylon suture can be used (Fig. 4-40*C*).

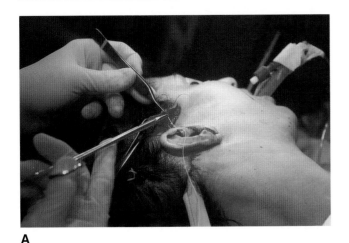

A

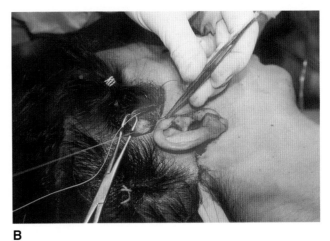

B

Sideburn restoration

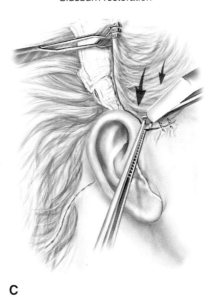

C

Figure 4-40   *Sideburn Restoration. **A** and **B**, Several buried stitches of 4-0 Vicryl suture are used to restore the sideburn to a natural height.*
***C,** Staples or a fine running stitch of 5-0 nylon suture is used for sideburn closure. Elevation of the sideburn should be no more than a few millimeters at most; otherwise, the second key anchor suture should be relocated.*

Using Lahey clamps, the *temporal skin tension vector* is the last to be set. This vector is set along a radial axis relative to the curved temporal incision (Fig. 4-41). The *third key anchor sutures* are terraced into the scalp, placed in buried fashion into the deep temporal fascia and temporalis muscle (Fig. 4-42*A*), and then into the temporoparietal fascia on the temporal flap (Fig. 4-42*B*).

These stitches are placed deeply into the scalp for good fixation (Fig. 4-42*C*). They are tied simultaneously under maximal tension (Fig. 4-42*D*). The skin bunching often noted in front of the temporal hairline is usually relieved after the temporal flap has been set by this method.

SETTING THE TEMPORAL LIFT

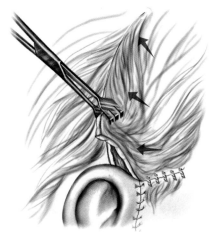

Vectors of tension

Figure 4-41 *The vectors of skin tension for the lateral temporal lift are set radial to the curved temporal incision.*

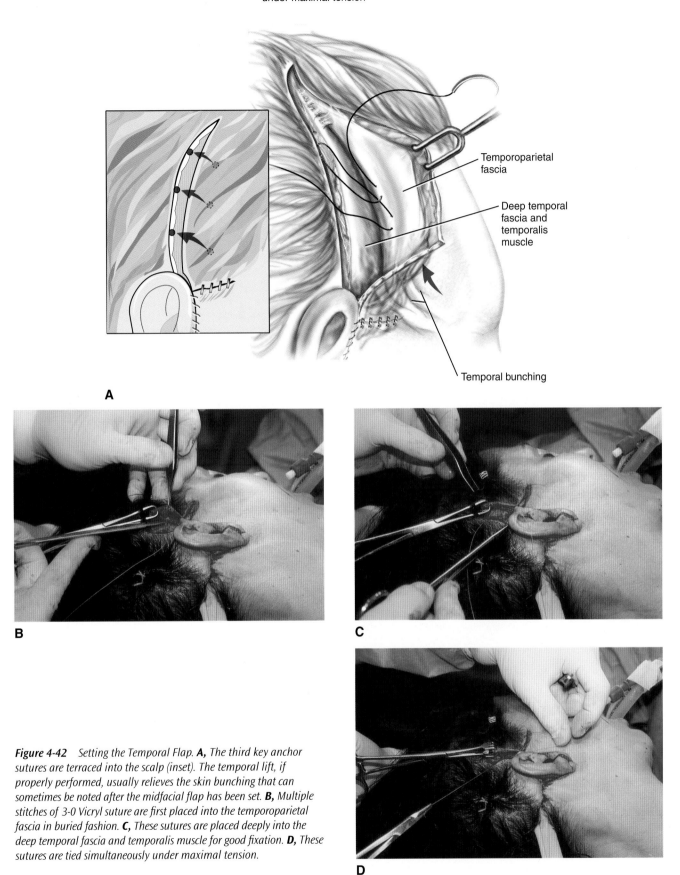

Placement of temporal sutures into deep temporal fascia and temporalis muscle under maximal tension

Temporoparietal fascia

Deep temporal fascia and temporalis muscle

Temporal bunching

A

B

C

D

Figure 4-42 *Setting the Temporal Flap.* **A,** *The third key anchor sutures are terraced into the scalp (inset). The temporal lift, if properly performed, usually relieves the skin bunching that can sometimes be noted after the midfacial flap has been set.* **B,** *Multiple stitches of 3-0 Vicryl suture are first placed into the temporoparietal fascia in buried fashion.* **C,** *These sutures are placed deeply into the deep temporal fascia and temporalis muscle for good fixation.* **D,** *These sutures are tied simultaneously under maximal tension.*

Scalp bunching is noted after the temporal lift has been set. This is relieved by a minor amount of sub-scalp dissection (Fig. 4-43*A*). Either a scalpel or a forceps alone can be used to lift and release the proximal scalp (Fig. 4-43*B*). Temporal and sideburn closure is performed with staples. Staples are much more hair follicle friendly than sutures. A smooth seam without scalp bunching should be achieved by this method (Fig. 4-43*C*). It is rare that resection of hair-bearing scalp is needed (Fig. 4-43*D*).

As a matter of fact, resection of hair-bearing skin should be avoided at all cost! A minor amount of scalp bunching will resolve within 4 to 6 weeks. If temporal fullness or bunching persists anterior to the hairline, a 2 mm flat-tipped cannula can be inserted through the sideburn incision and SAL of subcutaneous excess performed (Fig. 4-43*E*). The surgeon need not be concerned about injury to the frontal branch of the facial nerve as long as the cannula is kept within the superficial fat.

SETTING THE TEMPORAL LIFT AND RELIEVING SCALP AND TEMPORAL BUNCHING

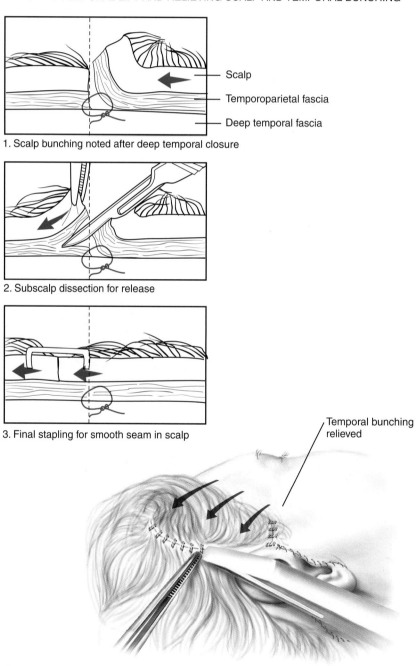

Scalp
Temporoparietal fascia
Deep temporal fascia

1. Scalp bunching noted after deep temporal closure

2. Subscalp dissection for release

3. Final stapling for smooth seam in scalp

Temporal bunching relieved

A

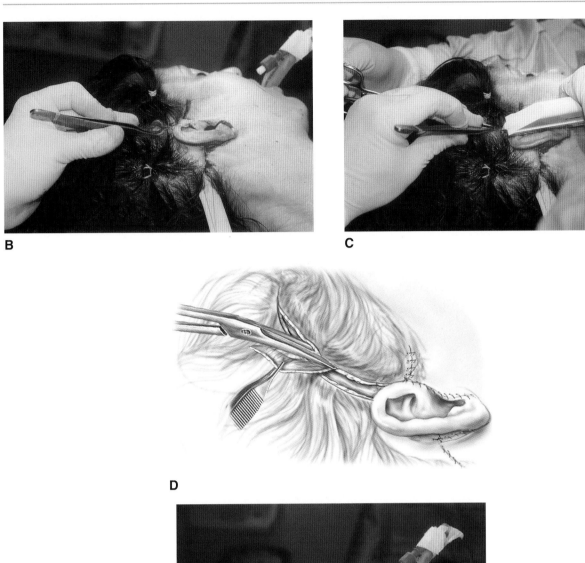

B

C

D

E

Figure 4-43   **A,** *Scalp bunching that is noted after the temporal lift has been set can be relieved by a minor amount of proximal subscalp dissection.* **Top,** *1–3: Technique.* **Bottom,** *Result.* **B,** *A forceps can be used to lift and release the proximal scalp.* **C,** *Final stapling can be performed without scalp bunching.* **D,** *Resection of hair-bearing scalp, as shown, is rarely needed if this method is followed.* **E,** *If temporal fullness persists anterior to the hairline, a 2 mm flat-tipped cannula can be inserted through the sideburn incision and SAL of subcutaneous excess performed.*

The *earlobe position* should be set a few millimeters "high" (Fig. 4-44*A*). Gravimetric and skin tensile forces associated with healing will lower the earlobe into proper position. Deep sutures should be avoided. The Rees or Gorney scissors is used to trim postauricular skin excess such that skin overlap in the sulcus is tension-free (Fig. 4-44*B*). The skin trim should be anterior enough that the earlobe drapes in a natural relaxed position after a skin stitch is placed (Fig. 4-44*C*). A scrunched-up and contorted lobe is just as unacceptable as the dreaded "pixie" lobe deformity in which the earlobe is set too low. Time spent setting the earlobe at proper height is time well spent. Earlobe height should not be determined until *after* all of the key anchor sutures have been placed with strong fixation and *after* all of the scalp incisions have been closed properly (Fig. 4-44*D*). If skin fixation above the earlobe is inadequate or if the amount of tension placed is too much for the suture material to withstand, inferior migration of the posterior auricular scar may result, dragging the earlobe along with it to a conspicuous location.

SETTING THE EARLOBE POSITION

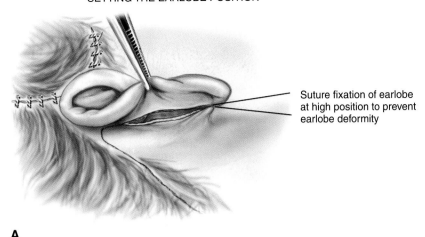

Suture fixation of earlobe
at high position to prevent
earlobe deformity

A

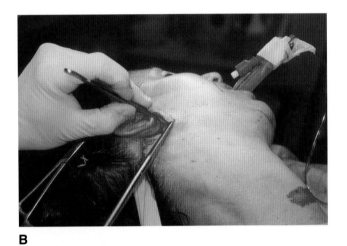

B

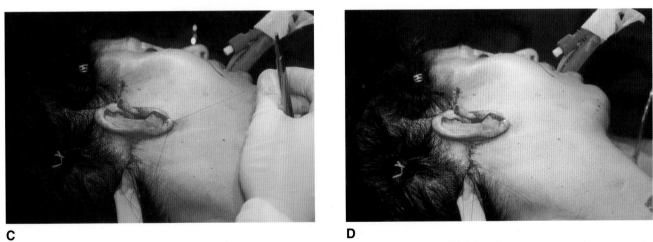

C   **D**

Figure 4-44 *Setting Earlobe Height.* ***A,*** *The position of the earlobe should be set a few millimeters "high."* ***B,*** *The Rees or Gorney scissors are used to trim postauricular skin excess such that skin flap overlap in the sulcus is tension-free.* ***C,*** *The earlobe drapes over the neck skin in a natural relaxed position after a skin stitch has been placed.* ***D,*** *Earlobe height should not be determined until after all of the key anchor sutures have been placed with good fixation and after the scalp incisions have been closed properly.*

After the earlobe position has been set, *postauricular skin closure* can be performed. This is performed with a simple running stitch of 3-0 plain suture (Fig. 4-45*A*). The suture line should be tension-free (Fig. 4-45*B*). It is unnecessary and fruitless to attempt taking a few bites of the ear cartilage with the suture if skin excision has been overshot and there is a skin gap. The 3-0 plain suture will not bear the tension necessary to fill the gap, resulting in splitting and inferior migration of the scar onto the neck. If the postauricular skin excision has been overshot and a skin gap results, it is far better to place a few buried stitches of 4-0 Vicryl into the fascia behind the ear and fix the suture line into the sulcus (Fig. 4-45*C*). In addition, the earlobe should have enough space that the post of an earring can sit comfortably without impinging on the neck skin or distorting the earlobe.

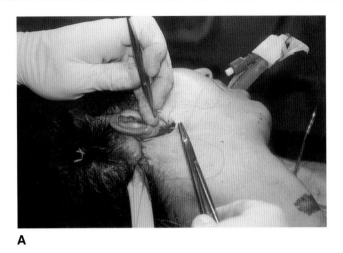

A

CLOSURE BEHIND THE EAR

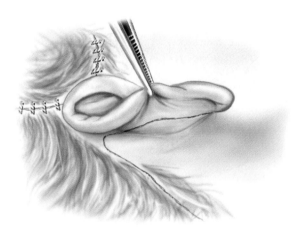

Tension-free subdermal closure

B

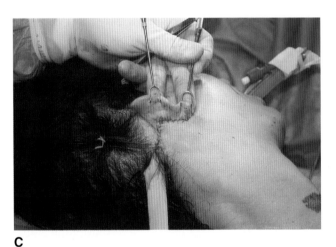

C

Figure 4-45 *Retroauricular Closure.* **A,** *After the earlobe position has been set, postauricular closure can be performed with a simple running stitch of 3-0 plain suture.* **B,** *The postauricular suture line should be tension-free.* **C,** *If the postauricular skin excision has been overshot and a gap results, it is better to place a few buried stitches of 4-0 Vicryl into the fascia behind the ear and fixate the suture line into the sulcus.*

The *preauricular skin closure* is the last suture line to be placed—all other suture lines should be trimmed, fixed, and closed before this most important and conspicuous of suture lines is closed (Fig. 4-46*A*). Previous markings often need to be adjusted. Rough trim allowing a few millimeters of overlap is performed initially with Rees or Gorney scissors (Fig. 4-46*B*). If a post-tragal approach has been chosen, the preauricular skin flap that covers the tragus should be defatted to full-thickness skin graft thickness to allow for tragal definition (Fig. 4-46*C*). If a pretragal approach has been chosen, this flap should be left thick and hearty with fat, because the most common secondary deformity associated with the pretragal approach is a depressed scar. The remainder of the preauricular flap should be finely trimmed so that closure can be performed with skin overlap (Fig. 4-46*D*). Tensile forces during healing will flatten this down, and a good seam will result. Excellent hemostasis at this point is essential—a minor hematoma under the preauricular flap can have devastating consequences! It is mandatory to avoid wide, depressed, or conspicuous scars along this suture line. Interrupted simple stitches of 5-0 nylon suture are placed for tacking, and final closure is performed with a running stitch of the same material (Fig. 4-46*E*). The completed closure, along with the proper subcutaneous position of the drain below the jawline, is illustrated in Figure 4-47*A* and *B*.

The *lipostructure* portion of the procedure is performed last. As described in the preceding overview, the objective of lipostructure when combined with one-layer subcutaneous facelift is not to recontour the entire face and neck with fat grafts but rather to correct residual furrows and folds once the skin has been tightened and the superficial fat has been repositioned. Laser resurfacing is also employed with lipostructure in an attempt to achieve these goals. The Coleman fat scaffolding technique is used for lipostructure. This technique employs centrifuged fat and Coleman needles of various sizes for fat deposition. The amount of fat deposition per region varies greatly, depending on the degree and number of residual facial folds, creases, and furrows. Primary lipostructure is most effective in regions of the face and neck that have not been undermined or liposuctioned (Fig. 4-48). These regions include the upper and lower lips, the nasolabial crease and marionette lines, the lateral lip commissures, the tear-trough above the orbital rim, the lateral chin, and the glabella, forehead, and brow furrows. Fat harvested during the liposculpture portion of the procedure is used, and if extra fat is necessary, fat is harvested from the inner knee region using a harvesting cannula. Ten milliliter Luer-Lok syringes are used for harvesting, and 1 mL Luer-Lok syringes are used for deposition. Stab incisions can be made in the nasal alar crease, commissural creases, and glabella furrows for grafting of the forehead, brow, naso-labial creases, marionette lines, upper and lower lips, and lateral chin. Only several milliliters of centrifuged fat is used per area, and slight overcorrection is desired. For heavy nasolabial folds, superficial SAL is used as well in an attempt to reduce the fold and elevate the crease. Closure of all stab wounds is performed using 6-0 nylon, especially in areas of concomitant laser resurfacing.

Dressings are applied after all wounds are closed. Rubber bands are removed, and the skin and hair washed gently with warm sudsy water to remove particulate and bloody material. A sterile gauze dressing is placed and the head wrapped. The posterior hairline suture line overlying the drain should be reinforced with Telfa gauze to prevent conspicuous bloodspotting from occurring through the dressing. The dressing should be taut and comfortable, not too tight, especially under the jawline and around the neck.

CLINICAL PEARLS

- The direction of the skin tension vectors and the sequencing of closure are paramount in achieving optimal results: the neck is set first, with closure along a skin tension vector that follows the jawline; the midface is set next, with closure along a skin tension vector that follows the axis of the ear; and the upper face is set last, with closure along an axis radial to the curved temporal incision.
- The three key deep dermal anchor sutures are placed before excess skin is trimmed. These sutures are placed to avoid migrating scars and avoid deformity to the ear and hairstyle.
- Earlobe and sideburn height should not be set until the key sutures have been placed and fixation has been verified.
- The earlobe position should be set a few millimeters "high"; gravimetric and the skin tensile forces associated with healing will lower the earlobe into proper position.
- Resection of hair-bearing scalp should be avoided at all costs.
- The preauricular suture line should be closed last—all hair-bearing suture lines should be trimmed, fixed, and closed beforehand.
- If a post-tragal approach has been chosen, the preauricular skin flap that covers the tragus should be defatted to full-thickness skin graft thickness to prevent tragal deformity; if a pretragal approach has been chosen, this flap should be left thick and hearty with fat to prevent a depressed preauricular scar.
- *Lipostructure* is the last part of the procedure. Lipostructure, in conjunction with laser resurfacing, is performed to correct residual lines, furrows, and folds. Lipostructure is more effective in regions of the face and neck that have not been undermined or liposuctioned.
- A Coleman fat scaffolding technique achieves the best long-term graft survival. This technique uses centrifuged fat and Coleman infiltration needles and syringes.
- For heavy nasolabial folds, superficial SAL and lipostructure are used in an attempt to reduce the fold and elevate the crease.

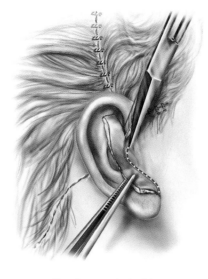

Rough preauricular trim

A

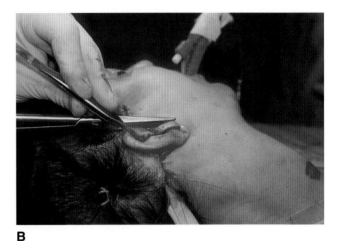

B

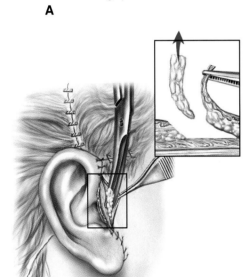

Preauricular defatting to full-thickness skin graft
thickness to allow for tragal definition

C

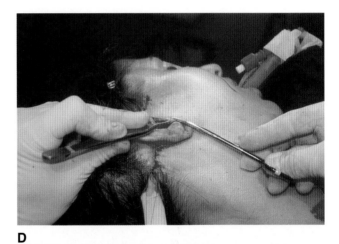

D

Figure 4-46 *Preauricular Closure.* ***A,*** *The preauricular suture line
should be the last one to be closed.* ***B,*** *Rough trim allowing a few
millimeters of overlap is performed initially with Rees or Gorney
scissors.* ***C,*** *If a post-tragal approach has been chosen, the
preauricular skin flap that covers the tragus should be defatted to full-
thickness skin graft thickness to allow for tragal definition.* ***D,*** *The
remainder of the preauricular flap should then be finely trimmed and
defatted so that closure can be performed with a minor amount of
skin overlap.* ***E,*** *Key interrupted simple stitches of 5-0 nylon suture
can be placed and closure performed with a running stitch of the
same material.*

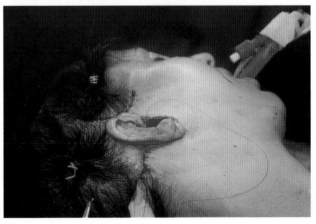

E

FINAL CLOSURE WITH DRAIN

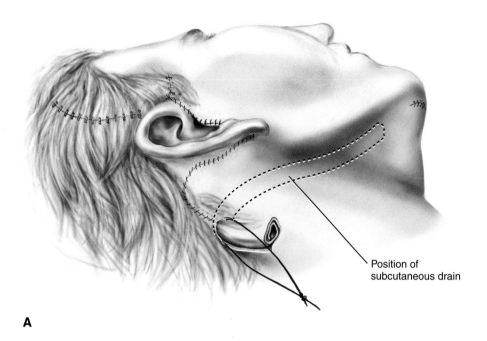

A

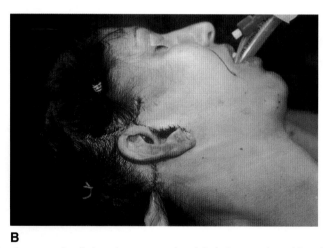

B

Figure 4-47 ***A*** *and* ***B,*** *The closure has been completed, the subcutaneous placed drain is properly positioned under the jawline, and the patient is now ready for lipostructure.*

Key References

Coleman S: Facial re-contouring with lipostructure. Clin Plast Surg 24:347, 1997.

Connell BF: Surgical technique of cervical lift and facial lipectomy. Aesth Plast Surg 5:43, 1981.

Hoefflin S: The extended supraplatysmal plane lift (ESP). Plast Reconstr Surg 101:494, 1998.

LaTrenta GS: Tumescent cervicofacial rhytidectomy. Aesthet Surg J 18:423, 1998.

LaTrenta GS: Does tumescent infiltration have a deleterious

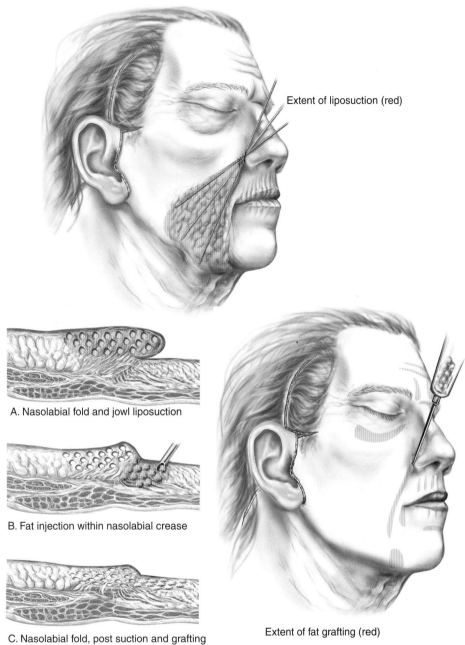

Extent of liposuction (red)

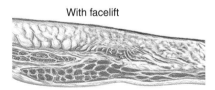

A. Nasolabial fold and jowl liposuction

B. Fat injection within nasolabial crease

C. Nasolabial fold, post suction and grafting

Extent of fat grafting (red)

With facelift

D. Nasolabial fold, post suction and grafting and facelift

Figure 4-48 *Lipostructure is the last step of the procedure. Lipostructure is used to correct residual furrows and folds in conjunction with laser resurfacing. The technique employed uses the Coleman fat scaffolding technique with centrifuged fat and Coleman needles of various sizes for fat deposition. A–D, Cross-sectional anatomy of nasolabial fold at different points in the procedure.*

effect on undermined skin flaps? Plast Reconstr Surg 104:2273, 1999.

LaTrenta GS, Talmor M: Tumescent cervicofacial rhytidectomy. Persp Plast Surg 15:47, 2001.

Rees TD, LaTrenta GS: Aesthetic Plastic Surgery, 2nd ed. Philadelphia, WB Saunders, 1994, pp 683-707.

Trepsat F: Volumetric face lifting. Plast Reconstr Surg 108:1358, 2002.

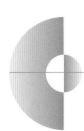

CHAPTER FIVE

Two-Layer Approaches to the Midface and Neck

The two-layer approach for facelift incorporates all of the elements of the one-layer approach, including superficial subcutaneous layer repositioning, skin tightening, small-cannula liposculpture, and lipostructure, but adds surgical reshaping of the deep subcutaneous layer to the procedure. The face and neck are composed of two quite different subcutaneous layers: the superficial and the deep. The superficial subcutaneous layer is superficial to the superficial fascia and most closely resembles a blanket of tightly woven fibrofatty tissue. It is evenly distributed throughout the face and neck. This blanket of compactly arranged and uniformly thick fat is dense with fibrous tissue, which holds it tightly to both the deep dermis and the superficial fascia. The deep subcutaneous layer is deep to the superficial fascia and superficial to the deep investing fascia. It is completely different from the superficial layer in both composition and distribution. Heavily laden with large fat globules in regions such as the anterior and middle cheek and the submental regions, and highly concentrated with fascia in regions such as the parotidomasseteric and temporoparietal regions and along the platysma muscle, it is also bereft of deep fat in the forehead, posterior cheek, and posterior neck and is thin and discontinuously distributed with fascia in the anterior cheek and submental triangle and over the jowls.

The deep subcutaneous layer more closely resembles a boxspring mattress. As the ligamentous supporting system and the musculofascial system lose their elasticity with aging, this boxspring mattress of deep subcutaneous tissue becomes less taut and firm and more bouncy and pliable. This is why the deep subcutaneous layer and the two-layer approach for rhytidectomy is so important in plastic surgery. As Dr. Sam Hamra has succinctly said, if subcutaneous dissection is the first generation of rhytidectomy, and subcutaneous dissection with limited SMAS/platysma surgery is the second generation of rhytidectomy, then two-flap subcutaneous and deep subcutaneous dissection is most certainly the third generation.

It is important to state at the outset that I believe there is no "best" deep subcutaneous plane procedure. The *lateral* midface deep plane approaches and the *anterior* neck deep plane approaches illustrated in this chapter provide the beginner as well as the seasoned surgeon with a solid foundation so that a "best patient fit" model can be easily adapted to the wide range of clinical practice problems. Midfacial approaches with access through the lower eyelid have purposely been omitted because the eyelid and the midface are separate and distinct anatomical regions that should not be surgically linked if at all possible, because of the inherent risk to the vulnerable and weaker lower eyelid when fixation of ptotic and heavier midfacial soft tissues either slackens or fails. In addition, subperiosteal approaches to the midface have also been omitted because aging of facial soft tissue proceeds far more rapidly at the skin surface level than at the subperiosteal level. After all, it is gravimetric displacement of ptotic and lax soft tissue, and not complete loss of the retaining ligaments at their sutural interfaces, that contributes most to the appearance of the aged face. Hence, I feel strongly that the subcutaneous approach is best for correction of aging.

The deep subcutaneous layer procedures illustrated, except for my personal approach, have been popularized and championed by a surgeon of considerable renown, and each procedure has its proponents. The illustrations provided in this chapter of other authors' procedures are not meant to be replicas of how each procedure is practiced by its "champion" surgeon but rather present adaptations of how I have interpreted, translated, and pursued their original ideas in my own practice of aesthetic face and neck surgery. For to paraphrase Albert Einstein, we are fortunate to have stood upon the shoulders of giants.

1) The two-layer approach incorporates all of the elements of the one-layer approach, including superficial subcutaneous layer repositioning, skin tightening, small-cannula liposculpture, and lipostructure, but adds surgical reshaping of the deep subcutaneous layer to the procedure.

2) With aging, the ligamentous supporting system and the musculofascial system lose their elasticity, allowing both the superficial and the deep subcutaneous tissues to become less taut and firm and more bouncy and pliable.

3) There is no "best" deep subcutaneous plane procedure; there is, however, a deep plane procedure that provides the best match for the patient's needs.

4) Trans-blepharoplasty midfacial approaches have been omitted because the eyelid and the midface are separate and distinct anatomical regions that should not be surgically linked because of the inherent risk to the vulnerable and much weaker lower eyelid if fixation of much heavier midfacial soft tissues slackens or fails.

5) Subperiosteal midfacial approaches have been omitted because aging of facial soft tissue proceeds far more rapidly at the skin surface level than at the subperiosteal level and because the deep subcutaneous approach is best for correction of aging.

THE SUPERFICIAL MUSCULOAPONEUROTIC SYSTEM AND THE PLATYSMA

Facial aging is easy to recognize but hard to define. Regardless, the two big anatomical offenders are (1) the true and false retaining ligaments and (2) the musculofascial system within the deep subcutaneous tissues. The retaining ligaments constitute the supporting system, and they can either emanate from the periosteum of the craniofacial skeleton at the sutural interfaces (true retaining ligaments) or form broad coalescences within the layers of the fascial planes of the cheeks (false retaining ligaments). The retaining ligaments ramify as they make their way through the mimetic musculature and the superficial and deep facial fascias. They eventually insert into the deep dermis of the skin, in this location many times their original size and thickness. Hence, it is primarily the retaining ligamentous system that holds the skin of the face and neck to the bone.

The superficial musculoaponeurotic system (SMAS) and the platysma muscle, along with the superficial mimetic musculature, form the deep subcutaneous musculofascial system of the face and neck. If the retaining ligaments can be visualized as forming the spokes of a wheel, thereby holding the wheel to the axle of the skeleton, the musculofascial system constitutes the wheel itself. It is the arrangement and sheer size of the musculofascial system, with its strengths and its weaknesses, its attachments and lack thereof, that are responsible for the many subcutaneous folds, grooves, and lines, and capacity for various expressions, in the human face. The SMAS and the platysma muscle, because of their relative lack of importance in facial animation, form the main surgical "building blocks" for deep layer techniques.

The SMAS and platysma can be likened to a tree. Although we mainly operate on the thick "surgical" fibrous trunklike layer of the superficial and deep fascia, the SMAS also has a rich and lush array of thinner fibrous tissue branches that sprout into the reticular dermis and along and through the blanket of superficial fat. Deep to this surgical trunk, the SMAS has a sparse but tough rootlike system that weaves around the large bedrock of the deep fat, through the tough roots of the deeper mimetic musculature, and around the tendrils of the neurovascular bundles. This rootlike system terminates in the deep investing fascia that covers the visceral musculature of the face and neck. It is this treelike pattern of branch, trunk, and root that gives the musculofascial system its tremendous surgical significance. And it is the precise arrangement and composition of each subcutaneous layer that give each of us our individual appearance. However, it is when this system slackens, from the relentless tug of time and the constant pull of gravimetric force, that the dreaded visage of age rears its unwanted head.

KEY POINTS

1) The two big anatomical offenders of facial aging are the true and false retaining ligaments and the musculofascial system within the deep subcutaneous tissues.

2) The retaining ligamentous system is primarily responsible for holding the skin of the face and neck to the bone.

3) Although the retaining ligaments form the spokes of the wheel, thereby holding the wheel to the axle of the skeleton, it is the musculofascial system that forms the wheel itself and that is primarily responsible for the many subcutaneous folds, grooves, lines, and expressions in the human face.

4) When the musculofascial system slackens, from the relentless tug of time and the constant pull of gravimetric force, the dreaded visage of age rears its unwanted head.

5) The SMAS and the platysma muscle, because of their relative lack of importance in facial animation, form the main surgical "building blocks" for deep layer techniques.

ONE-LAYER VERSUS TWO-LAYER TECHNIQUES

One-layer superficial subcutaneous procedures achieve two goals: (1) they tighten the skin and (2) they reposition the superficial fat. The amount of superficial fat that is repositioned is determined by the surgeon when the skin flaps are undermined. Hence, superficial layer surgery primarily corrects skin folding. How the skin is tightened and where the superficial fat is repositioned to are determined by the vectors used by the surgeon to reposition the flaps. Because the superficial fat is not separated from the skin flaps, one-layer techniques are inherently locked into "mono-block" vectors of movement (Fig. 5-1). Although the upper face, midface, and neck skin flaps can theoretically be repositioned along different vectors, they usually are not, because the optimal vector of movement for the superficial subcutaneous layer tends to parallel the axis of the ear. The closure sequence—the order of surgical maneuvers used for insetting and fixing the flaps into their new positions—can be varied only slightly, if at all, with one-layer techniques. The sequence generally proceeds from the ground up: the neck flap is inset and fixed in place first, the midface flap is inset and fixed in place next, and the upper facial flap is inset and fixed in place last.

Two-layer subcutaneous procedures achieve three goals: (1) they tighten the skin; (2) they reposition superficial fat, fascia, and deep fat; and (3) they bunch up and three-dimensionally rearrange fat, muscle, and fascia into different regions of the face *independent* of the skin flap. Hence, two-layer techniques actually *reshape* the subcutaneous tissues layers of the face and neck by correcting skin folding, tightening up musculofascial laxity, and repositioning and lifting ptotic soft tissue mass. How the skin and musculofascia are tightened and the ptotic soft tissue mass is lifted is determined by the vectors used by the surgeon to reposition the flaps. As with one-layer techniques, the superficial subcutaneous layer tends to have its optimal vector of movement along the axis of the ear. The deep subcutaneous layer, however, has a different optimal vector of movement (see Fig. 5-1). This vector is oriented along the *vertical* axis—because of gravity. Gravity is the force that causes soft tissues to descend over time. And the force of gravity is directly proportional to mass, which explains why patients with very heavy soft tissue mass in the midface and neck often demonstrate the most pronounced signs of aging.

True vertical repositioning of flaps is easy to achieve with two-layer techniques because skin flap transposition is achieved independent of deep plane repositioning. In the upper face and midface, vertical repositioning of the deep plane is easy to achieve; however, in the neck and over the curvature of the jawline, it is more difficult. This difficulty is solved if the vector of deep plane flap transposition is performed bidirectionally obliquely in the lower face and neck. The summation of these opposing vectors achieves near-vertical repositioning of the deep subcutaneous layer over the lower face and neck.

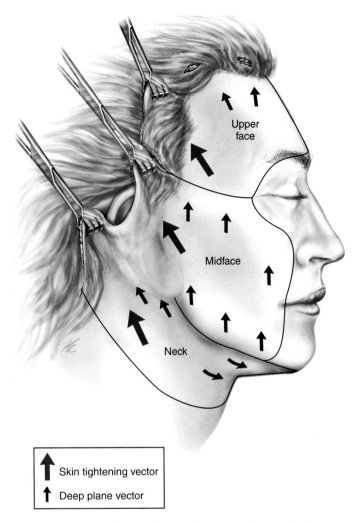

Figure 5-1 *Whereas the optimal vector of movement for superficial subcutaneous plane transposition (i.e., skin tightening and superficial fat repositioning) is obliquely oriented along the axis of the ear, the optimal vector of movement for the deep subcutaneous plane transposition (i.e., facial and neck reshaping) is oriented vertically in the upper and middle face and bidirectionally obliquely in the neck.*

Two-layer techniques provide far greater design flexibility for matching the patient's anatomical features of aging to procedures that optimize the patient's aesthetic potential. This is achieved primarily because the deeper subcutaneous tissues are repositioned independent of the skin. It is also achieved, however, because two-layer techniques offer far greater flexibility for the sequencing for closure. For example, in a patient who is pleased with her face and bothered primarily by the "turkey gobbler" appearance of her anterior neck, correction of the deep subcutaneous tissues in this region should be addressed first. The submental incision is the first incision made, with subsequent removal of excess superficial fat, direct excision of deep fat, resection of excess platysma, and "corset"-type platysmaplasty. After the high-priority anterior neck problem has been thoroughly addressed for the patient, the lateral-approach two-layer rhytidectomy can be performed. In contrast, in the patient who is bothered primarily by nasolabial and oromandibular grooves and folds, deep subcutaneous tissue fixation is best begun in the midface rather than in the neck, so that the deeper subcutaneous tissues of the midface can

be positioned as needed without being fought against and dragged down by deep anterior neck tissues that have been prematurely locked into position. In this patient, it is also important that the upper face be lifted and the deep upper tissues locked in initially to provide a solid foundation for suspension of the deep subcutaneous tissues in the midface. By allowing for a flexible closure sequencing, two-layer techniques provide greater facility for meeting higher standards of beauty for greater numbers of patients.

In order to achieve skin tightening, however, two-layer techniques must use a thinner skin flap than is acceptable with one-layer techniques. The deep subcutaneous layer flap is used as the primary vehicle for repositioning the superficial fat, fascia, and deep fat, so that the flap in two-layer techniques is subjected to great strain, especially if correction of skin folding is a high priority for the patient. This probably accounts for the greater tendency of aggressive two-layer techniques to cause minor skin sloughs than is seen with one-layer techniques. Hence, if correction of skin folding is the primary and only reason for the surgery, one-layer techniques are advised.

KEY POINTS

1) One-layer superficial subcutaneous procedures achieve two goals: they tighten the skin, and they reposition the superficial fat.

2) One-layer superficial subcutaneous procedures primarily correct *skin folding* and are advised if this is the primary and only reason for surgery.

3) The optimal vector of movement and the closure sequencing for one-layer subcutaneous procedures can be varied only slightly, if at all.

4) Two-layer subcutaneous procedures achieve three goals: they tighten the skin; they reposition superficial fat, fascia, and deep fat; and they bunch up and three-dimensionally rearrange fat, muscle, and fascia into different regions of the face *independent* of the skin flap.

5) Two-layer techniques actually *reshape* the subcutaneous tissues layers of the face and neck by correcting skin folding, tightening up musculofascial laxity, and repositioning and lifting ptotic soft tissue mass.

6) True vertical vectors of movement and flexible closure sequencing with two-layer techniques provide far greater design flexibility in matching the patient's anatomical features of aging to procedures that can optimize aesthetic potential.

INDICATIONS

The conceptual goals for deep subcutaneous plane surgery in the midface and neck can be simply stated: (1) to restore volume and add contour to the upper and middle face and (2) to reduce volume and sharply define the lower face and neck (Fig. 5-2). The actual goals for deep subcutaneous plane surgery include restoring cheekbone fullness; reducing any submalar hollow; softening any nasolabial, marionette, cheek, and neck folds; eradicating the jowl and restoring a clean and smoothly contoured jawline; removing any "waddle"

under the chin; and creating a smooth, well-defined cervicomental angle of near 120 degrees. Anatomically, although skin tightening and superficial fat repositioning are the goals primarily of one-flap superficial subcutaneous plane surgery, they are also achieved by two-flap techniques. However, they are performed *after* the midface volume has been restored, the ptotic soft tissue has been aesthetically repositioned, the musculofascial layer has been tightened, and the neckline slimmed down and better defined. Simply stated, the aim of deep layer surgery is to go from the square face of age to the oval face of youth.

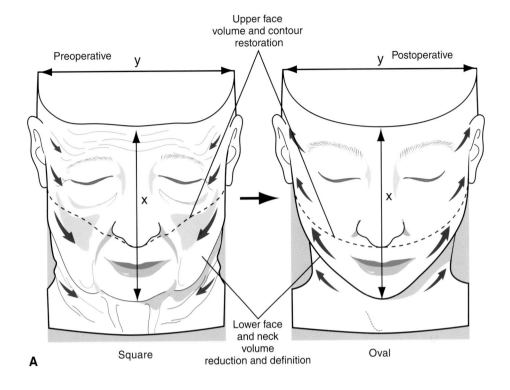

Upper face
volume and contour
restoration

Preoperative   y   y   Postoperative

x   x

Lower face
and neck
volume
reduction and definition

A   Square   Oval

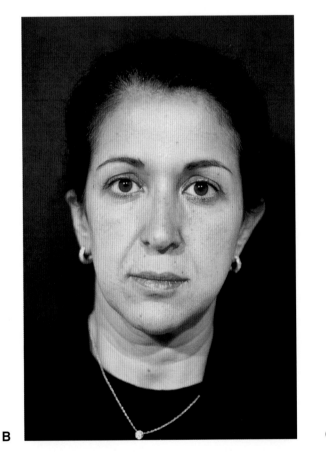

B

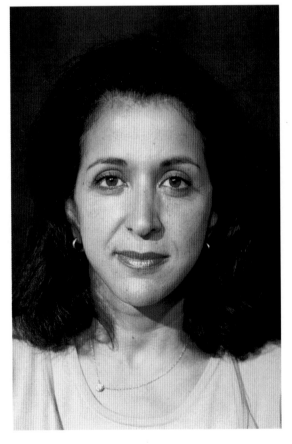

C

Figure 5-2   *The goals of deep subcutaneous plane surgery are twofold: (1) to restore volume and add pleasing contour to the upper face and midface and (2) to reduce volume and add definition to the lower face and neck. **A,** With these techniques, the square face of age is restored to the oval face of youth. **B,** This 47-year-old woman underwent deep plane rhytidectomy. **C,** Her postoperative appearance.*

The primary indication for deep subcutaneous plane surgery is to address facial and neck gravimetric ptosis of the deep subcutaneous tissues. Which technique is chosen is dependent on three factors: (1) the degree of *musculofascial laxity* in the midface and the neck, (2) the sheer size of the *ptotic soft tissue mass* in the midface and the neck, and (3) the depth, degree, and extent of nasolabial, oromandibular, cheek, and neck *skin folding* (Fig. 5-3).

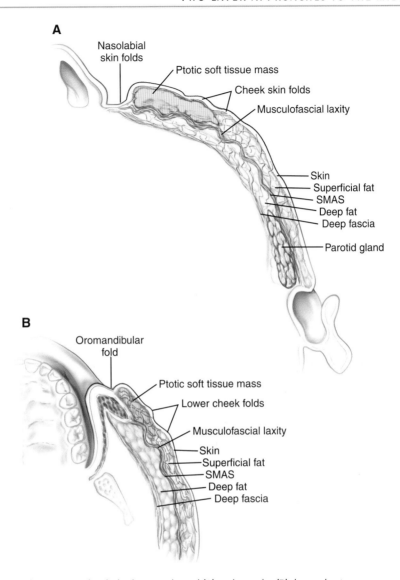

Figure 5-3   *The choice between lateral **(A)** and anterior **(B)** deep subcutaneous plane techniques for midface and neck rejuvenation depends on (1) the degree of facial and neck musculofascial laxity, (2) the sheer size of the ptotic soft tissue mass, and (3) the depth and extent of nasolabial, oromandibular, and neck skin folding.*

Musculofascial laxity is more easily demonstrated than described (Fig. 5-4). If the patient leans forward and brings the chin down toward the chest, the facial and neck soft tissues will at most simply bunch up if the musculofascial system is taut. If the musculofascial system is lax, however, the soft tissues will literally sag off the bone. Musculofascial laxity is related primarily to loss of ligamentous support and loss of elasticity within the musculofascial layer. Musculofascial laxity is easy to assess by placing the palm over the patient's face and gently elevating the subcutaneous layers. The degree of musculo-fascial laxity is proportional to the vertical excursion necessary to replace the ptotic soft tissues into their "best fit" position.

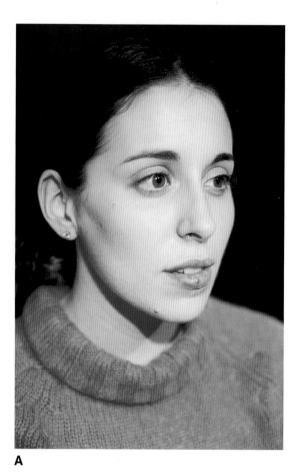

A

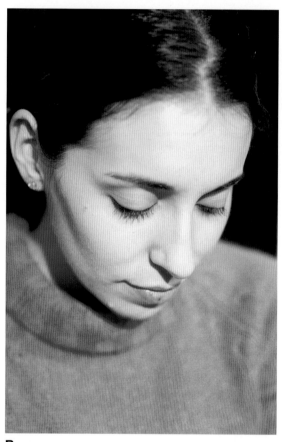

B

Figure 5-4　*Musculofascial Laxity. A simple test for assessing musculofascial laxity is to have the patient lean forward and bring the chin down to the chest.* ***A*** *and* ***B,*** *In the face of youth, when the musculofascial system is taut, the facial and neck soft tissues, if anything, may bunch up.*

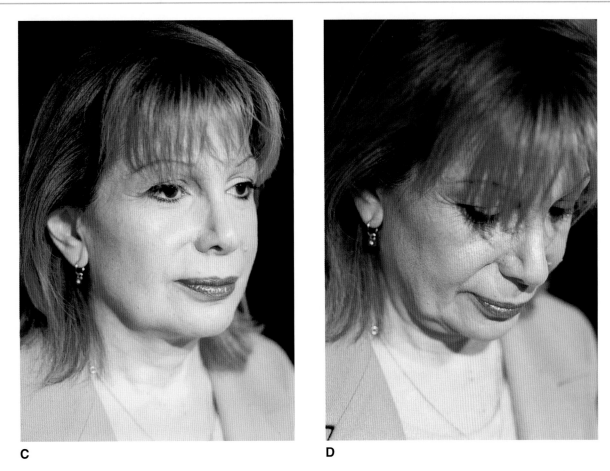

C

D

Figure 5-4, cont'd **C** and **D,** In the face of age, when musculofascial laxity is significant, the facial and neck soft tissues will literally sag off the bone.

Ptotic soft tissue mass is the thickness and sheer mass of the subcutaneous tissue identified as requiring "lifting" (Fig. 5-5). This concept was introduced in Chapter One when fat distribution and ligamentous support of the subcutaneous tissues in the human face were described. In the midface, for instance, cadaveric studies have found that one third of the total facial and neck fat mass is in the cheeks and that three quarters of deep facial and neck fat is in the anterior and middle cheeks alone. This fat mass was found to be poorly supported and farthest from major sources of ligamentous support. Ptotic soft tissue mass is caused by progressive gravitational descent of genetically prone facial and neck soft tissues. Ptotic soft tissue mass can range from very thin to very heavy. Much as for musculofascial laxity, it is assessed by placing the palm over the patient's face and gently elevating the subcutaneous layers. The degree of ptotic soft tissue mass is the volume and thickness of soft tissue that needs to be lifted with the surgical procedure.

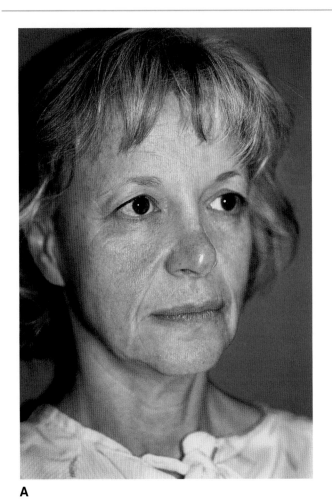

A

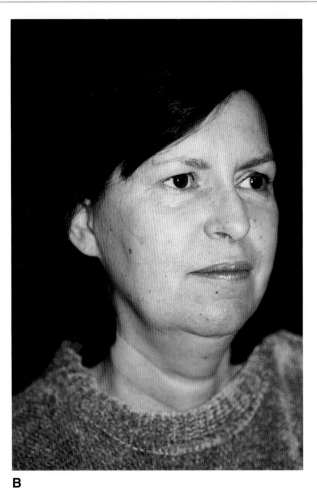

B

Figure 5-5   *Ptotic soft tissue mass is the volume of subcutaneous tissue, with respect to both thickness and bulk, identified by the surgeon and the patient as requiring "lifting." Although this mass is composed primarily of fat, fascia and mimetic musculature also add to its bulk. Ptotic soft tissue mass can range from very thin (**A**) to very heavy (**B**). It is easy to assess by lightly placing the palm over the patient's face and gently elevating the subcutaneous layers over the bone.*

Skin folds, in contrast to wrinkles, mimetic lines, and furrows, are redundant and overlapped subcutaneous tissue (Fig. 5-6). In contrast to ptotic soft tissue mass, skin folds are composed of skin and superficial fat only. Rapid weight gain or loss, excessive dynamic muscle tone, solar elastosis, genetic propensity, and, paradoxically, poor muscle tone cause the development of skin folding.

Skin folds, behaving much like folds of drapery, are mostly observed anteriorly, along the nasolabial, oromandibular, and cheek regions. This is due to the unique distribution of intrafascial coalescences that predominate in those regions of the face. There is enormous individual variability in skin folding in the human face and neck.

KEY POINTS

1) Conceptual goals for deep subcutaneous plane surgery are to restore volume and add contour to the upper and middle face and to reduce volume and sharply define the lower face and neck.

2) Actual goals for deep subcutaneous plane surgery include restoring cheekbone fullness; correcting any submalar hollow; softening any nasolabial, marionette, cheek, and neck folds eradicating the jowl and restoring a clean and smoothly contoured jawline; removing any "waddle" under the chin; and creating a smooth, well-defined cervicomental angle of near 120 degrees.

3) The primary indication for deep subcutaneous plane surgery is to correct facial and neck gravimetric ptosis of the deep subcutaneous tissues.

4) The technique chosen for deep subcutaneous plane surgery is dependent on three factors: the degree of musculofascial laxity in the midface and the neck, the sheer size of the ptotic soft tissue mass in the midface and the neck, and the depth, degree, and extent of nasolabial, oromandibular, cheek, and neck skin folding.

5) Musculofascial laxity is more easily demonstrated than described; if the musculofascial system is taut, in a patient who leans forward and brings the chin down toward the chest, the facial and neck soft tissues will at most simply bunch up; however, if the musculofascial system is lax, the soft tissues will literally sag off the bone.

6) Ptotic soft tissue mass is the volume of subcutaneous tissue, with respect to both thickness and bulk, identified by the surgeon as requiring "lifting."

7) Skin folds, in contrast to wrinkles, mimetic lines, and furrows, are redundant and overlapped subcutaneous tissue, composed primarily of skin and superficial fat.

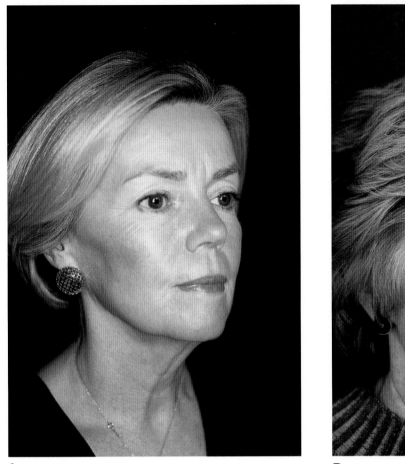

A

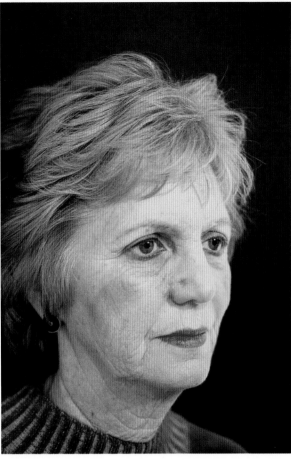

B

Figure 5-6 *Skin Folding. Skin folding is redundancy and overlapping of skin and superficial fat. Skin folds are observed mostly in the nasolabial, oromandibular, and cheek regions owing to the unique distribution of intrafascial coalescences that predominate in those regions of the face. There is wide individual variability, ranging from minor **(A)** to major **(B)** in both the depth and the degree of skin folding in the face and neck.*

TECHNIQUES

Lateral Approaches

Plication/Imbrication/Limited Lateral SMAS/Platysma Advancement Flap Techniques

Limited lateral SMAS/platysma flap elevation/fixation, with "lifting" of the anterior deep subcutaneous tissues by multiple strategically placed imbrication/plication sutures (Fig. 5-7), is the *simplest, most straightforward, and most commonly performed of the midfacial two-layer techniques.* It is also the least powerful of the lateral approaches.

This technique also has other limitations: (1) because it is not as powerful as other more extensive techniques, the patient should not have significant musculofascial laxity; (2) the patient needs to have a well-developed musculofascial layer so that the anterior plication/imbrication sutures can get enough purchase and not tear through; (3) the patient should have a lightly weighted anterior ptotic soft tissue mass, as this technique does not incorporate wide anterior undermining of ptotic soft tissue mass; and (4) because the anterior plication/imbrication sutures are used solely for deep tissue reshaping, skin fold correction is solely dependent on the skin tightening portion of the procedure.

Hence, the best candidates for plication/imbrication/limited lateral SMAS/platysma advancement flap techniques are patients with minimal to moderate musculofascial laxity, a lightly weighted anterior ptotic soft tissue mass, and minimal shallow nasolabial, oromandibular, and neck skin folding (Figs. 5-8 to 5-10).

KEY POINTS

1) The plication/imbrication/limited lateral SMAS/platysma advancement flap technique is the simplest, most straightforward, and most commonly performed of the midfacial two-layer techniques; however, it is also the least powerful.

2) The best candidates are patients who have a minimally lax musculofascial layer, a lightly weighted anterior ptotic soft tissue mass, and minimal shallow nasolabial, oromandibular, cheek and neck skin folding.

3) Patients need to have a well-developed musculofascial layer so that the anterior plication/imbrication sutures get enough purchase and do not tear through.

LIMITED SMAS/PLATYSMA ADVANCEMENT

SMAS/Platysma Plication/Imbrication

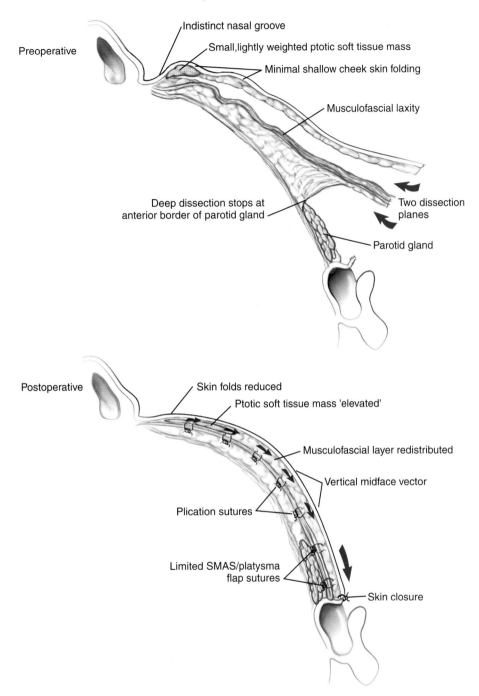

Figure 5-7 *Anterior Plication/Imbrication and Limited Lateral SMAS/Platysma Advancement. This is the simplest and most straightforward of the lateral approaches. It is best used for patients who have a lax but well-developed musculofascial layer, a lightly weighted ptotic soft tissue mass, and minimal shallow nasolabial, oromandibular, and neck skin folding.*

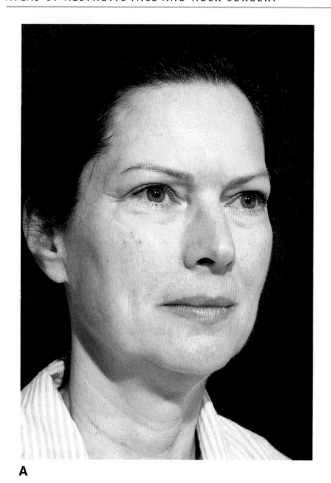

A

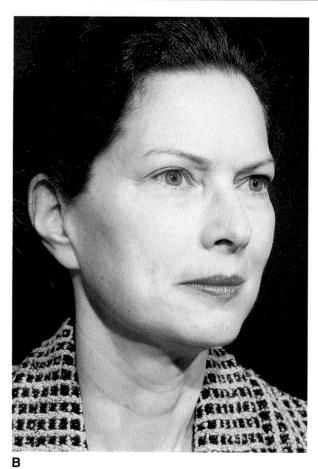

B

Figure 5-8 Anterior Plication/Imbrication and Limited Lateral SMAS/Platysma Advancement. **A,** This 54-year-old woman is an excellent candidate for this technique because she has a well-developed musculofascial layer with a good amount of laxity, seen primarily in the anterior regions of the midface and neck, yet possesses only a lightly weighted ptotic soft tissue mass and minor amounts of shallow skin folding. She also emphatically stated before her surgical procedure that she did not want to look like she had had a "facelift." **B,** Her postoperative appearance.

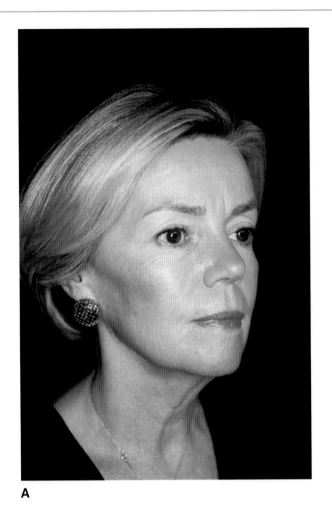

A

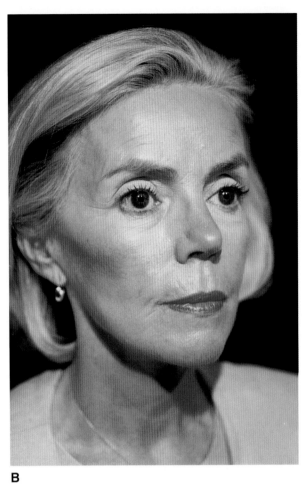

B

Figure 5-9 *Anterior Plication/Imbrication and Limited Lateral SMAS/Platysma Advancement. **A,** This 54-year-old woman was an excellent candidate for this technique because of her shallow, near-nonexistent nasolabial, oromandibular, and neck skin folding; her thick moderately lax anterior musculofascial layer; and her lightly weighted ptotic soft tissue mass. Medial platysma band resection and a "corset" platysmaplasty were necessary in the neck to deal with her excessive and lax platysma muscle. **B,** Her postoperative appearance.*

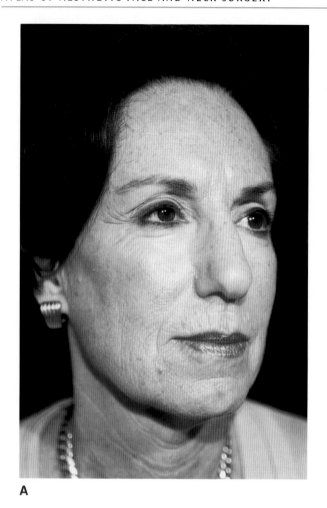

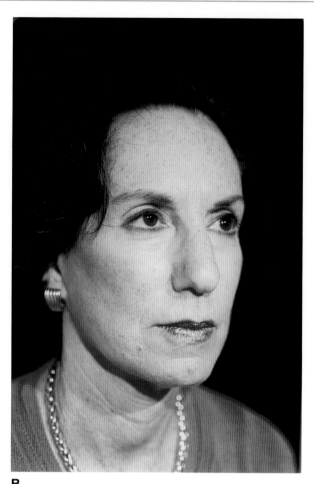

A

B

Figure 5-10   *Anterior Plication/Imbrication and Limited Lateral SMAS/Platysma Advancement.* **A,** *This 56-year-old woman is an excellent candidate for this technique because of her lightly weighted ptotic anterior soft tissue mass; her thickish, moderately lax anterior musculofascial layer; and her shallow skin folding.* **B,** *Her postoperative appearance. Upper blepharoplasty and dermabrasion to the upper lip were also performed.*

Technique

After the skin flaps have been raised and hemostasis has been obtained, the surgical plan for limited lateral SMAS/platysma advancement flap and anterior SMAS plication/imbrication is delineated (Fig. 5-11). The incision for the limited lateral SMAS/platysma advancement flap follows a lazy upside-down "L" pattern. The transverse portion of the incision is begun 1 cm below the zygomatic arch in order to avoid injury to the frontal branch of the facial nerve. The frontal branch of the facial nerve penetrates the superficial fascia immediately below the midportion of the zygomatic arch at a steep angle and obliquely courses over the arch within the temporoparietal fascia toward the forehead musculature. The vertical portion of the incision gently parallels and is within 1 cm of the skin incision. The incision line then dips posteriorly into the retrolobular sulcus around the earlobe and follows the lateral border of the platysma muscle for approximately 2 to 3 cm. Areas for the 4 or 5 anterior plication/imbrication sutures are marked as virtual anterior extensions of the transverse incision. These areas are approximately 1 cm apart in a pattern that roughly follows the course of the zygomaticus major muscle.

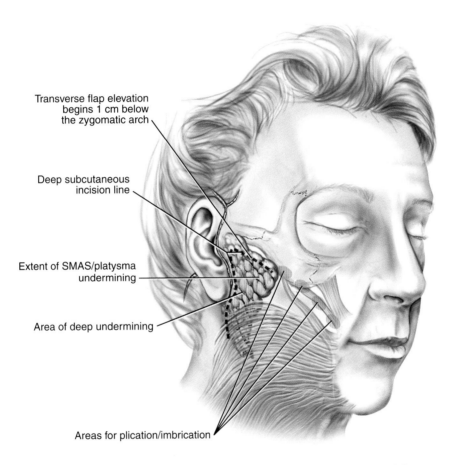

Transverse flap elevation begins 1 cm below the zygomatic arch

Deep subcutaneous incision line

Extent of SMAS/platysma undermining

Area of deep undermining

Areas for plication/imbrication

Figure 5-11 *The incision for the limited lateral SMAS/platysma advancement flap follows a lazy upside-down "L" pattern. The transverse portion of the incision is begun 1 cm below the zygomatic arch in order to avoid injury to the frontal branch of the facial nerve. The vertical portion of the incision gently parallels and is within 1 cm of the skin incision and dips posteriorly into the retrolobular sulcus to follow the lateral border of the platysma muscle for approximately 2 to 3 cm. The 4 or 5 anterior plication/imbrication sutures are placed approximately 1 cm apart in a pattern that roughly follows the course of the zygomaticus major muscle.*

Deep subcutaneous dissection is begun by elevating the platysma-auricular ligament (Fig. 5-12). A single-tooth Adson forceps grasps the ligament, which literally is a several-centimeter-square area of lateral platysma adherence to the underlying deep fascia. Using sharp dissection with a curved Gorney scissors, the ligament and the lateral platysma muscle are elevated. This maneuver creates a platysma/superficial fascial/subcutaneous fat flap over the neck and lower face. The Gorney scissors should hug the inferior surface of the platysma muscle in order to avoid injury to the marginal mandibular nerve. The marginal mandibular nerve exits the tail of the parotid gland and always courses below the angle of the jaw in the subplatysma plane, but its exit from the parotid gland can vary depending on the patient's parotid gland morphology. Once the platysma-auricular ligament is released, the platysma muscle flap is easy to release as far anteriorly and inferiorly as necessary. Subplatysma hemostasis should carefully be performed at this juncture.

The limited lateral SMAS flap is developed by sharp scalpel dissection down to the capsule of the parotid (Fig. 5-13). The meso-temporalis is developed over the zygomatic arch, which safely protects the frontal branch of the facial nerve within its borders. Sub-SMAS dissection then proceeds for several centimeters to the anterior border of the parotid gland. No facial nerve or sensory nerve branches should be visible at this point; if they are, the dissection plane has been carried too deep.

Lahey clamps are placed on the platysma-auricular ligament and the corner of the SMAS flap, and the vectors for flap transposition are determined (Fig. 5-14). In general, the vectors are more vertical for the SMAS flap in the midface and more oblique for the platysma flap in the neck. Several buried mattress stitches of 3-0 Mersilene suture are placed for SMAS flap fixation to the residual superficial fascia along the zygomatic arch and to the superficial temporal fascia laterally. After SMAS fixation has been completed, several buried mattress stitches of 3-0 Mersilene are placed for platysma flap fixation to the mastoid fascia and for several centimeters inferiorly to the deep cervical investing fascia. If any contour irregularities exist at this point, they should be resected and smoothed with a buried stitch of 4-0 Mersilene suture.

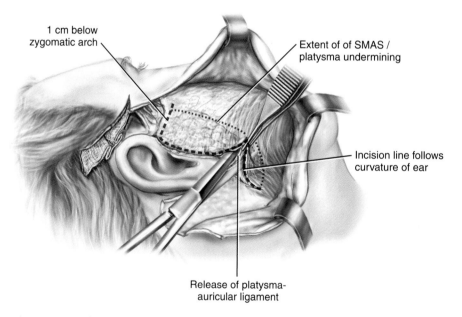

1 cm below zygomatic arch

Extent of of SMAS / platysma undermining

Incision line follows curvature of ear

Release of platysma-auricular ligament

Figure 5-12 *A single-tooth Adson forceps grasps the platysma-auricular ligament, which literally is a several-centimeter-square area of lateral platysma adherence to the underlying deep fascia. Using sharp dissection with a curved Gorney scissors, the ligament and the lateral platysma muscle are elevated to begin flap undermining. Beware: The marginal mandibular nerve exits the tail of the parotid gland and always courses below the angle of the jaw in the subplatysma plane.*

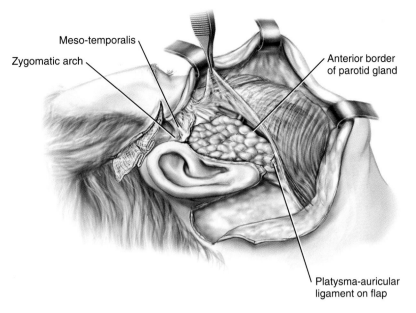

Meso-temporalis

Zygomatic arch

Anterior border
of parotid gland

Platysma-auricular
ligament on flap

Figure 5-13 *The limited lateral SMAS flap is developed by sharp scalpel dissection down to the capsule of the parotid. The meso-temporalis is developed over the zygomatic arch, which safely protects the frontal branch of the facial nerve within its borders. Sub-SMAS dissection then proceeds for several centimeters to the anterior border of the parotid gland. No facial nerve or sensory nerve branches should be visible.*

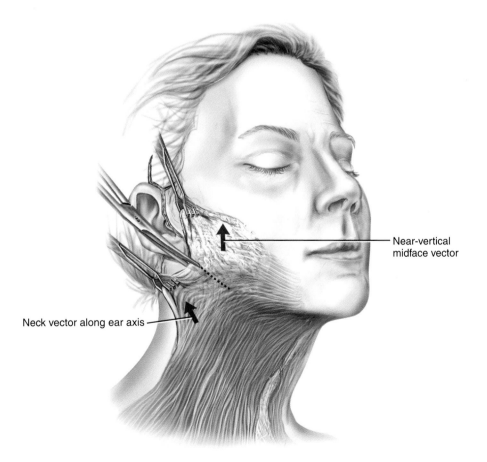

Near-vertical
midface vector

Neck vector along ear axis

Figure 5-14 *Lahey clamps are placed on the platysma-auricular ligament and the corner of the SMAS flap, and the vectors for flap transposition are determined. In general, the vectors are more vertical for the SMAS flap in the midface and more oblique for the platysma flap in the neck.*

Residual musculofascial laxity anterior to the parotid is evident as anterior bunching of soft tissue and is best addressed by placement of several anterior plication/imbrication sutures (Fig. 5-15). This anterior bunching especially becomes evident as the lateral advancement flap is transposed under tension and fixed into its new position. The pattern of the plication/imbrication sutures roughly follows the path of the zygomaticus major muscle. This muscle arises on the inferolateral surface of the zygomatic body and obliquely courses across the cheek to the nasolabial groove. The 4 or 5 plication/imbrication sutures are strategically sited several centimeters apart.

The vector for the plication/imbrication sutures is purely *vertical* (Fig. 5-16). In using the limited lateral SMAS/platysma flap, simple buried stitches of 4-0 Mersilene suture are placed. Great care must be taken in placing the sutures superficial enough that injury to the zygomatic and buccal branches of the facial nerve is avoided. Four or five of these sutures are placed from lateral to medial and tied as they are inset (Fig. 5-17). Any contour irregularities can be resected and smoothed down with simple buried stitches of 4-0 Mersilene suture.

CLINICAL PEARLS

- The incision for the limited lateral SMAS/platysma advancement flap follows a lazy upside-down "L" pattern, with its transverse incision placed 1 cm below the zygomatic arch in order to avoid injury to the frontal branch of the facial nerve.
- During the platysmaplasty portion of the procedure, the Gorney scissors should hug the inferior surface of the platysma muscle in order to avoid injury to the densely adherent marginal mandibular nerve, which is always subplatysmal.
- Sub-SMAS/platysma dissection proceeds and halts at the anterior border of the parotid gland.
- The vectors for the limited flap transposition are more vertical for the midfacial SMAS flap and more oblique for the platysma flap in the neck.
- Residual musculofascial laxity anterior to the parotid is evident as anterior bunching of soft tissue and is best addressed by 4 or 5 anterior buried plication/imbrication sutures placed with a purely vertical vector.
- Great care must be taken in placing the plication/imbrication sutures superficial enough that injury to the zygomatic and buccal branches of the facial nerve is avoided, as these nerves can often balloon into a more superficial and vulnerable position after the lateral SMAS/platysma flap has been tightened.

Anterior bunching

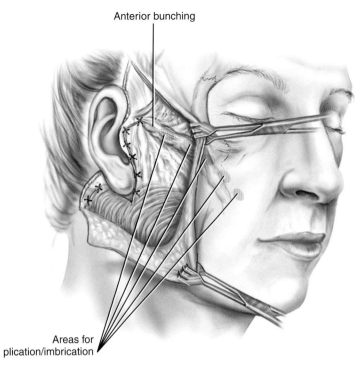

Areas for
plication/imbrication

Figure 5-15 *Several buried mattress stitches of 4-0 Mersilene suture are placed for SMAS flap fixation to the residual superficial fascia along the zygomatic arch and to the superficial temporal fascia laterally. After SMAS fixation has been completed, several buried mattress stitches of 4-0 Mersilene are placed for platysma flap fixation to the mastoid fascia and for several centimeters inferiorly to the deep cervical investing fascia. Residual musculofascial laxity anterior to the parotid is evident as anterior bunching of soft tissue.*

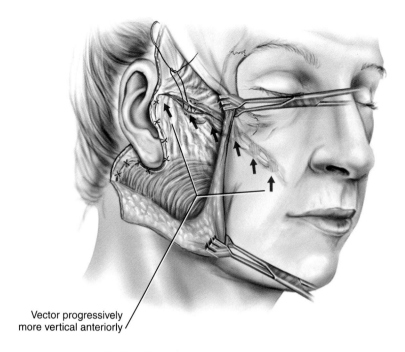

Vector progressively
more vertical anteriorly

Figure 5-16 *Anterior bunching especially becomes evident as the lateral advancement flap is transposed under tension and fixated into its new position. The placement of the plication/imbrication sutures roughly follows the path of the zygomaticus major muscle. These 4 or 5 plication/imbrication sutures are strategically sited several centimeters apart. The vector for the plication/imbrication sutures is purely vertical, and simple buried stitches of 4-0 Mersilene suture are placed.*

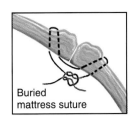

Buried
mattress suture

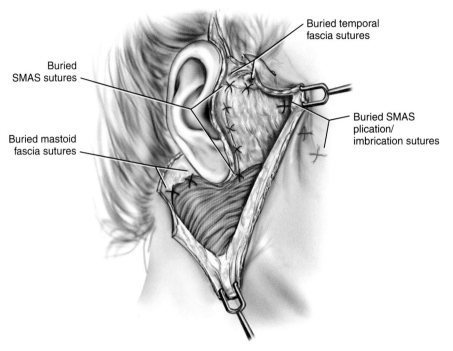

Buried temporal
fascia sutures

Buried
SMAS sutures

Buried SMAS
plication/
imbrication sutures

Buried mastoid
fascia sutures

Figure 5-17 *Great care must be taken to place the plication/imbrication sutures superficial enough that injury to the zygomatic and buccal branches of the facial nerve is avoided. Four or five of these sutures are placed from lateral to medial and tied as they are inset. Any contour irregularities can be resected and smoothed down with simple buried stitches of 4-0 Mersilene suture.*

Resective Techniques: Lateral SMAS/Platysma-ectomy

A well-designed resection of lateral SMAS and platysma muscle, along with musculofascial tightening achieved by a deep subcutaneous suture line of considerable strength and durability, is the strongest method for *tightening* the deeper subcutaneous tissues of the lateral midface and neck (Fig. 5-18). When combined with a properly performed skin-tightening superficial layer procedure, it optimally corrects *musculofascial and skin folding*. When the vector for "lifting" is directed obliquely upward, resective techniques can also lift a lightly weighted and ptotic soft tissue mass, thereby reshaping the face and neck. The technique, however, requires that the patient's musculofascial layer be very lax; otherwise, the deep subcutaneous tissues will simply bunch up and not be optimally reshaped.

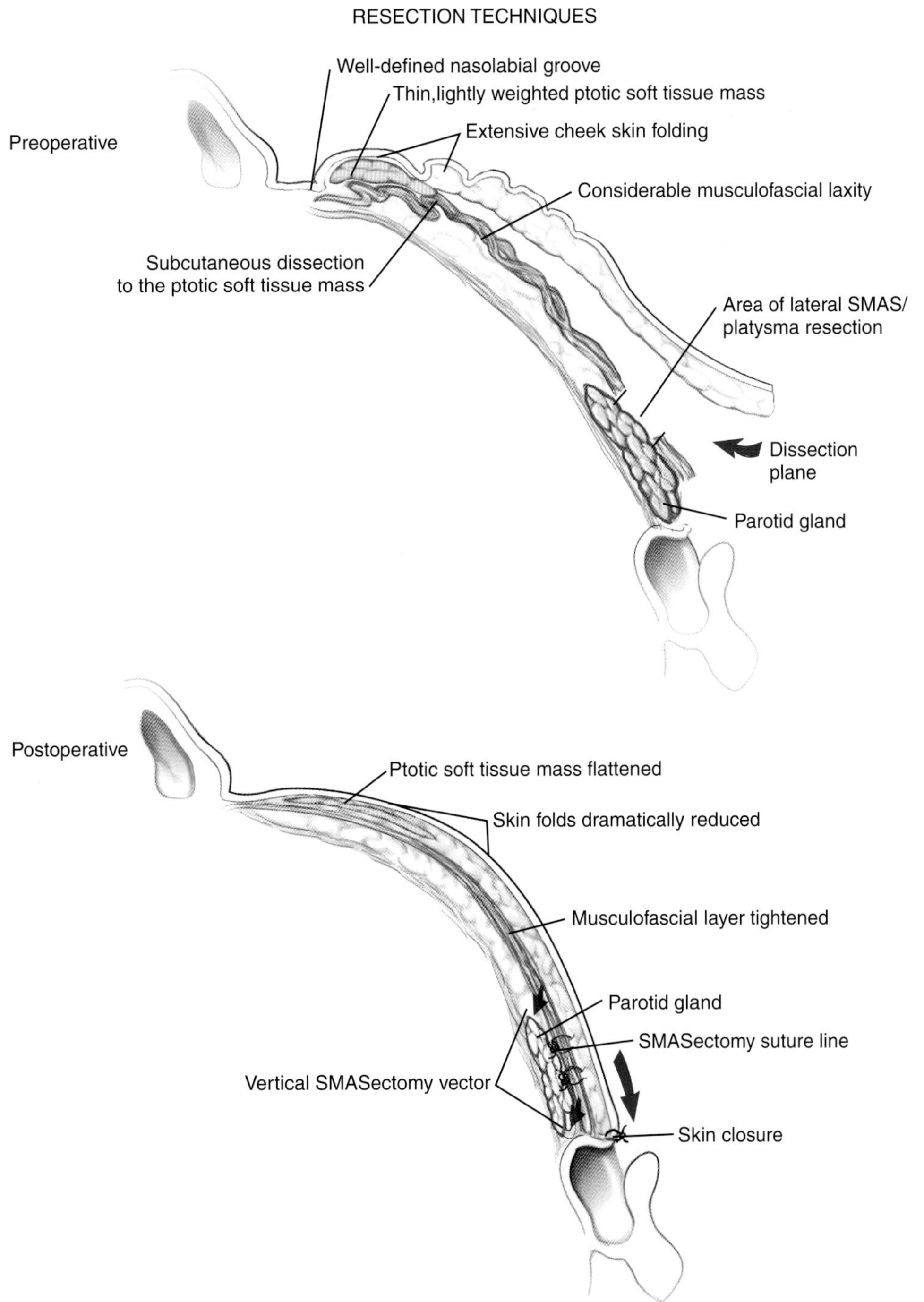

RESECTION TECHNIQUES

Preoperative

Well-defined nasolabial groove
Thin, lightly weighted ptotic soft tissue mass
Extensive cheek skin folding
Considerable musculofascial laxity
Subcutaneous dissection to the ptotic soft tissue mass
Area of lateral SMAS/platysma resection
Dissection plane
Parotid gland

Postoperative

Ptotic soft tissue mass flattened
Skin folds dramatically reduced
Musculofascial layer tightened
Parotid gland
SMASectomy suture line
Vertical SMASectomy vector
Skin closure

Figure 5-18 *Resective Techniques: Lateral SMAS/Platysma-ectomy. This is the best technique to use in patients with extensive shallow skin folds in the nasolabial, oromandibular, and neck regions. Optimally, these patients also have considerable laxity of the musculofascial layer and a lightly weighted ptotic soft tissue mass.*

Resective techniques are not without other limitations: (1) the musculofascial resection must be aligned along the appropriate axis to avoid the creation of "lateral sweep"; (2) the SMAS/platysma tissues should have enough tensile strength that the suture line does not tear through; (3) the patient needs to have considerable musculofascial laxity for the technique to be effective; and finally, (4) the patient should not have heavy ptotic soft tissue mass in the anterior midface and neck, or the sutures will have too much tension placed upon them and either tear through or rip the underlying musculofascial tissue.

Hence, the best candidates for resective techniques have a very lax musculofascial layer (Fig. 5-19); a small, lightly weighted anterior ptotic soft tissue mass (Fig. 5-20); and extensive shallow skin folding in the nasolabial, cheek, oromandibular, and neck regions (Fig. 5-21).

KEY POINTS

1) Resective techniques constitute the strongest method for *tightening* the deeper subcutaneous tissues of the lateral midface and neck.

2) When a deep subcutaneous plane resective technique is combined with a properly performed skin-tightening procedure, extensive shallow musculofascial and skin folding are optimally corrected.

3) The best candidates for resective techniques are patients who have a very lax musculofascial layer, a lightly weighted ptotic soft tissue mass, and extensive shallow skin folding in the nasolabial, cheek, oromandibular, and neck regions.

4) Patients must have a very lax musculofascial layer; otherwise, the deep subcutaneous tissues will simply bunch up and not be optimally reshaped.

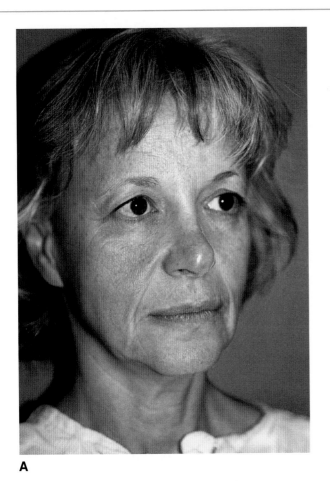

A

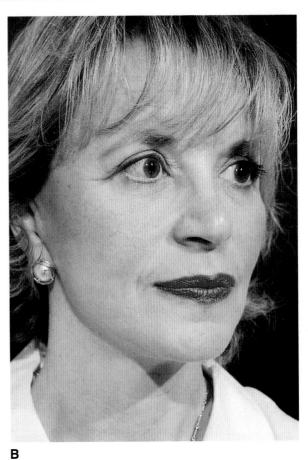

B

Figure 5-19 *Resective Techniques: Lateral SMAS/Platysma-ectomy.* **A,** *This thin-framed 55-year-old woman was an excellent candidate for this technique because of her well-developed anterior musculofascial layer, with considerable laxity, minimally weighted anterior ptotic soft tissue mass, and extensive shallow nasolabial, oromandibular, and neck skin folding.* **B,** *Her postoperative appearance.*

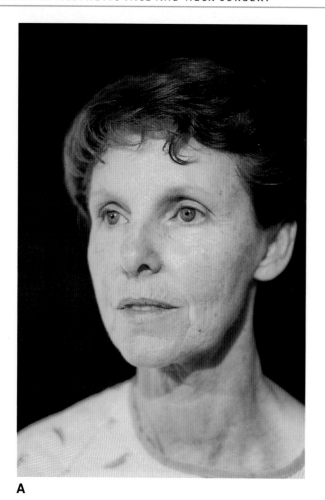

A

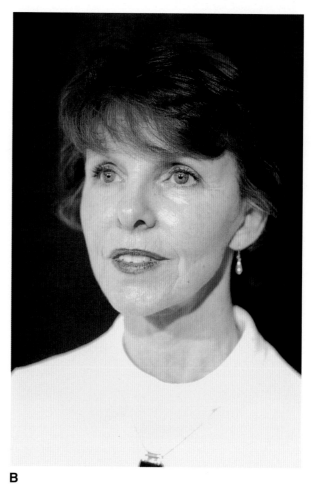

B

Figure 5-20 *Resective Techniques: Lateral SMAS/Platysma-ectomy.* **A,** *This 57-year-old woman was an excellent candidate for the resective technique because of her lightly weighted ptotic anterior soft tissue mass; her extensive shallow skin folding in the nasolabial, cheek, perioral, and oromandibular regions; and her considerable skin and musculofascial laxity. She also underwent simultaneous perioral laser resurfacing.* **B,** *Her postoperative appearance.*

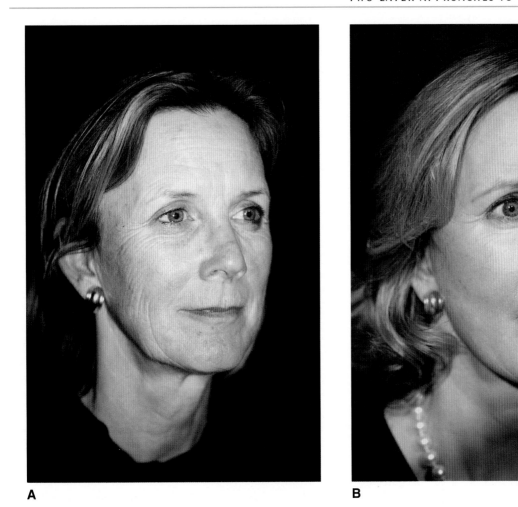

A   **B**

Figure 5-21   *Resective Techniques: Lateral SMAS/Platysma-ectomy.* **A,** *This thin 56-year-old athletic woman with considerable solar elastosis exhibited very extensive shallow cheek skin folding, a thick lax anterior musculofascial layer, and a very light minimally ptotic soft tissue mass. She was an excellent candidate for a resective technique. She also underwent simultaneous forehead and perioral laser resurfacing.* **B,** *Her postoperative appearance.*

Technique

After the skin flaps have been raised and hemostasis has been obtained, the surgical plan for the lateral SMAS/platysma resection is delineated on the deep layer (Fig. 5-22). The area for the resection should stay within the borders of the parotid gland such that injury to the facial nerve is avoided at all cost. The upper portion of the resection begins at least 1 cm below the zygomatic arch, thereby avoiding injury to the frontal branch of the facial nerve. The frontal branch of the facial nerve penetrates the superficial fascia immediately below the midportion of the zygomatic arch at a steep angle and obliquely courses over the arch within the temporoparietal fascia toward the forehead musculature. The lower portion of the resection is angled slightly into the retrolobular sulcus and follows the posterior border of the platysma muscle and the platysma-auricular ligament. This path avoids injury to the marginal mandibular nerve, which always lies deep to the tail of the parotid gland and always courses below the angle of the jaw in the subplatysma plane. The central and widest portion of the resection should stay within the borders of the parotid gland and not wander beyond the anterior border of the gland. The zygomatic and buccal branches of the facial nerve become more superficial anterior to the parotid gland and are vulnerable to injury if a blind resective technique is carried out without careful dissection of the parotido-masseteric fascia in this region. The optimal axis for the deep subcutaneous tissue resection is aligned on a more vertical plane than the axis of the nasolabial fold. The configuration for the resection is best when it follows an upwardly tilted half-moon shape, with the curved side facing the anterior border of the parotid gland. The tilted half-moon shape for resection allows for a steeper, more vertical repositioning of the more lax upper SMAS tissue

and a more oblique repositioning of the less lax platysma muscle. If the axis of the resective plane is made parallel to or less steep than the axis of the nasolabial fold, nasolabial fold correction is optimized at the cost of creating a lateral sweep to the lower face. Lateral sweep is a postsurgical sequela created by overtightening the subcutaneous layers of the lower face in relation to the midface. Lateral sweep is easy to recognize as a drapery-like sweep of bunched-up midfacial soft tissue and skin that mars an otherwise pleasing postoperative result.

Deep subcutaneous resection of SMAS is easy to perform over the body of the parotid gland while the SMAS is elevated with a single-tooth Adson forceps; the excess SMAS is resected with a Gorney scissors (Fig. 5-23). Resection of the SMAS proceeds down to the external capsule of the parotid gland, which often is difficult to distinguish from the gland itself. Resection of the lateral platysma is much more difficult and is greatly aided by tenting the platysma-auricular ligament with a single-tooth Adson forceps, while a curved Gorney scissors resects progressive deeper and deeper slices of fascia and platysma until the subplatysma space becomes evident. If difficulty is encountered with the resection, the ligament and the lateral platysma muscle can be developed as a small lateral platysma/superficial fascial/subcutaneous fat flap and then the excess resected. During development of the flap, the Gorney scissors should hug the inferior surface of the platysma muscle in order to avoid injury to the marginal mandibular nerve. The marginal mandibular nerve exits the tail of the parotid gland and always courses below the angle of the jaw in the subplatysma plane, but its exit from the parotid gland can vary depending on the patient's parotid gland morphology. Subplatysma and sub-SMAS hemostasis should carefully be performed at this juncture.

Figure 5-22 The area for the resection should stay within the borders of the parotid gland such that injury to the facial nerve is avoided at all cost. The upper portion of the resection begins at least 1 cm below the zygomatic arch, thereby avoiding injury to the frontal branch of the facial nerve. The lower portion of the resection is angled slightly into the retrolobular sulcus and follows the posterior border of the platysma muscle. The central and widest portion of the resection should stay within the borders of the parotid gland. The optimal axis for the deep subcutaneous tissue resection is aligned on a more vertical plane than the axis of the nasolabial fold. The configuration for the resection is best when it follows an upwardly tilted half-moon shape, with the curved side facing the anterior border of the parotid gland. The tilted half-moon shape for resection allows for a steeper, more vertical repositioning of the more lax upper SMAS tissue and a more oblique repositioning of the less lax platysma muscle.

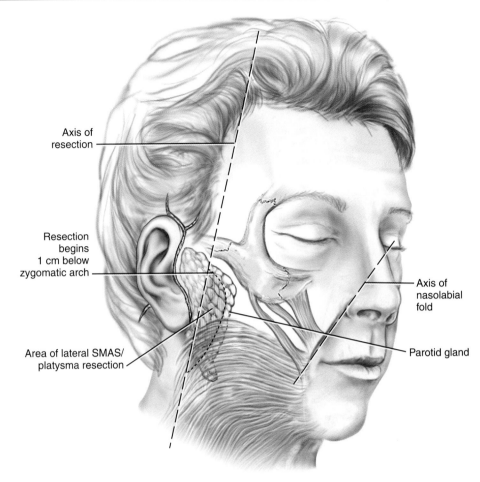

Figure 5-23 Deep subcutaneous resection of SMAS is easy to perform over the body of the parotid gland while the SMAS is elevated with single-tooth Adson forceps; the excess SMAS is resected with a Gorney scissors. Resection of the SMAS proceeds down to the external capsule of the parotid gland. Resection of the lateral platysma is much more difficult and is greatly aided by tenting the platysma-auricular ligament with a single-tooth Adson forceps while a curved Gorney scissors resects progressively deeper and deeper slices of fascia and platysma until the subplatysma space becomes evident.

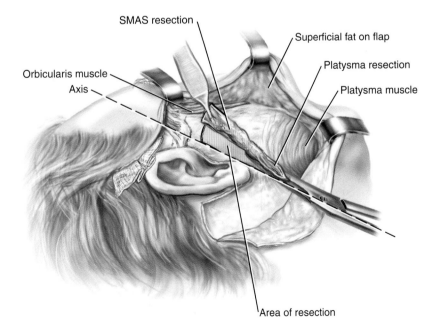

In general, the vectors for transposition of tissues are more vertical in the upper midfacial SMAS region of the resection and more oblique in the lower facial and neck platysma region of the resection (Fig. 5-24). Great care must be exercised in controlling the depth of these sutures along the anterior suture line, where the zygomatic and buccal facial nerve branches can become more superficial and more vulnerable to a tension or traction injury. Several buried mattress stitches of 3-0 Mersilene suture are placed for SMAS flap fixation to the residual superficial fascia and to the superficial temporal fascia laterally. After SMAS fixation has been completed, several buried mattress stitches of 3-0 Mersilene are placed for platysma flap fixation to the residual superficial fascia and to the mastoid fascia and for several centimeters inferiorly to the deep cervical investing fascia (Fig. 5-25). If any contour irregularities exist at this point, they should be resected and smoothed with a buried stitch of 4-0 Mersilene suture.

CLINICAL PEARLS

- The upper portion of the resection begins at least 1 cm below the zygomatic arch, thereby avoiding injury to the frontal branch of the facial nerve.
- The area for the resection stays within the border of the parotid gland; the incision is best configured as an upwardly tilted half-moon, with the curved side facing the anterior border of the parotid gland. This allows for vertical repositioning of the more lax upper SMAS tissue and oblique repositioning of the less lax platysma muscle.
- Resection of the excess SMAS and platysma muscle should be very carefully performed and is aided by tenting the tissues with a single-tooth Adson forceps and slowly resecting progressively deeper and deeper slices of excessive fascia and platysma until the sub-SMAS/platysma space becomes evident.
- The optimal axis for the resection is a more vertical plane than the axis of the nasolabial fold; if the axis of the resective plane is made parallel to or less steep than the axis of the nasolabial fold, nasolabial fold correction is optimized at the cost of creating a lateral sweep to the lower face.
- Great care must be exercised in controlling the depth of the fixation sutures along the anterior suture line, because the zygomatic and buccal facial nerve branches become more superficial and more vulnerable to a tension or traction injury in that location.

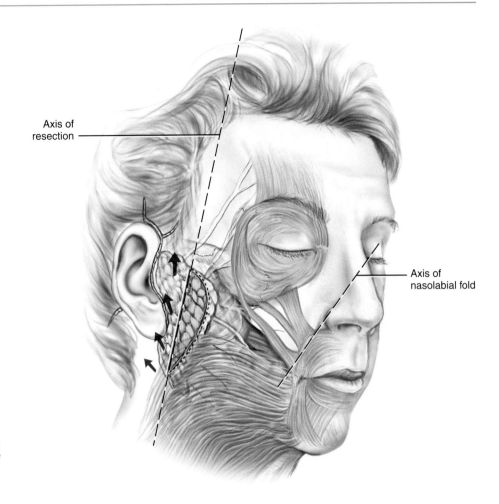

Axis of resection

Axis of nasolabial fold

Figure 5-24 *The vectors for transposition of tissues are more vertical in the upper midfacial SMAS region of the resection and more oblique in the lower facial and neck platysma region of the resection. Great care must be exercised in controlling the depth of these sutures along the anterior suture line, where the zygomatic and buccal facial nerve branches can become more superficial and more vulnerable to a tension or traction injury.*

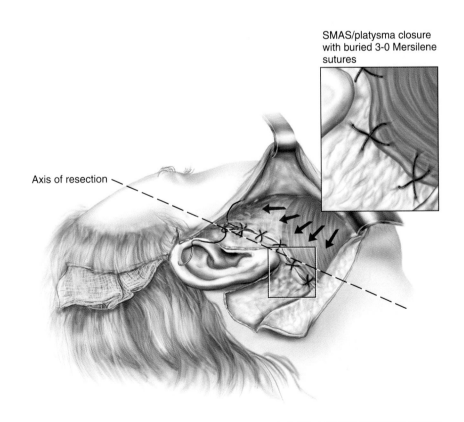

SMAS/platysma closure with buried 3-0 Mersilene sutures

Axis of resection

Figure 5-25 *Several buried mattress stitches of 3-0 Mersilene suture are placed for SMAS flap fixation to the residual superficial fascia and to the superficial temporal fascia laterally and for platysma flap fixation to the residual superficial fascia and to the mastoid fascia.*

Extended Lateral SMAS/Platysma Advancement Flap Technique

This technique involves extending the anterior musculofascial dissection of the limited SMAS/platysma advancement flap technique well beyond the anterior border of the parotid and over the zygomaticus major muscle body (Fig. 5-26). Rather than rely on multiple, anterior plication and imbrication sutures to "lift" ptotic anterior deep soft tissue, the extended technique develops an extensive and versatile lateral and anterior deep subcutaneous tissue flap independent of the skin flap. Because the patient's anterior ptotic soft tissue mass remains adherent to the deep plane flap, *heavy ptotic soft tissue mass in the anterior midface and neck is optimally corrected by this technique.* The extended SMAS/platysma technique reshapes the deep subcutaneous tissues by layering widely *undermined* musculofascial layers. In patients with extensive submalar hollows and those with relative malar deficiency, augmentation can be effected with the excess lateral musculofascial tissue normally discarded by this technique. The

shortcoming of this technique, however, is that, by layering extensively undermined tissues, the musculofascial layer loses much of the viscoelastic property it possesses in situ, and tightening of the musculofascial layer becomes compromised. Hence, extreme laxity of the musculofascial layer is not optimally corrected by this technique.

This technique also has other limitations: (1) it is inherently tedious and time-consuming, with a steep learning curve; (2) the patient needs to have a well-developed anterior musculofascial layer to which the ptotic soft tissue mass is densely adherent; otherwise, the flap will literally fall apart in the surgeon's hands when tension is applied laterally; (3) results are dependent on how far anterior the dissection is performed; and (4) because the musculofascial flap is used primarily for repositioning of ptotic anterior soft tissue mass, and not to tighten the superficial subcutaneous tissues, skin fold correction is dependent on the skin-tightening portion of the procedure.

EXTENDED SMAS/PLATYSMA

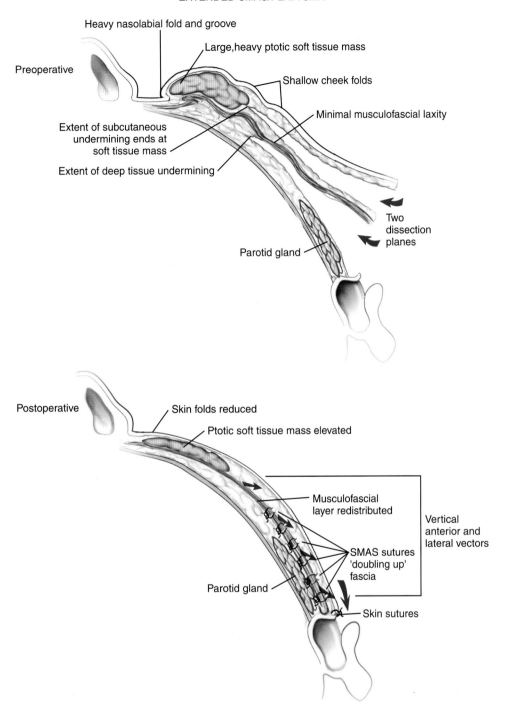

Figure 5-26 *Extended Lateral SMAS/Platysma Advancement Flap. This is the best technique for patients with heavy ptotic anterior soft tissue mass without a significant degree of musculofascial laxity. If the musculofascial layer is of good quality, then heavy skin folds and deep grooves in the nasolabial, oromandibular, and neck regions can be greatly reduced by this technique.*

Hence, the best candidates for the extended SMAS/platysma technique have a heavy ptotic anterior soft tissue mass without a significant degree of musculofascial laxity (Figs. 5-27 and 5-28). If the musculofascial layer is of good quality, then heavy skin folds and deep grooves in the nasolabial, oromandibular, and neck regions can be reduced by this technique (Fig. 5-29). If the anterior musculofascial layer is thin and discontinuous, then skin fold correction is solely dependent on the skin-tightening portion of the procedure (Fig. 5-30).

KEY POINTS

1) The extended SMAS/platysma technique incorporates an extensively undermined and versatile lateral and anterior deep subcutaneous tissue flap that is independent of the skin flap yet remains adherent to the patient's ptotic soft tissue mass.

2) Heavy ptotic soft tissue mass in the anterior midface and neck is optimally corrected by this technique.

3) The shortcoming of the extended SMAS/platysma technique is that, by layering extensively undermined tissues, the musculofascial layer loses much of the viscoelastic property it possesses in situ, and tightening of the musculofascial layer becomes compromised. Hence, extreme laxity of the musculofascial layer is not optimally corrected by this technique.

4) Continuity must be maintained between the malar SMAS and the cheek SMAS such that the extended SMAS flap can be transposed under tension and without tears.

5) The best candidates for the extended SMAS/platysma technique have a heavy ptotic anterior soft tissue mass without a significant degree of musculofascial laxity and without heavy skin folds and deep grooves in the nasolabial, oromandibular, and neck region.

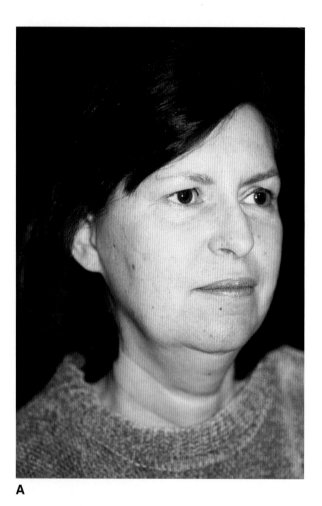

A

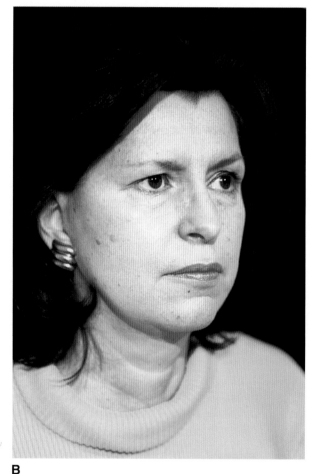

B

Figure 5-27 *Extended Lateral SMAS/Platysma Advancement Flap.* **A,** *This 56-year-old woman suffered from a heavy ptotic anterior soft tissue mass. She had surprisingly little musculofascial laxity; with significant laxity, her anterior soft tissue mass would have hung considerably and her skin folds would have etched deep grooves. This patient is an excellent candidate for extended musculofascial techniques. She also underwent extensive subplatysma defatting and a full anterior "corset" platysmaplasty.* **B,** *Her postoperative appearance.*

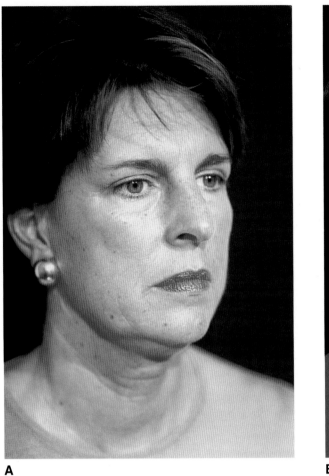
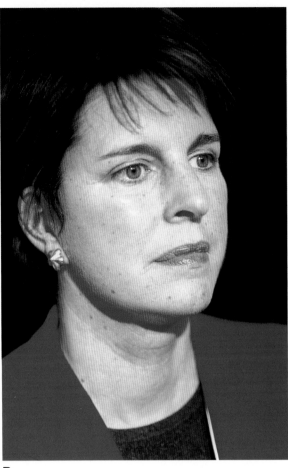

A

B

Figure 5-28 *Extended Lateral SMAS/Platysma Advancement Flap.* **A,** *This 54-year-old woman suffered from a moderately heavy ptotic anterior soft tissue mass and a mild degree of midfacial musculofascial laxity, which caused some shallow skin folding in the nasolabial, perioral, cheek, and oromandibular regions. A limited anterior "corset" platysmaplasty, submental subplatysma fat excision, and upper blepharoplasty was also performed.* **B,** *Her postoperative appearance.*

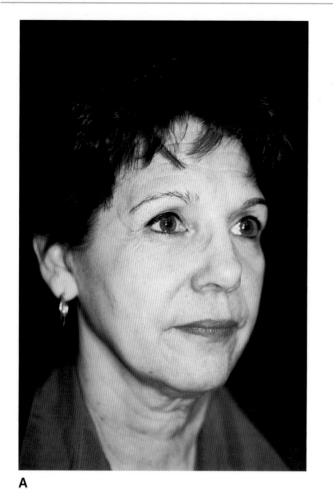

A

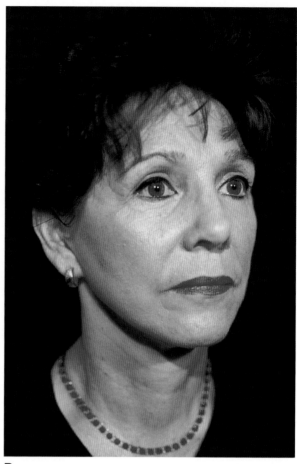

B

Figure 5-29 Extended Lateral SMAS/Platysma Advancement Flap. **A,** This 54-year-old woman suffered from a moderately heavy ptotic anterior soft tissue mass with a mild degree of musculofascial laxity, which caused thick nasolabial, oromandibular, and neck skin folding. She also underwent limited anterior platysmaplasty, endoscopic brow lift, lower blepharoplasty, and simultaneous laser resurfacing in the forehead, lower eyelid, and perioral regions. **B,** Her postoperative appearance.

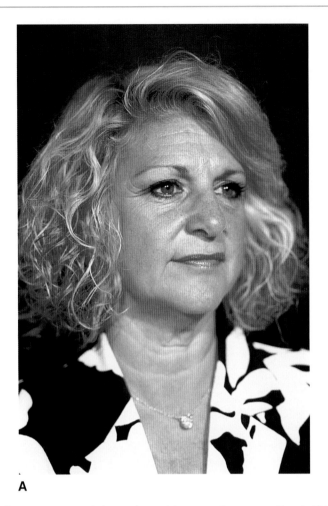

A

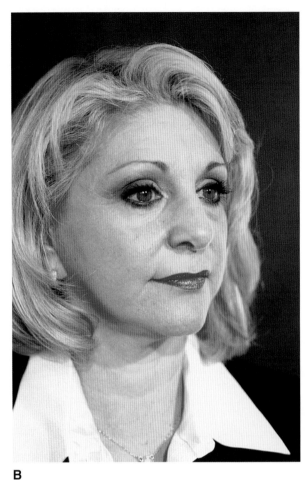

B

Figure 5-30 *Extended Lateral SMAS/Platysma Advancement Flap.* **A,** *This 56-year-old woman suffered from a heavy ptotic anterior soft tissue mass and considerable musculofascial laxity, which etched deep nasolabial, oromandibular, and neck skin folds and grooves into her face. She also underwent a full anterior "corset" platysmaplasty, an endoscopic brow lift, upper and lower blepharoplasty, and extensive simultaneous forehead and perioral laser resurfacing.* **B,** *Her postoperative appearance.*

Technique

After the skin flaps have been raised and hemostasis has been obtained, the surgical plan for the extended SMAS/platysma advancement flap is delineated (Fig. 5-31). The incision is similar to yet far larger than the one used for the limited lateral SMAS/platysma advancement flap. In general, the incision follows a lazy upside-down extended "L" pattern. The transverse portion of the incision is always begun 1 cm below the zygomatic arch in order to avoid injury to the frontal branch of the facial nerve. The frontal branch of the facial nerve penetrates the superficial fascia immediately below the midportion of the zygomatic arch at a steep angle and obliquely courses over the arch within the temporoparietal fascia toward the forehead musculature. The transverse incision follows the lower border of the zygomatic arch until it reaches the zygomatic body, where the incision is carried over the malar eminence and then downward for a variable distance towards the nasolabial fold. The vertical portion of the incision gently parallels and is within 1 cm of the skin incision. The incision line then dips posteriorly into the retrolobular sulcus around the earlobe and follows lateral border of the platysma muscle for approximately 5 to 6 cm below the mandibular border.

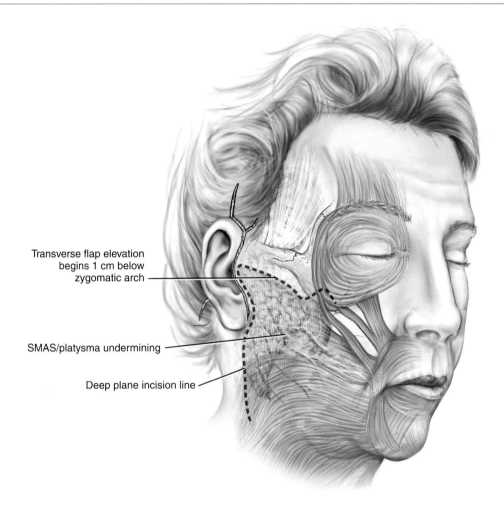

Transverse flap elevation
begins 1 cm below
zygomatic arch

SMAS/platysma undermining

Deep plane incision line

Figure 5-31 *Planned Incisions for Extended Lateral SMAS/Platysma-ectomy. The incisions follow a similar yet far larger pattern than the one used for the limited lateral SMAS/platysma advancement flap. The transverse portion of the incision is always begun 1 cm below the zygomatic arch in order to avoid injury to the frontal branch of the facial nerve. The transverse incision follows the lower border of the zygomatic arch until it reaches the zygomatic body, where the incision is carried over the malar eminence and then downward for a variable distance toward the nasolabial fold. The vertical portion of the incision gently parallels and is within 1 cm of the skin incision. The incision line then dips posteriorly into the retrolobular sulcus around the earlobe and follows the lateral border of the platysma muscle for approximately 5 to 6 cm below the mandibular border.*

It is easiest to begin the extended SMAS/platysma procedure with the subplatysma dissection (Fig. 5-32). A single-tooth Adson forceps grasps the platysma auricular ligament, which literally is a several-centimeter-square area of lateral platysma adherence to the underlying deep fascia. Using sharp dissection with a curved Gorney scissors, the ligament and the lateral platysma muscle are elevated. This maneuver creates a platysma/superficial fascial/subcutaneous fat flap over the neck and lower face. The Gorney scissors should hug the inferior surface of the platysma muscle in order to avoid injury to the marginal mandibular nerve. The marginal mandibular nerve exits the tail of the parotid gland and always courses below the angle of the jaw in the subplatysma plane, but its exit from the parotid gland can vary depending on the patient's parotid gland morphology. Once the platysma-auricular ligament is released, the platysma muscle flap is undermined for approximately 5 to 6 cm inferior to the mandibular body and for approximately 3 to 4 cm anterior to the tail of the parotid gland. Subplatysma hemostasis should carefully be performed at this juncture.

The extended SMAS flap is begun by sharp scalpel dissection down to the capsule of the parotid (Fig. 5-33). The meso-temporalis is developed over the zygomatic arch, which safely protects the frontal branch of the facial nerve within its borders. Sub-SMAS dissection is easiest over the body of the parotid but eventually encounters the fibers of the orbicularis and the zygomaticus major. These muscles are important landmarks in the anterior dissection, because the flap is developed along the superficial surfaces of these muscles. The zygomatic facial nerve branches lie deep to the bellies of these muscles.

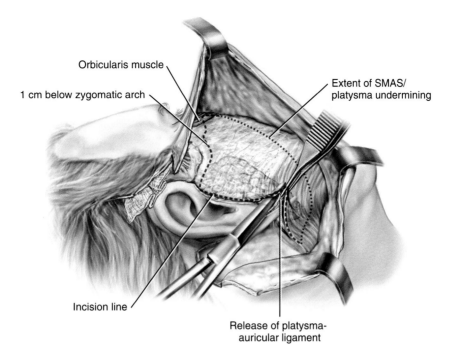

Figure 5-32 *It is easiest to begin the extended SMAS/platysma procedure by beginning with the subplatysma dissection. A single-tooth Adson forceps grasps the platysma-auricular ligament, which literally is a several-square-centimeter area of lateral platysma adherence to the underlying deep fascia. Using sharp dissection with a curved Gorney scissors, the ligament and the lateral platysma muscle are elevated. Once the platysma-auricular ligament is released, the platysma muscle flap is undermined for approximately 5 to 6 cm inferior to the mandibular body and for approximately 3 to 4 cm anterior to the tail of the parotid gland.*

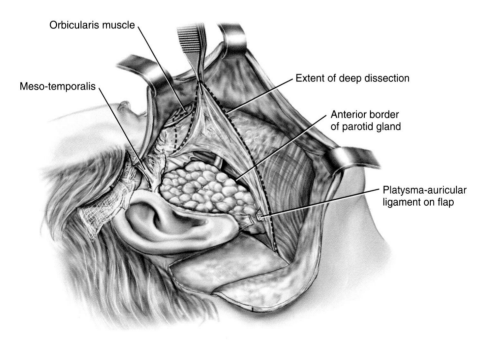

Figure 5-33 *The extended SMAS flap is begun by sharp scalpel dissection down to the capsule of the parotid. The meso-temporalis is developed over the zygomatic arch, which safely protects the frontal branch of the facial nerve within its borders. Sub-SMAS dissection is easiest over the body of the parotid, sub-SMAS dissection eventually encounters the fibers of the orbicularis and the zygomaticus major. These muscles are important landmarks in the anterior dissection because the flap is developed along the superficial surfaces of these muscles. The zygomatic facial nerve branches lie deep to the bellies of these muscles.*

Once the zygomatic body is encountered, the transverse dissection is carried up and over the malar eminence, with care taken to stay superficial to the orbicularis muscle, and then obliquely downward toward the cheek until the zygomaticus minor is encountered (Fig. 5-34). It is extremely important to maintain continuity between the malar SMAS and the cheek SMAS, such that flap transposition can be accomplished under tension and without a tear in the flap. To achieve this, the malar SMAS should be freed from the malar eminence, and inferiorly, several of the spiky masseteric-cutaneous ligaments should be divided with a combination of sharp and blunt dissection. This midfacial dissection exposes the parotidomasseteric fascia and the buccal fat pad. The facial nerve branches deep to the parotid masseteric fascia are visible at this point. Dissection medial to the zygomaticus minor is unnecessary and inherently problematic. The facial nerve becomes more superficial and more vulnerable to injury as it passes over the body of the masseter, and the cheek SMAS begins to thin as fat becomes an ever increasing component of the anterior ptotic soft tissue mass. Hence, for both safety and biomechanical concerns, no further anterior dissection is performed.

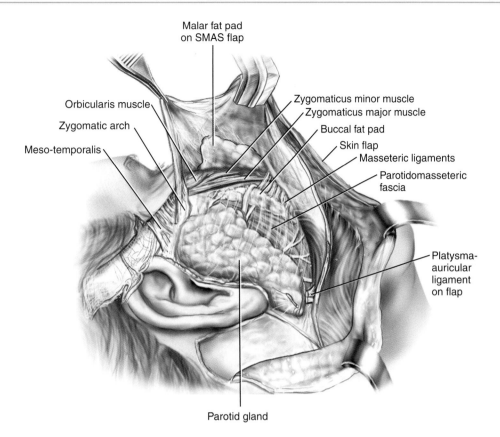

Malar fat pad
on SMAS flap

Orbicularis muscle

Zygomatic arch

Meso-temporalis

Zygomaticus minor muscle
Zygomaticus major muscle

Buccal fat pad

Skin flap

Masseteric ligaments

Parotidomasseteric
fascia

Platysma-
auricular
ligament
on flap

Parotid gland

Figure 5-34   *Once the zygomatic body is encountered, the transverse dissection is carried up and over the malar eminence and then obliquely downward toward the cheek until the zygomaticus minor is encountered. It is extremely important to maintain continuity between the malar SMAS and the cheek SMAS, such that flap transposition can be accomplished under tension and without a tear in the flap. Several of the spiky masseteric-cutaneous ligaments should be divided with a combination of sharp and blunt dissection. This midfacial dissection exposes the parotidomasseteric fascia and the buccal fat pad. The facial nerve branches deep to the parotid masseteric fascia are visible at this point. Dissection medial to the zygomaticus minor is unnecessary and inherently problematic.*

Lahey clamps are placed on the platysma-auricular ligament and the corner of the SMAS flap, and the best vector for midfacial flap transposition is determined (Fig. 5-35). In general, the optimal vector for the midfacial SMAS flap transposition is vertical in the midface. The SMAS/platysma/superficial fat flap is "V" cut with a Gorney scissors, and the vectors for both the SMAS and the platysma flap are determined. The optimal vector for the neck platysma flap is oblique. Several buried mattress stitches of 3-0 Mersilene suture are placed for SMAS flap fixation to the residual superficial fascia along the zygomatic arch and to the superficial temporal fascia

laterally after the excess is resected (Fig. 5-36). The lateral excess SMAS/superficial fat can be doubled over in order to create better fixation and a thicker flap for suturing, or, if the patient has extensive submalar hollows and relative malar deficiency, can be layered to increase midfacial volume After the SMAS flap has been fix in place, several mattress stitches of 3-0 Mersilene are placed for platysma flap fixation to the mastoid fascia and for several centimeters inferiorly to the deep cervical investing fascia. If any contour irregularities exist at this point, they should be resected and smoothed with a buried stitch of 4-0 Mersilene suture.

CLINICAL PEARLS

- It is easiest to begin the extended SMAS/platysma procedure with the subplatysma dissection.
- The orbicularis oculi and the zygomaticus major are the landmarks for the malar and cheek SMAS dissection, and the musculofascial flap is developed along their superficial surfaces.
- The malar SMAS should be freed entirely from the malar eminence after dividing several of the masseteric-cutaneous ligaments with a combination of sharp and blunt dissection.
- Undermining medial to the zygomaticus minor is unnecessary and inherently problematic because the facial nerve branches

become more superficial and vulnerable and because the anterior cheek SMAS begins to thin as fat becomes an ever-increasing component of the anterior ptotic soft tissue mass.
- The optimal vector for the midfacial SMAS flap transposition is vertical in the midface and for the platysma flap is bidi-rectionally oblique in the neck.
- The lateral excess SMAS/superficial fat can be doubled over in order to create better fixation and a thicker flap for suturing, or, if the patient has extensive submalar hollows and relative malar deficiency, can be layered to increase midfacial volume.

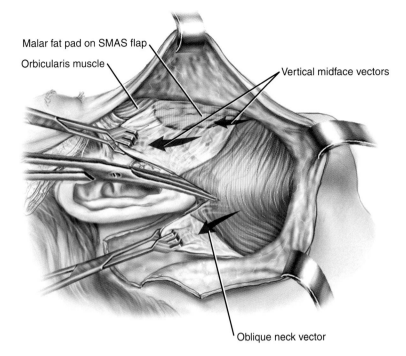

Malar fat pad on SMAS flap

Orbicularis muscle

Vertical midface vectors

Oblique neck vector

Figure 5-35 *Lahey clamps are placed on the platysma-auricular ligament and the corner of the SMAS flap, and the best vector for midfacial flap transposition is determined. In general, the optimal vector for the midfacial SMAS flap transposition is vertical in the midface. The SMAS/platysma/superficial fat flap is "V" cut with a Gorney scissors, and the vectors for both the SMAS and the platysma flap are determined. The optimal vector for the neck platysma flap is oblique.*

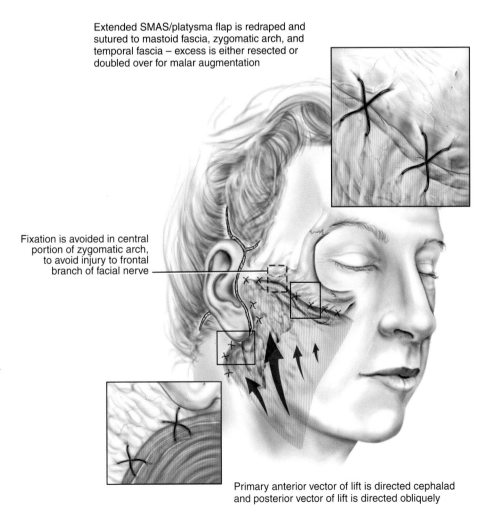

Extended SMAS/platysma flap is redraped and sutured to mastoid fascia, zygomatic arch, and temporal fascia – excess is either resected or doubled over for malar augmentation

Fixation is avoided in central portion of zygomatic arch, to avoid injury to frontal branch of facial nerve

Primary anterior vector of lift is directed cephalad and posterior vector of lift is directed obliquely

Figure 5-36 *Several buried mattress stitches of 3-0 Mersilene suture are placed for SMAS flap fixation to the residual superficial fascia along the zygomatic arch and to the superficial temporal fascia laterally after the excess is either resected or doubled over to create a thicker flap for suturing. Alternatively, if the patient has extensive submalar hollows and relative malar deficiency, the doubled-over portion can be layered to augment midfacial volume. After fixation of the SMAS flap has been accomplished, several mattress stitches of 3-0 Mersilene are placed for platysma flap fixation to the mastoid fascia and for several centimeters inferiorly to the deep cervical investing fascia.*

Combination Techniques

I have developed a technique that combines resection of SMAS/platysma lateral to the anterior border of the parotid gland with an extended sub-SMAS/platysma dissection medial to the anterior border of the parotid gland. It is occasionally complemented by several strategically placed anterior plication/imbrication sutures, when needed.

The procedure is begun with resection of the lateral SMAS/platysma within the border of the parotid gland, with the incision configured as an upwardly tilted half-moon, with the curved side facing the anterior border of the parotid gland. An extended sub-SMAS/platysma dissection is performed anteriorly well over the zygomaticus major muscle body. Hence, a versatile *independent* anterior deep subcutaneous tissue flap encompassing the patient's ptotic soft tissue mass is also included in order to correct the ptotic soft tissue mass. By combining the lateral resection with extensive anterior undermining, this technique takes the viscoelastic tension and subsequent stretch/relaxation response and, rather than "wasting" it laterally, applies it along the medial border of the parotid gland where musculofascial laxity is the greatest and where the patient's ptotic soft tissue mass is situated. Hence, a combination of considerable musculofascial laxity and heavy ptotic anterior soft tissue mass can be optimally corrected by this technique.

One of the shortcomings of this technique is that redundant lateral musculofascial tissue is resected, and not layered as in the extended flap technique. Hence, this technique is not advised for patients who require augmentation of the submalar or malar region in tandem with reshaping.

Hence, combination techniques are best for patients with considerable musculofascial laxity (Figs. 5-37 and 5-38), those with heavy ptotic soft tissue mass in the anterior midface and neck (Fig. 5-39), and those with extensive shallow anterior skin folding (Fig. 5-40). As with the extended SMAS technique, if the anterior musculofascial layer is thin and discontinuous, then skin fold correction will be solely dependent on the skin-tightening portion of the procedure.

KEY POINTS

1) Combination techniques combine resection of SMAS/platysma lateral to the anterior border of the parotid gland with an extended sub-SMAS/platysma dissection medial to the anterior border of the parotid gland and add several strategically placed plication/imbrication sutures when necessary.

2) By combining the lateral resection with extensive anterior undermining, this technique takes the viscoelastic tension and subsequent stretch/relaxation response and, rather than "wasting" it laterally, applies it along the medial border of the parotid gland where musculofascial laxity is the greatest and where the patient's ptotic soft tissue mass is situated.

3) Considerable musculofascial laxity as well as heavy ptotic soft tissue mass in the face can be corrected by this technique.

4) This technique is not advised for patients who require augmentation of the submalar or malar region in tandem with reshaping.

5) Continuity must be maintained between the malar SMAS and the cheek SMAS such that the extended SMAS flap can be transposed under tension and without tears.

6) Combination techniques are best for patients with considerable musculofascial laxity, with moderate to heavy ptotic soft tissue mass in the anterior midface and neck, and with extensive shallow anterior skin folding.

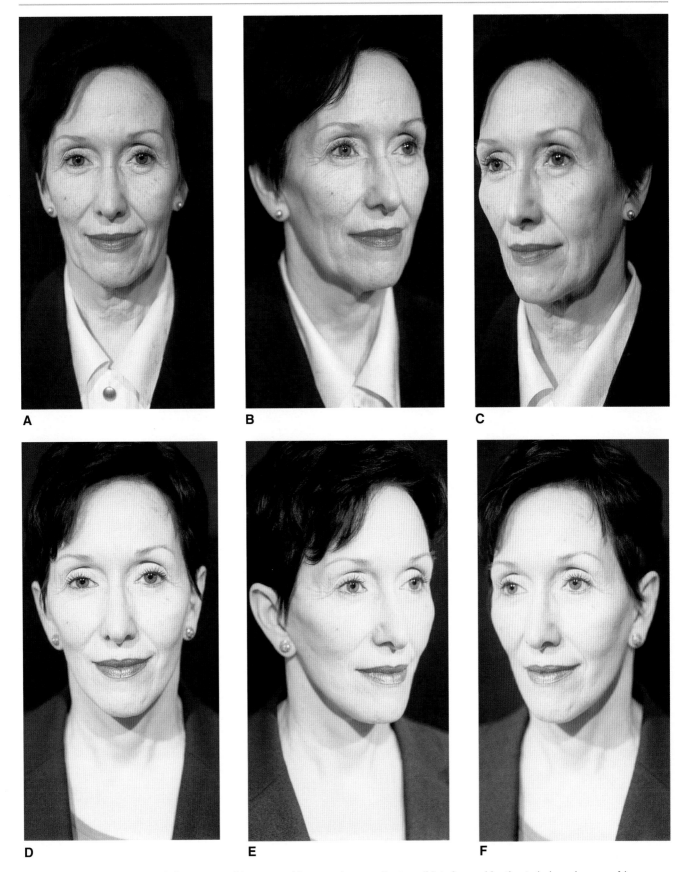

Figure 5-37 *Combination Techniques.* **A–C,** *This 58-year-old woman is an excellent candidate for combination techniques because of her considerable musculofascial laxity, her lightly weighted anterior soft tissue mass, and her shallow nasolabial, cheek, neck, and perioral skin folding. She also underwent a lower blepharoplasty.* **D–F,** *Her postoperative appearance.*

Technique

The combined technique does not require a separate illustration section because of the striking similarities it has with the other techniques that have been previously illustrated in great detail. Several clinical pearls, however, are pertinent.

CLINICAL PEARLS

- The combined technique is begun with some form of anterior platysmaplasty performed through a submental approach followed by raising the skin flaps through periauricular incisions, with care taken to ensure that subcutaneous tunneling is performed to join the lateral and anterior neck dissections.
- In contrast to pure resective techniques, the curved side of the upwardly tilted half-moon resection should face the ear, and the straight side shouldface the anterior border of the parotid gland.
- If difficulty is encountered with the resection, the platysma-auricular ligament and the lateral platysma muscle can be developed as a small flap.
- Undermining for the extended SMAS/platysma flap is begun along the anterior border of the parotid gland.
- The superficial surfaces of the orbicularis oculi and the zygomaticus major muscles are landmarks for the extended SMAS anterior dissection.
- The malar SMAS should be freed entirely from the malar eminence after division of several of the masseteric-cutaneous ligaments with a combination of sharp and blunt dissection.
- Undermining medial to the zygomaticus minor is unnecessary and inherently problematic because the facial nerve branches become more superficial and vulnerable and because the anterior cheek SMAS begins to thin as fat becomes an ever-increasing component of the anterior ptotic soft tissue mass.
- Insetting and fixation with this technique follow the following transposition sequence: vertical vector midfacial SMAS flap transposition, "V" cut, lateral vector preauricular SMAS transposition, bidirectional oblique platysma flap transposition, lateral vector inferior platysma flap transposition.
- When patients have severe musculofascial laxity, residual anterior bunching medial to the zygomaticus minor can encountered, and several anterior plication/imbrication sutures can be placed to inset this residual excess along a purely vertical vector.

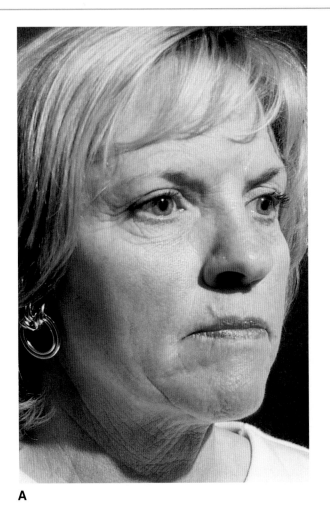

A

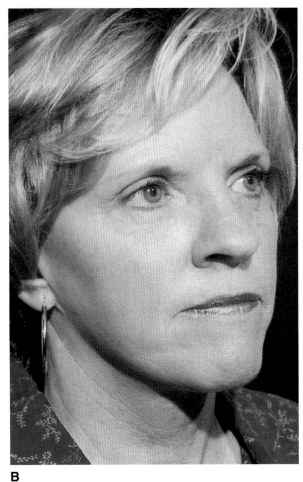

B

Figure 5-38 *Combination Techniques.* ***A,*** *This 58-year-old woman was also an excellent candidate for combination techniques because she had a considerably lax musculofascial layer, extensive shallow skin folding in the perioral, cheek, and neck regions, and a moderately heavy ptotic soft tissue mass. She also underwent anterior limited "corset" platysmaplasty, upper and lower blepharoplasty, and extensive simultaneous laser resurfacing.* ***B,*** *Her postoperative appearance.*

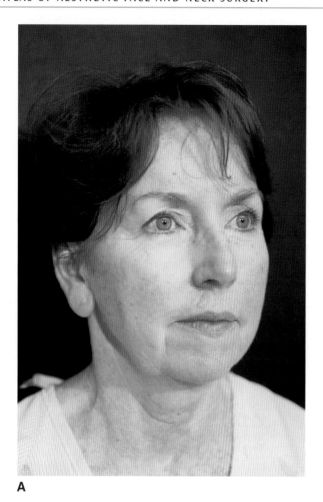

A

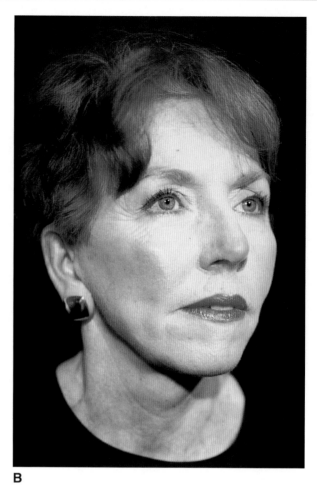

B

Figure 5-39 *Combination Techniques.* ***A,*** *This 50-year-old woman had a heavy ptotic midfacial and neck soft tissue mass, considerable lower facial and neck musculofascial laxity, and extensive shallow skin folding in the jowls, cheek, and neck regions. An anterior "corset" platysmaplasty was also performed, along with lower blepharoplasty.* ***B,*** *Her postoperative appearance.*

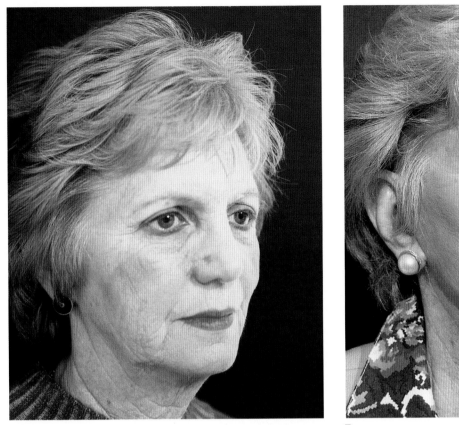
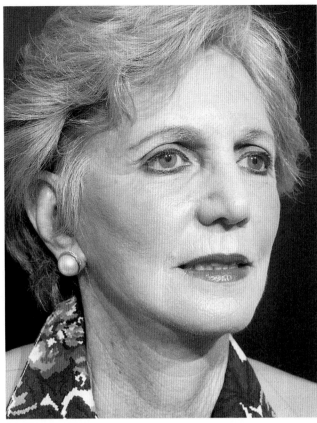

A

B

Figure 5-40   *Combination Techniques.* **A,** *This tall, thin 63-year-old woman was an excellent candidate for a combination technique because of her extensive shallow facial and neck skin folding, her considerably lax musculofascial layer, and her heavy ptotic soft tissue mass. She also underwent temporal lift, lower blepharoplasty, and simultaneous forehead and perioral laser resurfacing.* **B,** *Her postoperative appearance.*

Deep Plane Technique

The deep plane technique is unique (Fig. 5-41). Although the anterior musculofascial dissection is performed well beyond the anterior border of the parotid and over the zygomaticus major muscle body, much as in the extended SMAS/platysma flap technique, the deep plane technique combines a thick, widely undermined one-layer *midfacial* transposition flap with a bidirectionally oblique two-layer neck procedure. The patient's anterior ptotic soft tissue mass is left intimately connected to the midfacial skin flap. Unlike in most of the previously described techniques, anterior skin fold correction is not solely dependent on the skin-tightening portion of the procedure. The midfacial flap is repositioned obliquely upward along a vector perpendicular to the axis of the nasolabial fold. Because the midfacial flap is thick and hearty, it can be transposed and inset under extraordinary tension. This allows *optimal correction for patients with deep, heavy nasolabial, oro-mandibular, and cheek skin folds.*

The deep plane technique, however, also has its drawbacks: (1) like the extended flap technique, the deep plane technique is inherently tedious and time-consuming, with has a steep learning curve; (2) because the SMAS layer and the skin layer have different viscoelastic properties, each requiring different applied tensile forces in order to achieve an optimal stretch/relaxation response, the deep plane technique (which, by definition, does not separate the SMAS flap from the skin flap), provides only suboptimal improvement for patients with considerable midfacial musculofacial laxity; (3) because the patient's anterior ptotic soft tissue mass is not separately dissected and repositioned along a different vector from that for the skin flap, heavy ptotic soft tissue mass is suboptimally corrected by this technique; and (4) as with the extended flap technique, the surgical results are dependent on how far anterior the deep plane dissection is performed.

DEEP PLANE MIDFACE TECHNIQUE

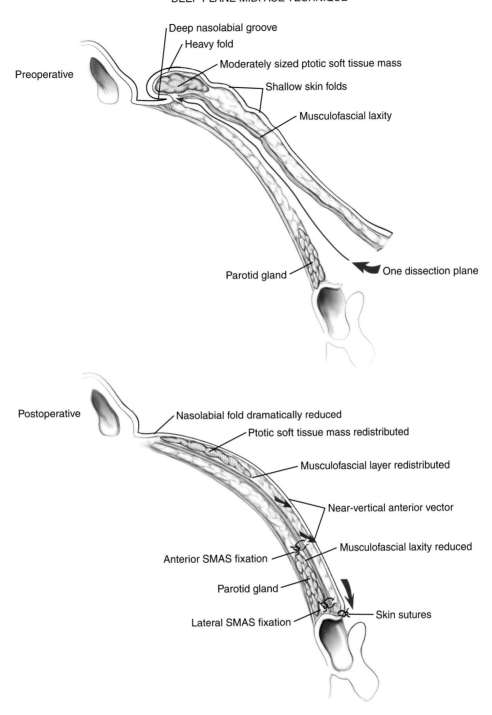

Figure 5-41 *Deep Plane. This is the best technique for patients whose primary complaints are heavy skin folds and deep grooves in the nasolabial, oromandibular, and neck regions. To take advantage of the techniques strengths, patients should have a lightly weighted ptotic anterior soft tissue mass and a nild degree of musculofascial laxity.*

Hence, the most optimal candidates for the deep plane technique are patients whose primary complaint is the presence of heavy skin folds and deep grooves in the nasolabial, oromandibular, cheek, and neck regions (Fig. 5-42), especially if the ptotic anterior soft tissue mass is lightly weighted and they do not exhibit a considerable degree of musculofascial laxity in their midface (Fig. 5-43). When patients do have considerable musculofascial laxity, the surgeon must make every effort to inset the facial flap along a purely vertical vector (Fig. 5-44).

KEY POINTS

1) The deep plane technique is unique in that a thick widely undermined one-layer *midfacial* transposition flap is combined with a bidirectionally oblique two-layer neck procedure, allowing the patient's anterior ptotic soft tissue mass to be left intimately connected to the midfacial skin flap.

2) Because the midfacial flap is thick and hearty, it can be transposed and inset under extraordinary tension.

3) The best patients for the deep plane technique are those whose primary complaints are those with heavy skin folds and deep grooves in the nasolabial, oromandibular, and cheek regions, especially if their ptotic anterior soft tissue mass is lightly weighted and they do not exhibit considerable musculofascial laxity.

4) When patients do have considerable musculofascial laxity, one must make every effort to inset the midfacial flap along a purely vertical vector.

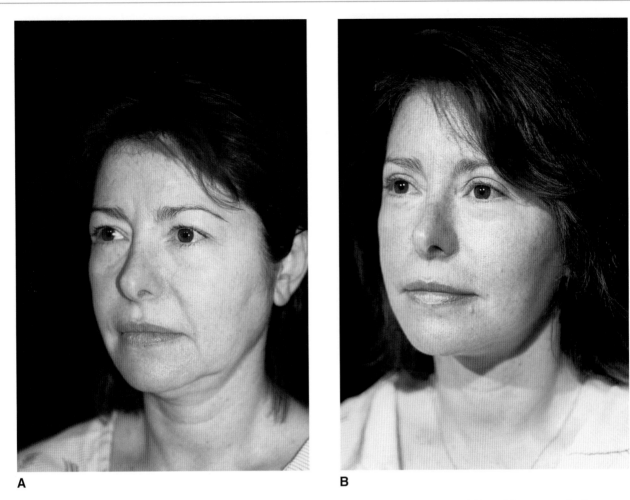

A

B

Figure 5-42 *Deep Plane Technique.* **A,** *This 53-year-old woman complained primarily about heavy folds and deep grooves in the nasolabial and oromandibular regions.* **B,** *The deep plane midfacial technique was instrumental in correcting this unsightly cosmetic problem for her. In addition, upper and lower blepharoplasty was performed.*

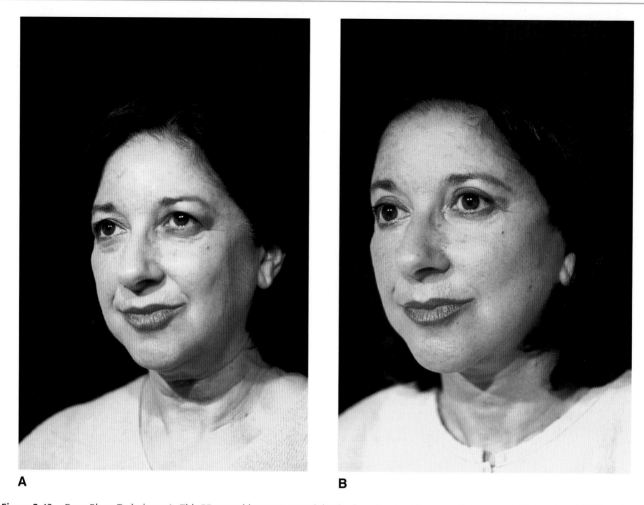

A   **B**

Figure 5-43   *Deep Plane Technique.* **A,** *This 55-year-old woman complained primarily about heavy and deep nasolabial and neck folds and grooves. She had a lightly weighted ptotic soft tissue mass and the musculofascial laxity in her midface was nominal. Upper and lower blepharoplasty and limited "corset" platysmaplasty complemented the deep plane midfacial lift.* **B,** *Her postoperative appearance.*

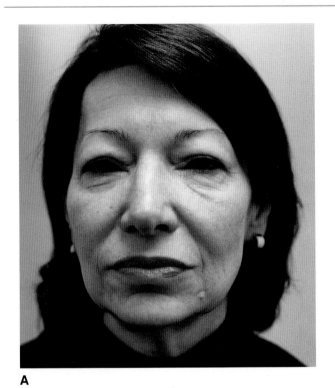

A

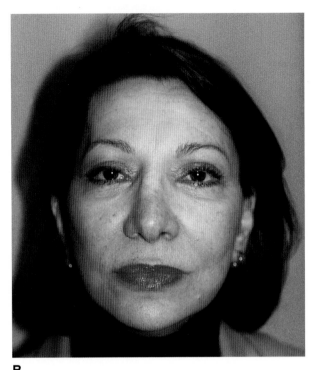

B

Figure 5-44 *Deep Plane Technique.* **A,** *This 50-year-old woman complained primarily of a deep nasolabial groove and heavy nasolabial fold. She had considerable musculofascial laxity, and her ptotic soft tissue mass was moderately weighted.* **B,** *The deep plane midfacial technique, performed along a vector more vertical than normal, greatly reduced her deep skin folding as well as her anterior musculofascial laxity. Upper and lower blepharoplasty with arcus marginalis release was performed as well.*

Technique

With the deep plane technique, the facial skin flap and the SMAS flap are one and the same. The midfacial dissection is performed through an extended transverse sideburn and pretrichal incision *after* an anterior "corset" platysmaplasty is completed through a submental approach and after the lower facial and neck skin flaps have been undermined through the preauricular and postauricular incisions, with care taken to create a subcutaneous tunnel between the lateral and anterior skin flaps. Lateral preparotid subcutaneous dissection is carried down to approximately 1 cm below the zygomatic arch, thereby avoiding injury to the frontal branch of the facial nerve (Fig. 5-45). The frontal branch of the facial nerve penetrates the superficial fascia immediately below the midportion of the zygomatic arch at a steep angle and obliquely courses over the arch within the temporoparietal fascia toward the forehead musculature. Preservation of the meso-temporalis is vital in order to prevent injury to the nerve. Once the meso-temporalis has been preserved 1 cm below the zygomatic arch, deep subcutaneous dissection can be carried down to the capsule of the parotid gland.

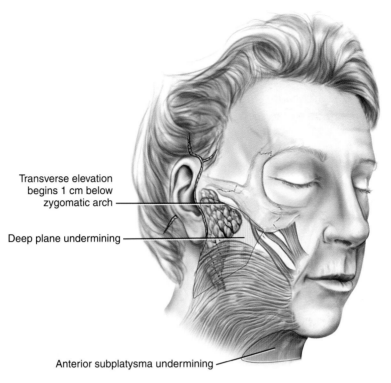

Transverse elevation
begins 1 cm below
zygomatic arch

Deep plane undermining

Anterior subplatysma undermining

Figure 5-45   *With the deep plane technique, midfacial dissection is performed through an extended transverse sideburn and pretrichal incision after an anterior "corset" platysmaplasty is completed through a submental approach and after the lower facial and neck skin flaps have been undermined through the preauricular and postauricular incisions. Lateral preparotid subcutaneous dissection is carried down to approximately 1 cm below the zygomatic arch to preserve the meso-temporalis and to prevent injury to the frontal branch of the facial nerve. The extent of deep plane undermining is similar to that achieved by the extended SMAS and combined techniques.*

The transverse portion of the dissection begins the procedure and follows nearly the same pattern as the extended SMAS technique (Fig. 5-46). Anterior sub-SMAS dissection eventually encounters the fibers of the orbicularis and the zygomaticus major. These muscles are the landmarks of the anterior dissection, since the flap is developed along the superficial surfaces of these muscles. The zygomatic facial nerve branches lie deep to the bellies of these muscles. Once the zygomatic body is encountered the transverse dissection is carried up and over the malar eminence, with care taken to stay superficial to the orbicularis muscle. At this point, usually further anterior cheek dissection is limited by tethering from below. A single-tooth Adson forceps grasps the platysma-auricular ligament, which literally is a several-centimeter-square area of lateral platysma adherence to the underlying deep fascia. Using sharp dissection with a curved Gorney scissors, the ligament and the lateral platysma muscle are elevated. The Gorney scissors should hug the inferior surface of the platysma muscle in order to avoid injury to the marginal mandibular nerve. The marginal mandibular nerve exits the tail of the parotid gland and always courses below the angle of the jaw in the sub-platysma plane, but its exit from the parotid gland can vary depending upon the patient's parotid gland morphology. Once the platysma-auricular ligament is released, the platysma muscle flap is easy to release for approximately 3 to 5 cm anteriorly and for 2 to 4 cm inferior to the border of the mandible and can easily be connected to the preparotid SMAS flap. The anterior dissection then is obliquely angled downward toward the cheek until the zygomaticus minor is encountered. The malar SMAS should be freed from the malar eminence, and inferiorly, several of the spiky masseteric-cutaneous ligaments should be divided with a combination of sharp and blunt dissection. This midfacial dissection exposes the parotidomasseteric fascia and the buccal fat pad. The facial nerve branches deep to the parotidomasseteric fascia are visible at this point. Dissection medial to the zygomaticus minor is unnecessary and inherently problematic. The facial nerve becomes more superficial and more vulnerable to injury as it passes over the body of the masseter, and the cheek SMAS begins to thin as fat becomes an ever-increasing component of the anterior ptotic soft tissue mass. Hence, for both safety and biomechanical concerns, no further anterior dissection is performed.

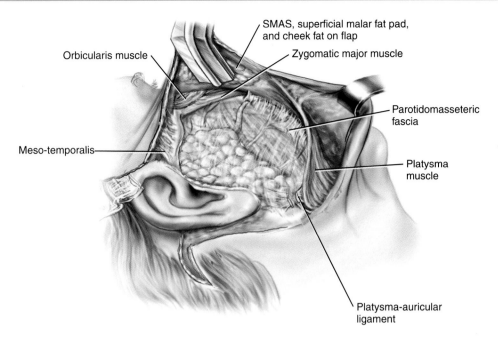

Orbicularis muscle

SMAS, superficial malar fat pad, and cheek fat on flap

Zygomatic major muscle

Parotidomasseteric fascia

Meso-temporalis

Platysma muscle

Platysma-auricular ligament

Figure 5-46 *The transverse portion of the dissection begins 1 cm below the arch and eventually encounters the fibers of the orbicularis and the zygomaticus major. These muscles are important landmarks in the anterior dissection. Once the zygomatic body is encountered, the transverse dissection is carried up and over the malar eminence, with care taken to stay superficial to the orbicularis muscle. Further anterior cheek dissection is limited by tethering from the platysma-auricular ligament. Using sharp dissection with a curved Gorney scissors, the ligament and the lateral platysma muscle are elevated. Once the platysma-auricular ligament is released, the platysma muscle flap is easy to release for approximately 3 to 5 cm anteriorly, for 2 to 4 cm inferior to the border of the mandible. The anterior dissection then is obliquely angled downward toward the cheek until the zygomaticus minor is encountered. Several of the spiky masseteric-cutaneous ligaments should be divided with a combination of sharp and blunt dissection. This midfacial dissection exposes the parotidomasseteric fascia and the buccal fat pad. The facial nerve branches deep to the parotidomasseteric fascia are visible at this point. Dissection medial to the zygomaticus minor is unnecessary and inherently problematic.*

Lahey clamps are placed on the platysma flap and the corner of the skin/SMAS flap (Fig. 5-47). The platysma flap is inset initially into the mastoid fascia along a bidirectional oblique vector at 180 degrees to the vector of the anterior "corset" platysmaplasty. Several mattress stitches of 3-0 Mersilene are placed for fixation of the lateral platysmaplasty flap to the mastoid fascia and for several centimeters inferiorly to the deep cervical investing fascia. This creates the buttresses to support the tension necessary for a suspension bridge-type platysmaplasty in the neck. Once the platysmaplasty is complete, several deep plane sutures are placed into the zygomatic body for fixation of the SMAS of the skin/SMAS flap for *vertical* midfacial flap transposition. This is performed with several buried mattress stitches of 3-0 Mersilene suture. If any dimpling is noted, the sutures are removed and replaced at a deeper level in the SMAS flap. If any contour irregularities are noted, they should be resected and smoothed with a buried stitch of 4-0 Mersilene suture.

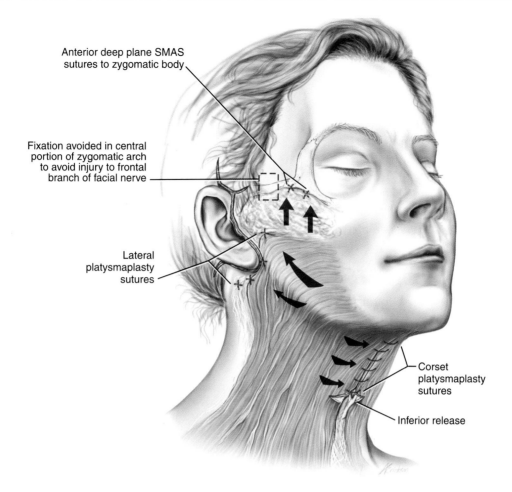

Anterior deep plane SMAS
sutures to zygomatic body

Fixation avoided in central
portion of zygomatic arch
to avoid injury to frontal
branch of facial nerve

Lateral
platysmaplasty
sutures

Corset
platysmaplasty
sutures

Inferior release

Figure 5-47 *The platysma flap is inset initially into the mastoid fascia along a bidirectional oblique vector at 180 degrees to the vector of the anterior "corset" platysmaplasty with several mattress stitches of 3-0 Mersilene suture. Several deep plane sutures are placed into the zygomatic body for fixation of the SMAS of the skin/SMAS flap for vertical midfacial flap transposition, using a similar stitch. If any dimpling is noted, the sutures are removed and replaced at a deeper level in the SMAS flap.*

Lahey clamps are then placed on the corner of the skin/SMAS flap such that the deep plane facial flap can be closed under extraordinary tension (Fig. 5-48). The vector for this flaps transposition is as vertical as possible. A buried mattress stitch of 2-0 Mersilene suture is placed as deeply as possible into the skin/SMAS flap after the excess is resected to fix the flap into the superficial temporal fascia. Several deeply placed buried stitiches of 3-0 Mersilene suture complement and buttress the skin/SMAS flap fixation to the superficial temporal fascia. The sideburn is then restored by bringing the hair-bearing flap down to meet the skin/SMAS flap. The subcutaneous neck flap and skin closure can then be completed.

ANTERIOR APPROACHES

Anterior approaches performed through a positioned cosmetically acceptable submental incision are necessary if (1) a well-defined cervicomental angle has not been established or residual anterior neck bulging is noted after the lateral approach has been closed, (2) significant anterior platysma banding or extensive platysma anterior excess is noted preoperatively, or (3) an extensive subplatysmal fat collection is noted preoperatively. Unlike lateral deep plane approaches, which are either/or techniques, anterior deep plane techniques are hierarchical in nature. They range from simple subplatysma fat resection and suture plication of the platysma to extensive subplatysma fat resection, to full anterior neck "corset" platysmaplasty, to full bridging interlocking suture suspension. Of utmost importance to keep in mind before beginning anterior neck deep plane recontouring is to preserve a relatively thick and uniform blanket of superficial fat. This minimizes contour irregularities from the deep plane procedure and provides suppleness to the skin of the neck. It should also be emphasized that over-resection of neck fat in the vain hope that anterior deep plane procedures can be avoided is counterproductive and can also have long-term adverse sequelae that are difficult to correct (Fig. 5-49).

CLINICAL PEARLS

- The midfacial dissection is performed through an extended transverse sideburn and pretrichal incision *after* an anterior "corset" platysmaplasty is completed through a submental approach and after the lower facial and neck skin flaps have been undermined through the preauricular and postauricular incisions, with care taken to create a subcutaneous tunnel between the lateral and anterior skin flaps.
- Once the meso-temporalis has been preserved 1 cm below the zygomatic arch, deep subcutaneous dissection can be carried down to the capsule of the parotid gland.
- Deep subcutaneous dissection of the lower face and neck is far easier to perform after the platysma-auricular ligament has been released.
- Anterior sub-SMAS dissection is performed over the superficial surfaces of the orbicularis oculi and the zygomaticus major muscles, which are landmarks for the deep plane anterior dissection.
- Deep plane dissection medial to the zygomaticus minor is unnecessary and inherently problematic.
- Deep subcutaneous insetting and fixation with this technique follow the following transposition sequence: platysma flap transposition initially into the mastoid fascia along a bidirectional oblique vector opposite to the "corset" platysmaplasty vector, midfacial deep plane flap transposition next along a vertical vector into the zygomatic body, followed finally by transposition of the lateral deep plane facial flap under extraordinary tension along a vector as vertical as possible.

EXTRAORDINARY LATERAL TENSION CLOSURE
OF DEEP PLANE FACIAL FLAP

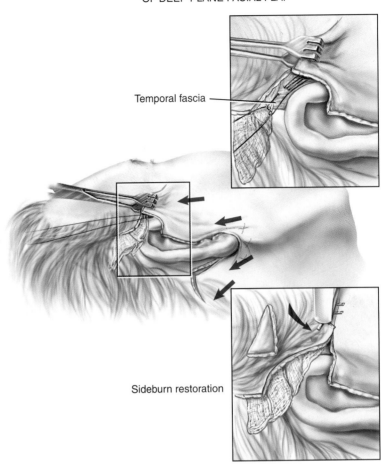

Temporal fascia

Sideburn restoration

Figure 5-48 Lahey clamps are placed on the corner of the skin/SMAS flap such that the deep plane facial flap can be closed under extraordinary tension. The vector for this flap is as vertical as possible. A buried mattress stitch of 2-0 Mersilene suture is placed as deeply as possible into the skin/SMAS flap after the excess is resected, for fixation of the flap to the superficial temporal fascia. Several deeply placed buried stitiches of 3-0 Mersilene suture complement and buttress the skin/SMAS flap fixation to the superficial temporal fascia. The sideburn is then restored by bringing the hair-bearing flap down to meet the skin/SMAS flap.

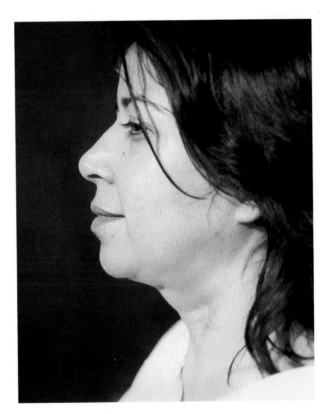

Figure 5-49 Over-resection of neck fat in the vain hope of avoiding the need for a deep plane procedure in the neck can have adverse sequelae that are difficult to correct. This 48-year-old prospective patient had undergone overaggressive cervical SAL a year earlier by another surgeon that resulted in a large left anterior cervical contour defect. She presented now for facial rejuvenation surgery.

There is no question that in many patients, satisfactory anterior deep plane recontouring can be achieved without an open anterior approach—that is, with superficial submental liposuction and lateral platysmaplasty alone (Fig. 5-50). These are usually youngish patients with minor collections of submental fat (Fig. 5-51), or middle-aged patients with minimal platysma laxity and no submental fat excess (Figs. 5-52 and 5-53). However, when patients have extensive subplatysma fat compartments, or inelastic and deeply folded cervical skin, or winglike flaps of platysma muscle at rest, the open anterior approach is unavoidable. This should be discussed with the patient preoperatively.

The hierarchical approach for deep plane recontouring in the anterior neck includes (1) subplatysma fat resection and platysma plication, (2) limited "corset" platysmaplasty with inferior release, (3) anterior platysma resection with "corset" platysmaplasty and inferior release, (4) full "corset" platysmaplasty with inferior release, and (5) the use of transverse neck interlocking suspension sutures with "corset" platysmaplasty and inferior release.

KEY POINTS

1) Anterior approaches are necessary if a well-defined cervicomental angle has not been established or residual anterior neck bulging is noted after the lateral approach has been closed, if significant anterior platysma bands or extensive platysma anterior excess is noted preoperatively, or if an extensive subplatysmal fat collection is noted preoperatively.

2) Of utmost importance before beginning anterior neck deep plane recontouring is to preserve a relatively thick and uniform blanket of superficial fat.

3) Anterior deep plane techniques are hierarchical in nature, as follows: subplatysma fat resection and platysma plication; limited "corset" platysmaplasty with inferior release; anterior platysma resection with "corset" platysmaplasty and inferior release; full "corset" platysmaplasty with inferior release; and last, the use of transverse neck interlocking suspension sutures with "corset" platysmaplasty and inferior release.

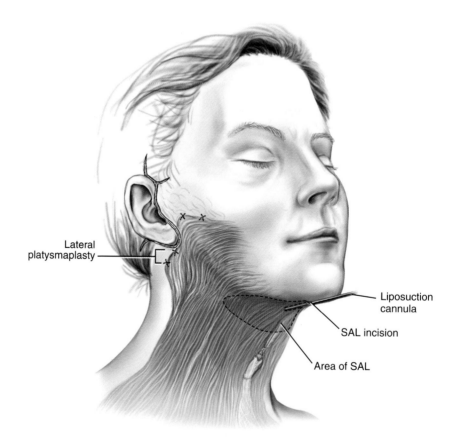

Lateral platysmaplasty

Liposuction cannula

SAL incision

Area of SAL

Figure 5-50 *In patients with minor to moderate collections of superficial submental fat, minor anterior platysma mauscle laxity, and supple cervical skin, as in this case, adequate anterior deep plane recontouring can be achieved with superficial submental liposuction and lateral platysmaplasty alone.*

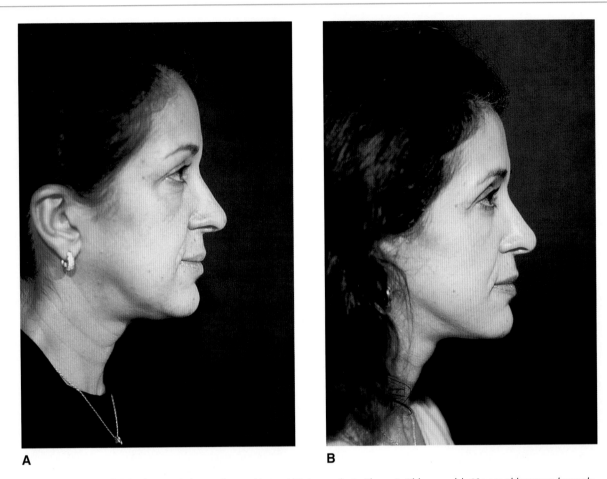

A   **B**

Figure 5-51 *Superficial Submental Liposuction and Lateral Platysmaplasty Alone.* **A,** *This youngish 46-year-old woman has only minor amounts of submental fat and very supple cervical skin.* **B,** *Cervical liposuction and lateral platysmaplasty-assisted rhytidectomy redraped her neck without the need for an open anterior approach.*

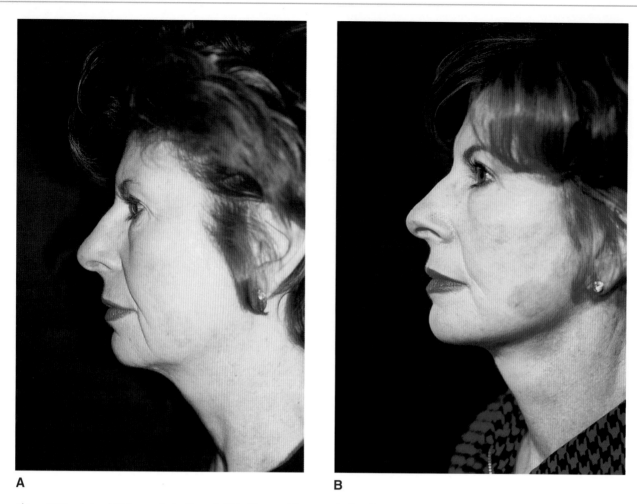

A   B

Figure 5-52 *Lateral Platysmaplasty Alone.* **A,** *This 56-year-old woman had undergone cervical liposuction 10 years previously. She was bereft of superficial fat in her neck and had supple cervical skin with a minor degree of anterior platysma laxity.* **B,** *Lateral platysmaplasty-assisted rhytidectomy recontoured her neck without the need for an open anterior approach.*

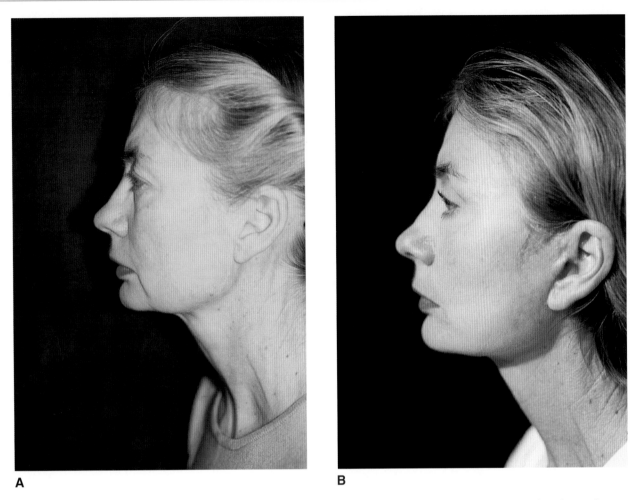

A

B

Figure 5-53 Lateral Platysmaplasty Alone. **A,** This 53-year-old woman has very supple skin for her age and only a minor degree of platysma muscle laxity. **B,** Minor anterior platysma banding at rest was corrected by a lateral plastysmaplasty-assisted rhytidectomy alone.

Subplatysma Fat Resection and Anterior Platysma Plication

If underappreciated preoperatively, large subplatysmal fat compartments become evident as residual anterior neck bulging after the lateral approach has been completed (Fig. 5-54). Wide subcutaneous undermining in the supraplatysmal plane over the area of the bulging is initially performed through a submental curvilinear incision. The incision should be approximately 2 to 3 cm in length, should be centered over the origin of the platysma muscle, and should not be detectable when the patient is viewed either in repose or in profile. Extensive subplatysma fat usually splays apart the platysma raphe; hence, an anterior platysmaplasty is necessary for optimal cervical recontouring. Subplatysma fat resection is more safely performed under direct vision, either by open suction-assisted lipectomy (SAL) or sharply, and is greatly aided by using either a fiberoptic retractor or an endoscope. Closed SAL of the deep subplatysma fat compartment should be avoided for the following reasons: (1) there is a tendency toward either over-resection or under-resection of subplatysma fat, and (2) there is inherent risk of injury to the marginal mandibular nerve, which occasionally can dip below the mandibular border anteriorly. Subplatysma fat is optimally resected conservatively and in a sculptural manner respecting the submental and cervical contours. After an adequate amount of subplatysma fat has been removed and hemostasis obtained, a simple anterior platysma muscle plication can be performed if the platysma muscle has good elasticity and is not

excessive (Figs. 5-55 and 5-56). Excessive resection of subplatysma fat should be avoided at all cost because soft tissue depressions in the submental region are extremely difficult to repair. Plication is performed with several buried simple stitches of 3-0 Mersilene suture. Plication sutures do not reef up excess platysma, so if there is any question about the quality of the platysma muscle or its relative excess, then the next level of complexity—the "corset" platysmaplasty—becomes necessary.

CLINICAL PEARLS

- The submental incision should be approximately 2 to 3 cm in length, should be centered over the origin of the platysma muscle, and should not be detectable when the patient is viewed either in repose or in profile.
- Subplatysma fat resection is more safely performed under direct vision by either sharp dissection or open SAL than by closed SAL.
- Closed SAL in this region should be avoided because there is a tendency toward either over-resection or under-resection of subplatysma fat, and because there is inherent risk of injury to the marginal mandibular nerve, which occasionally can dip below the mandibular border anteriorly.
- Subplatysma fat is optimally resected conservatively and in a sculptural manner respecting the submental and cervical contours.
- Excessive resection of subplatysma fat should be avoided at all cost because soft tissue depressions in the submental region are extremely difficult to repair.
- A simple anterior platysma muscle plication can be performed if the platysma muscle has good elasticity and is not excessive.

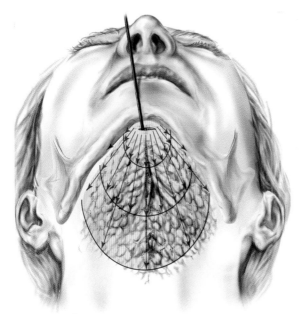

A Area of superficial fat suction

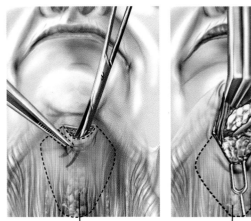

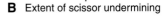

B Extent of scissor undermining

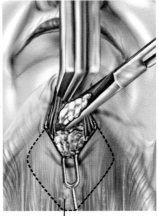

C Area of subplatysma fat removal under direct vision

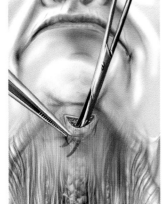

D Anterior platysma plication

Figure 5-54 *When patients have residual anterior neck bulging, the usual culprit is an excessively large subplatysma fat compartment. Subplatysma fat can splay apart the anterior platysma muscle; therefore, anterior platysmaplasty becomes necessary for optimal cervical recontouring. When the platysma muscle has good elasticity, anterior platysma muscle plication is achieved with simple buried stitches of 3-0 Mersilene suture.*

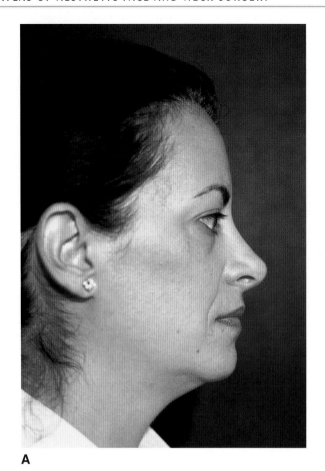

A

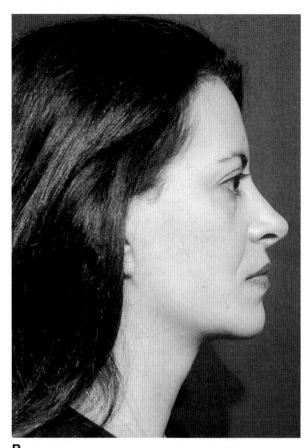

B

Figure 5-55 *Subplatysma Fat resection and Anterior Platysma Plication.* **A,** *This 40-year-old woman had residual anterior neck bulging after the lateral SMAS/platysma-ectomy.* **B,** *Resection of the excess portion of her subplatysma fat compartment along with anterior platysma plication improved her neck contours. Her platysma muscle was of excellent quality.*

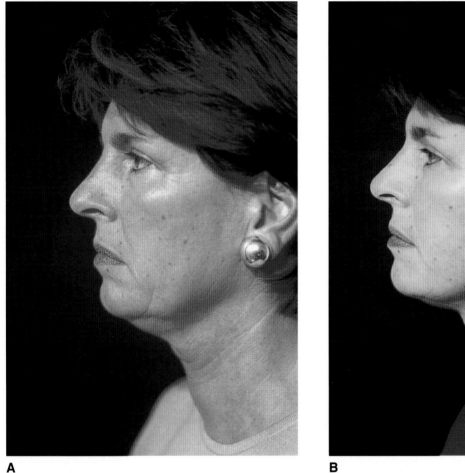

A

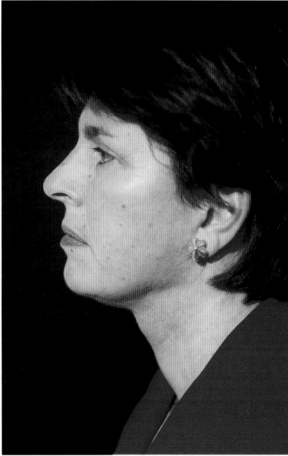

B

Figure 5-56 *Subplatysma Fat Resection and Anterior Platysma Plication.* **A,** *This 50-year-old woman had a heavy ptotic subplatysma fat compartment, which splayed apart her platysma muscles. Resection of the excess portion of her subplatysma fat compartment and anterior platysma plication were performed.* **B,** *Her postoperative appearance. The laxity of the platysma was underappreciated, and a better cervical recontouring would have been achieved if a "corset" platysmaplasty had been performed.*

Limited "Corset" Platysmaplasty with Inferior Release

When the platysma muscle has been found to have significant laxity, reefing up of the anterior excess becomes necessary (Fig. 5-57). This type of platysmaplasty is called a "corset" because of its cinching effect on the neckline (Figs. 5-58 and 5-59). The "corset" platysmaplasty is combined with a midline resection of subplatysma fat when a ptotic and excessive subplatysma fat compartment is present (Figs. 5-60 and 5-61). Subplatysma fat is optimally resected conservatively with a midline trough when "corset" platysmaplasty is to be employed so that a midline bulge from the "corset" itself is not inadvertently created. In many patients it is only necessary to perform the "corset" from the platysma muscle origin behind the chin to the new cervicomental angle near the hyoid bone. In order to prevent a secondary "bowstring" deformity, a transverse 1 to 2 cm release of the platysma muscle over the hyoid bone near the new cervicomental angle is necessary. The limited "corset" platysmaplasty is performed with running over-and-over anterior mattress stitch of 3-0 Mersilene suture. This stitch can be rerun anteriorly, if necessary, and tied in buried fashion under the chin. Minor irregularities can be corrected with several buried stitches of 4-0 Vicryl suture.

CLINICAL PEARLS

- When the platysma muscle has considerable laxity, reefing up of the anterior excess from the platysma muscles origin below the chin to the hyoid bone becomes necessary.
- The limited "corset" platysmaplasty is performed with running over-and-over anterior mattress stitch of 3-0 Mersilene suture, which can be rerun anteriorly if necessary.
- If concomitant subplatysma fat is to be resected, the resection should be conservatively performed with a midline trough in order to avoid secondary deformity.
- To prevent "bowstring" deformity of the "corset," a transverse 1 to 2 cm release of the platysma muscle over the hyoid bone near the new cervicomental angle is necessary.

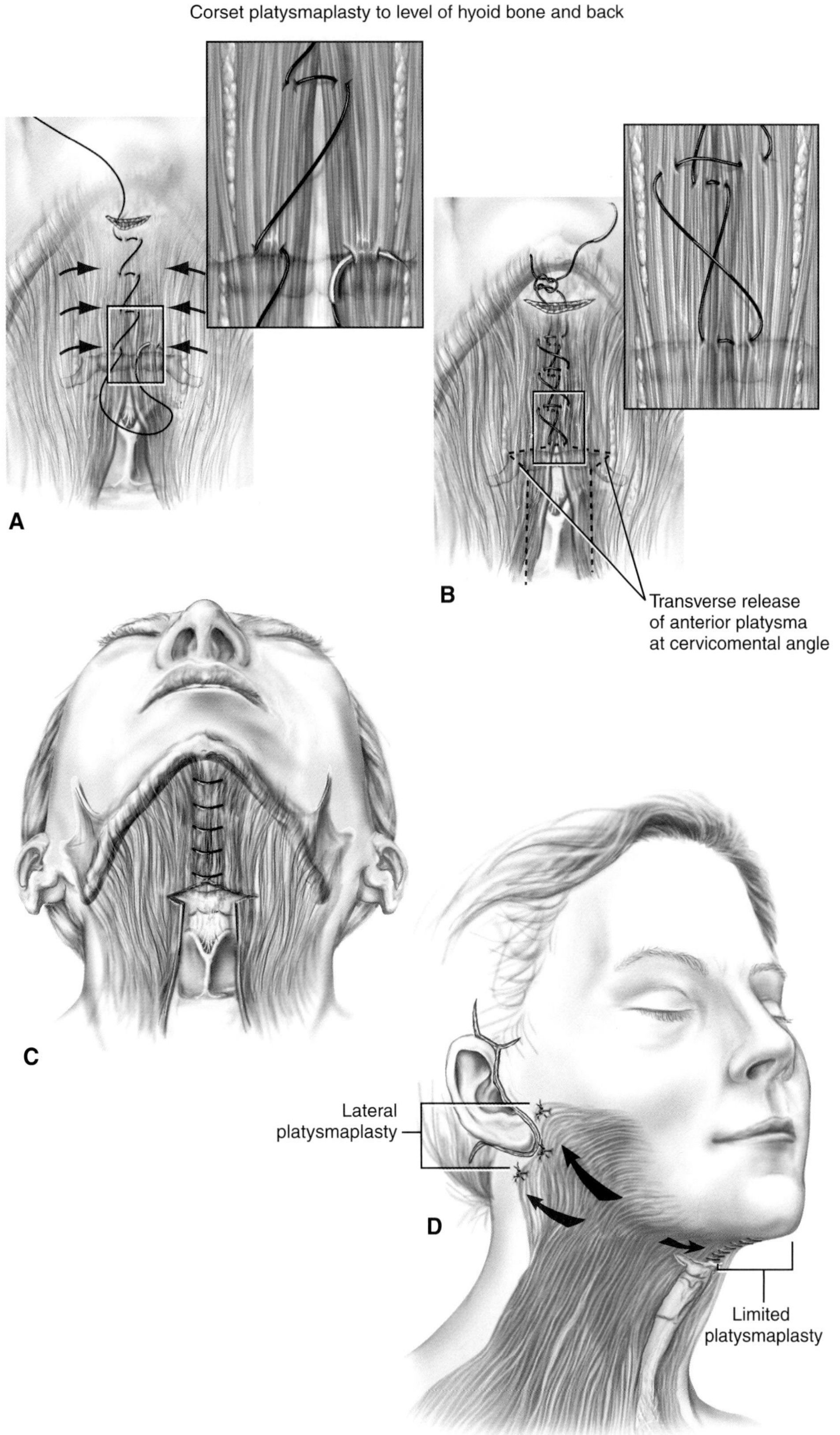

Corset platysmaplasty to level of hyoid bone and back

Figure 5-57 *When significant laxity of the platysma muscle is present, reefing up of the excess platysma muscle is necessary. This type of platysmaplasty, usually performed with a running back-and-forth anterior mattress stitch of 3-0 Mersilene suture, is called a "corset" because of its cinching effect on the neckline. The limited "corset" platysmaplasty ends at the hyoid bone and is often performed with subplatysma fat resection.*

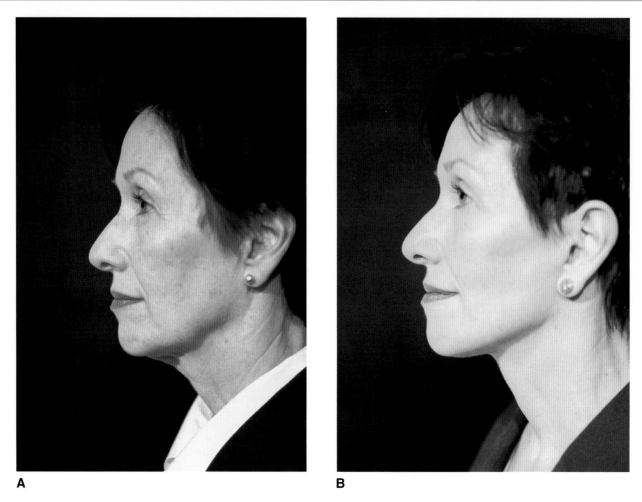

A

B

Figure 5-58 *Limited Anterior "Corset" Platysmaplasty with Inferior Release.* **A,** *This 58-year-old woman had anterior platysma laxity above the hyoid bone with greater laxity on the right.* **B,** *A "corset" platysmaplasty ending at the hyoid bone reefed up the excessive and lax platysma muscle.*

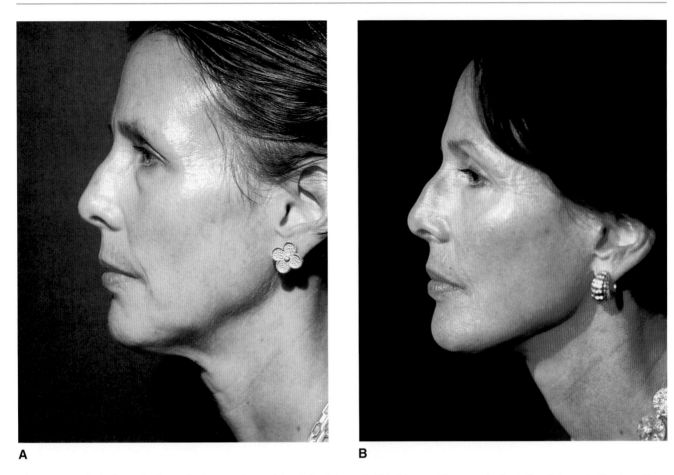

A

B

Figure 5-59 *Limited Anterior "Corset" Platysmaplasty with Inferior Release.* ***A,*** *This 54-year-old woman had anterior platysma laxity above the hyoid bone with greater laxity on the left.* ***B,*** *A "corset" platysmaplasty ending at the hyoid bone reefed up the excessive and lax platysma muscle.*

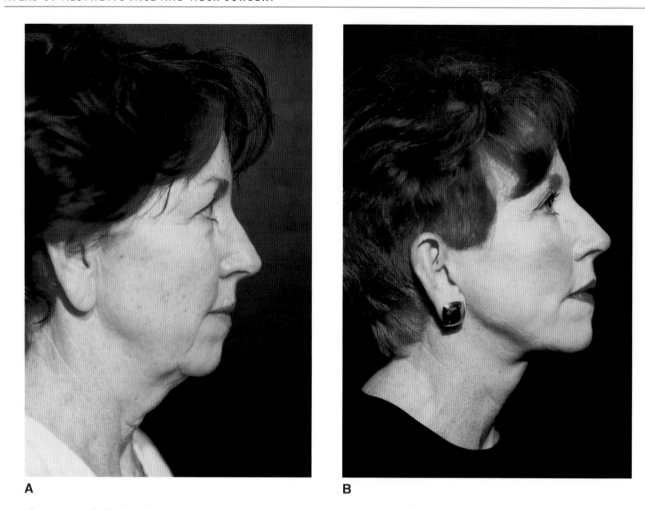

A
B

Figure 5-60 *Limited Anterior "Corset" Platysmaplasty with Inferior Release.* ***A,*** *This 56-year-old woman had extensive subplatysma fat and anterior platysma laxity above the hyoid bone. Extensive subplatysma fat resection along the anticipated line of her platysmaplasty and anterior limited "corset" with inferior release was performed.* ***B,*** *Her postoperative appearance.*

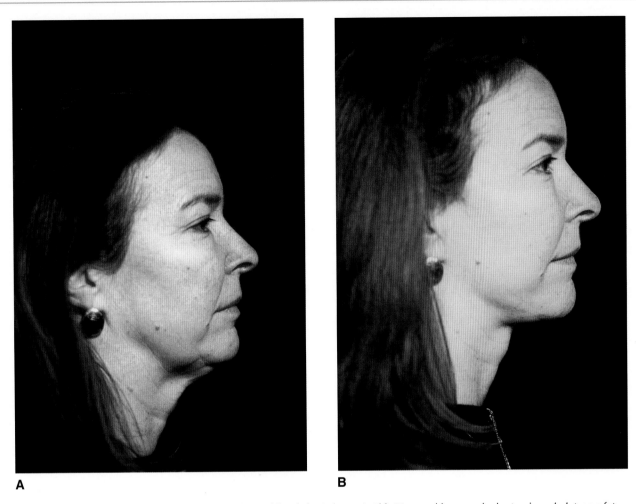

A **B**

Figure 5-61 *Limited Anterior "Corset" Platysmaplasty with Inferior Release. **A,** This 55-year-old woman had extensive subplatysma fat and anterior platysma laxity above the hyoid bone. Extensive subplatysma fat resection and limited anterior "corset" platysmaplasty with inferior release were performed. **B,** Her postoperative appearance.*

Anterior Platysma Resection

If laxity of the platysma is severe, it is best to resect the anterior platysma excess in strips 1 to 2 cm wide rather than to bunch up the excess, thereby creating a thick bowstring of muscle (Fig. 5-62). After the anterior excess platysma muscle has been resected and hemostasis judiciously performed, the neckline is recontoured with a "corset" platysmaplasty and inferior release. Resection of the excessive anterior platysma muscle should be tailored

to the patient's needs—that is, if the excess is solely between the chin and the hyoid bone, then resection of platysma muscle excess should be restricted to that region only (Fig. 5-63). If, however, the excess platysma muscle extends the full length of the neck, then resection should proceed over the full length of the neck (Figs. 5-64 and 5-65). Hemostasis should be extensive and meticulously performed when resection proceeds below the level of the hyoid bone.

CLINICAL PEARLS

- If laxity of the platysma is severe, it is best to resect the anterior platysma excess in strips 1 to 2 cm wide rather than to bunch up the excess, creating a thick bowstring of muscle.
- Resection of the excessive anterior platysma muscle should be tailored to the patient's needs and extended the full length of the neckline if necessary.

- After the anterior excess platysma muscle has been resected and hemostasis judiciously performed, the neckline should be recontoured with a "corset" platysmaplasty and inferior release.

Platysma Resection with Anterior Corset and Inferior Release

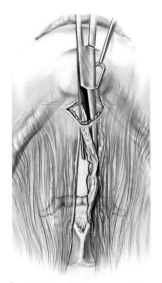

A Anterior platysma resection

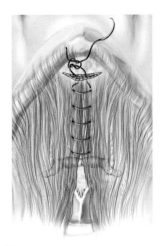

B Corset to level of hyoid bone

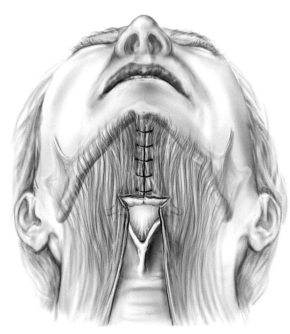

C Inferior release at hyoid bond

Figure 5-62 *If laxity of the platysma is severe, it is best to resect the anterior platysma excess, rather than bunching up the excess to create a visible and thick midline "bowstring." Strips of anterior platysma muscle 1 to 2 cm wide are resected, and the neck is recontoured with a limited "corset" platysmaplasty, with inferior release at the level of the hyoid bone.*

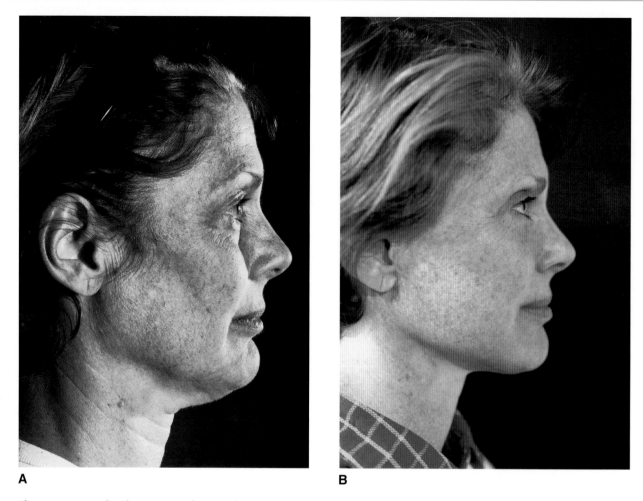

A   B

Figure 5-63 *Anterior Platysma Resection.* ***A,*** *This 50-year-old woman had severe excess anterior platyma above the level of the hyoid bone. Reefing up of the excess muscle would have created a thick midline bowstring.* ***B,*** *Anterior platysma resection and limited "corset" platysmaplasty with inferior release proved to be a much better option, as evident at her 5-year follow-up evaluation.*

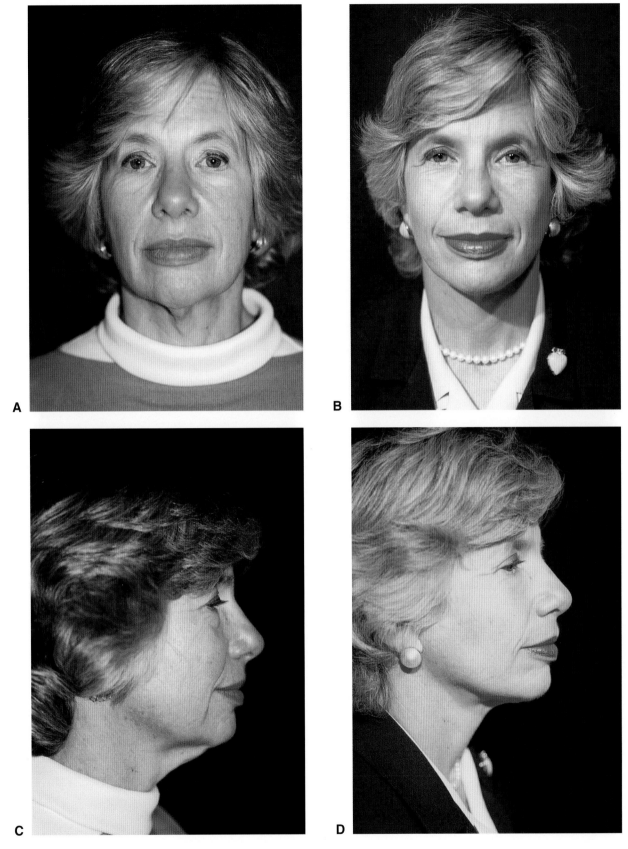

Figure 5-64 *Anterior Platysma Resection.* ***A*** *and* ***C,*** *This 58-year-old woman had extensive anterior platysma muscle excess extending the full length of the platysma muscle. Anterior platysma resection the full length of the platysma muscle was performed along with an anterior "corset" platysmaplasty.* ***B*** *and* ***D,*** *Her postoperative appearance.*

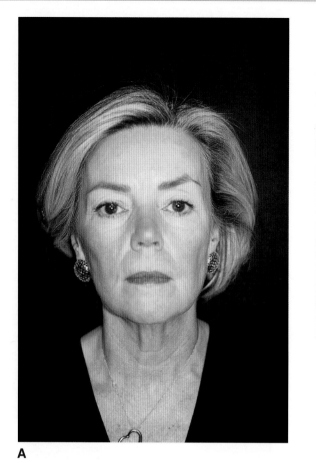

A

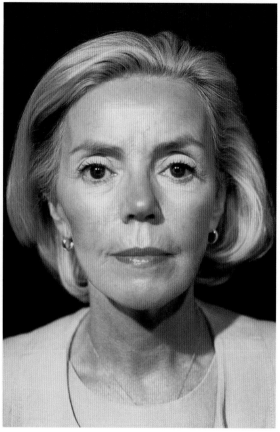

B

Figure 5-65 *Anterior Platysma Resection.* **A** *and* **C,** *This 54-year-old woman had extensive platysma muscle excess without any decussation of platysma muscle fibers. Extensive anterior platysma muscle resection and "corset" platysmaplasty with inferior release were performed.* **B** *and* **D,** *Her postoperative appearance.*

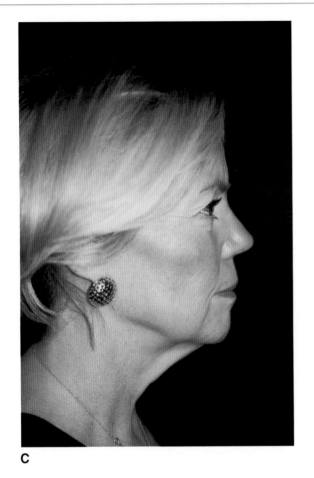

C

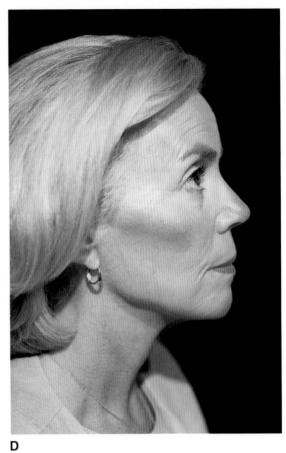

D

Figure 5-65, cont'd

Full "Corset" Platysmaplasty

When platysma muscle laxity extends the full length of the neckline and the platysma muscle is not excessive enough to justify resection, a full "corset" platysmaplasty is best (Fig. 5-66). Invariably the best candidates for a full "corset" are thick-necked patients who appear to have "low" hyoid bones but who in reality have extensive subplatysma fat collections and lack of platysma muscle decussation (Figs. 5-67 and 5-68). The normal hyoid bone location is either above or at the inferior border of the chin in the lateral view. If the hyoid is below the level of the inferior chin, the cervicomental angle becomes obliterated by the geniohyoid musculature. A truly "low" hyoid is not surgically correctable, and the patient should be informed preoperatively of this anatomical limitation in achieving optimal cervical recontouring (Fig. 5-69).

Full Corset Procedure

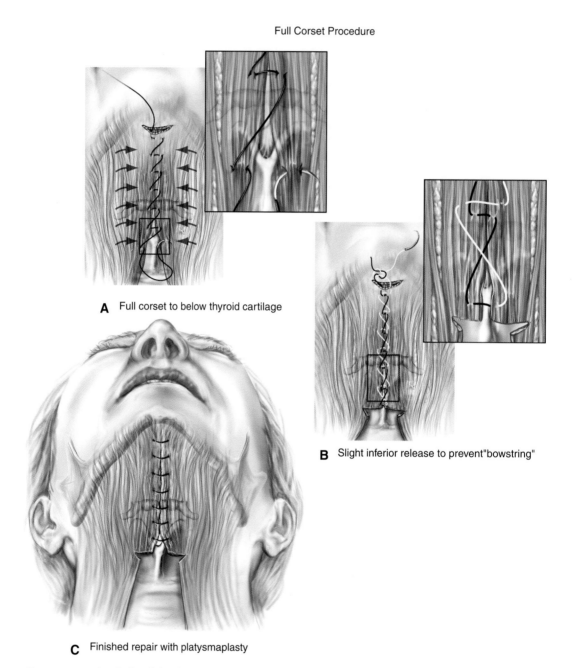

A Full corset to below thyroid cartilage

B Slight inferior release to prevent "bowstring"

C Finished repair with platysmaplasty

Figure 5-66   *When laxity of the platysma muscle extends its entire length, yet muscle tissue is not so excessive as to be amenable to resection, a full "corset" platysmaplasty is best. Invariably the best candidates for a full "corset" are thick-necked patients with extensive subplatysma fat collections and platysma muscle divarications extending the full length of the muscle, as in this case. Inferior release is performed at the level of the thyroid cartilage in order to prevent a bowstring.*

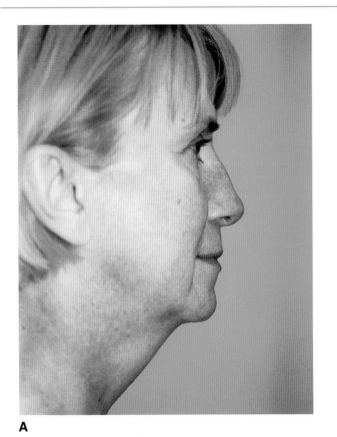

A

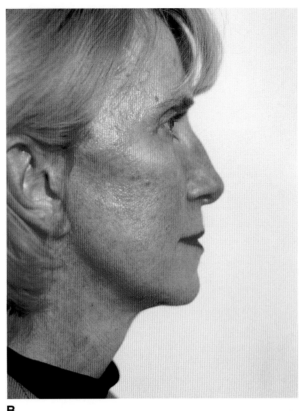

B

Figure 5-67 *Full "Corset" Platysmaplasty.* **A,** *This 54-year-old woman with supple skin appears to have a "low" hyoid bone below the level of her chin. In reality she has extensive subplatysma fat and platysma muscle laxity extending the full length of the muscle, giving her a "bull neck" appearance.* **B,** *Extensive subplastysma fat resection and a full "corset" plastysmaplsty to the level of her thyroid cartilage slimmed her neck and better defined her cervicomental angle.*

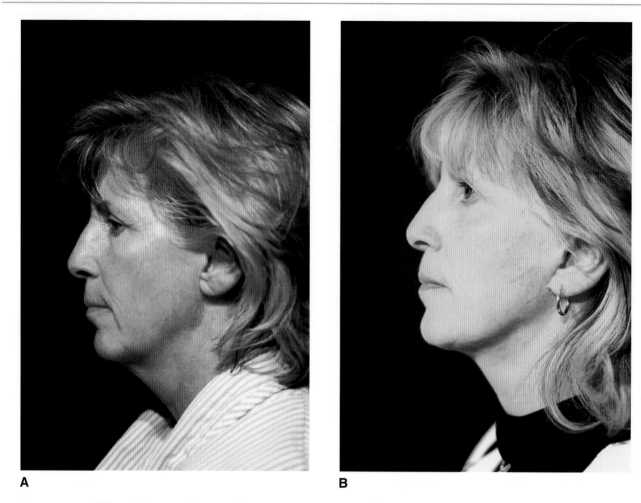

A **B**

Figure 5-68   *Full "Corset" Platysmaplasty.* ***A,*** *This 56-year-old woman also appeared to have a "low" hyoid, when in reality it was at the level of the lower border of her chin. In actuality she had extensive subplatysma fat and playtsma muscle laxity extending the full extent of the muscle.* ***B,*** *A full "corset" platysmaplasty after aggressive resection of subplatysma fat gave her neck more definition and created a cervicomental angle that approached the aesthetic ideal.*

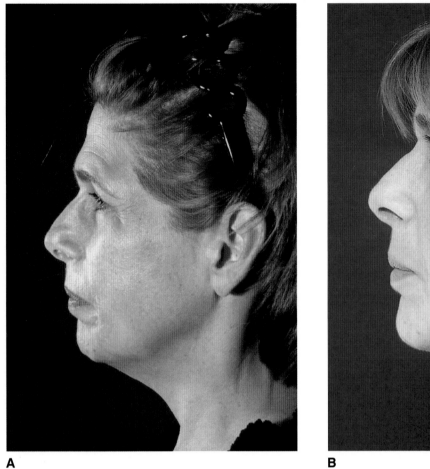

A

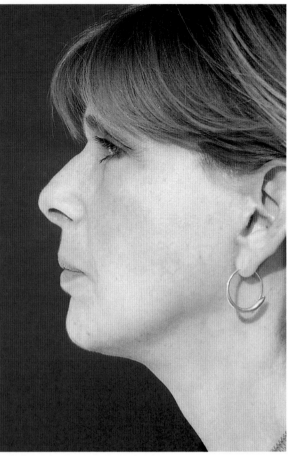

B

Figure 5-69   *Full "Corset" Platysmaplasty.* ***A,*** *This 58-year-old woman did have a "low" hyoid bone, which extended well below her chin.* ***B,*** *Even with extensive subplatysma defatting and a full anterior "corset," her cervicomental angle could not be angulated any more acutely than her low hyoid would allow. In such cases the patient should be informed preoperatively of this anatomical limitation to achieving optimal cervical recontouring.*

A full "corset" platysmaplasty extends from the platysma muscle origin to the thyroid cartilage. A 1- to 2-cm inferior platysma muscle release is necessary in order to prevent a secondary bowstring deformity. The inferior release is set at the level of the thyroid cartilage. When the release is sufficient, a cervicomental angle of sufficient angularity is created in the proper location. Rarely, a very "difficult" neck may be encountered that requires extensive subplatysma muscle defatting and resection of a 1- to 2-cm strip of platysma muscle over its entire length, followed by a full "corset" platysmaplasty (Fig. 5-70).

CLINICAL PEARLS

- When platysma muscle laxity extends the full length of the neckline and the platysma muscle is not excessive enough to justify resection, a full "corset" platysmaplasty is best.
- The best candidates for a full "corset" are thick-necked patients who appear to have "low" hyoid bones but who really have extensive subplatysma fat collections and lack of platysma muscle decussation.
- When a full "corset" is used, the inferior release is set at the level of the thyroid cartilage.
- Rarely, a very difficult neck may be encountered that requires extensive subplatysma muscle defatting and resection of a 1- to 2-cm strip of platysma muscle over its entire length, followed by a full "corset" platysmaplasty.

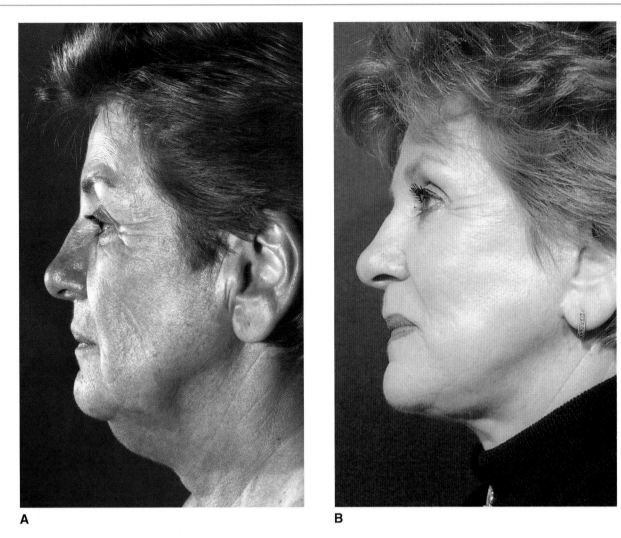

A   **B**

Figure 5-70   *Full "Corset" Platysmaplasty.* **A,** *This 64-year-old woman epitomizes the "difficult neck"—tissue laden with ptotic pre-and subplatysma fat, severe platysma muscle excess and laxity extending the full length of the muscle, and stretched, inelastic cervical skin.* **B,** *Even with conservative preplatysma defatting, aggressive subplatysma defatting and cervical skin resection, and anterior platysma muscle resection and full "corset" platysmaplasty, cervical recontouring was improved but not superlative.*

Suspension Sutures

There are times one finds that even with a full "corset" platysmaplasty the neckline is not properly recontoured and the cervicomental angle is not well defined. There may even be residual bulges in paramedian locations in the neck. On close examination, the platysma muscle is seen to be thin, its fibers literally tearing apart as the "corset" is tightened, and the entire span of the platysma muscle has a moth-eaten appearance. In such cases, interlocking suspension sutures spanning the full width of the neck become necessary (Fig. 5-71). Suspension sutures consist of a pair of vertical and horizontal mattress stitches of 2-0 Prolene suture interlocked at the level of the hyoid bone along the full "corset" and tightened to the mastoid fascia in order to create a new cervicomental angle.

SUSPENSION SUTURES

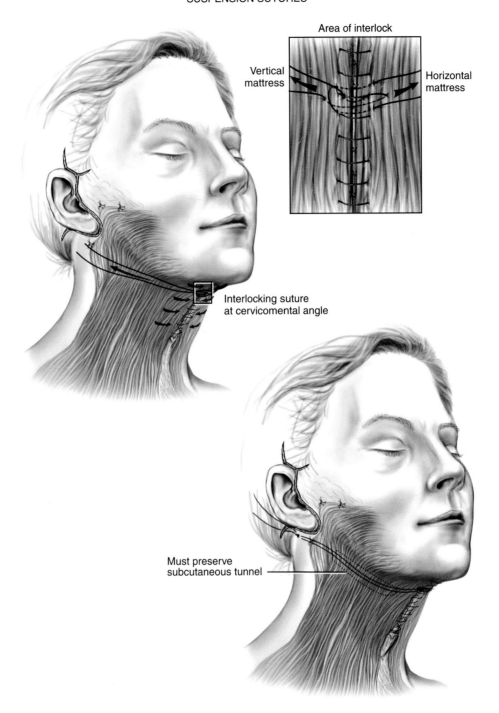

Area of interlock

Vertical mattress

Horizontal mattress

Interlocking suture
at cervicomental angle

Must preserve
subcutaneous tunnel

Figure 5-71 *When the platysma muscle is judged to be of such poor quality that a full "corset" platysmaplasty cannot properly recontour and define the neckline, placement of interlocking suspension sutures spanning the full width of the neck becomes necessary. Vertical and horizontal mattress stitches of 2-0 Prolene suture are interlocked over the hyoid bone along the full "corset" to create a new cervicomental angle. Of utmost importance is to preserve a subcutaneous tunnel in the neck, to place them in an accessible location into the mastoid fascia adjacent to the postauricular suture line, and not to tighten them excessively.*

Of utmost importance in choosing suspension sutures are several details: (1) with the lateral approach, the surgeon must anticipate the need for suspension sutures before closing because the sutures need to be placed through a subcutaneous tunnel, which should be carefully created along the proposed location of the new cervicomental angle; (2) the suspension sutures should be placed deep into the mastoid fascia in a accessible location adjacent to the postauricular suture line in the event that they require removal postoperatively; (3) the suspension sutures should be tied under "passive" tension, that is, a degree of tension that creates an optimal cervicomental angle and reduces cervical bulging with the patient in the recumbent position, not a degree of tension that deforms the normal anatomical relationships in the anterior neck or strangulates the patient; and (4) when well placed, suspension sutures do not require an inferior release of the "corset" because they themselves prevent secondary bowstring formation.

Patients who require suspension sutures are older and have extensive inelastic anterior cervical skin excess (Fig. 5-72) and extensive laxity of their platysma musculature (Fig. 5-73). Many of these patients do not mind the look of the slightly "overcorrected" neckline resulting with use of suspension sutures. In fact, many of them desire the look achieved by this method. Patients should be informed preoperatively that if this technique does not meet their desired goals, the suspension sutures can be removed 6 weeks postoperatively with a minor procedure. So that this minor procedure remains minor, it is imperative to use a monofilament permanent suture and to place the mastoid suspension sutures in an accessible location adjacent to the postauricular suture line.

CLINICAL PEARLS

- Suspensions sutures consist of a pair of vertical and horizontal mattress stitches of 2-0 Prolene suture interlocked at the level of the hyoid bone along a "corset" platysmaplasty and tightened to the mastoid fascia in order to create a new cervicomental angle.
- Patients that require suspension sutures are older, have extensive inelastic anterior cervical skin excess, and extensive laxity of their platysma musculature.
- Several details are important when employing suspension sutures: (1) they need to be placed through a subcutaneous tunnel, which should be carefully created along the proposed location of the new cervicomental angle; (2) they should be placed deep into the mastoid fascia in an accessible location adjacent to the postauricular suture line; (3) they should be tied under "passive" tension; and (4) when well placed, they do not require an inferior release of the "corset," since they themselves prevent secondary bowstring formation.
- Patients should be informed preoperatively that if this technique does not meet their desired goals, the suspension sutures can be removed 6 weeks postoperatively with a minor procedure.

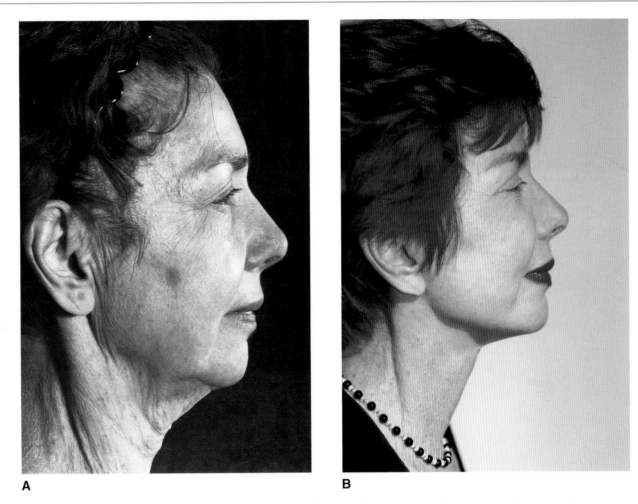

A　　　　　　　　　　　　　　　　　　　　　**B**

Figure 5-72　*Suspension Sutures.* **A,** *This 70-year-old woman had extensive inelastic cervical skin excess and a "moth-eaten" platysma muscle, which a full "corset" platysmaplasty did not optimally address.* **B,** *Interlocking midline suspension sutures placed along the anticipated cervicomental angle greatly assisted in properly recontouring her neck. The resulting "overdone look" is typical of this technique and should be emphasized preoperatively to patients.*

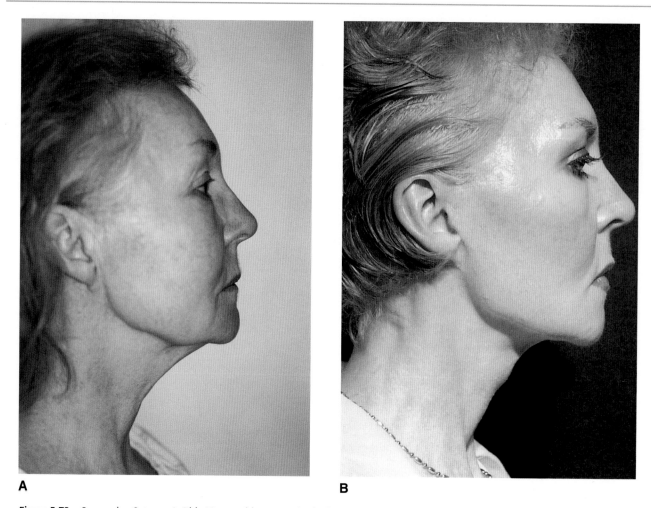

A **B**

***Figure* 5-73** *Suspension Sutures.* **A,** *This 69-year-old woman also had a poor-quality platysma muscle that a full "corset" did not optimally address.* **B,** *Interlocking suspension sutures spanning the full width of her neck greatly improved her neck recontouring results.*

References

Aston S, Thorne C: Contemporary rhytidectomy. In Rees TD, LaTrenta GL (eds): Aesthetic Plastic Surgery, 2nd ed. Philadelphia, WB Saunders, 1994.

Baker D: Lateral SMASectomy. Plast Reconstr Surg 100:509, 1997.

Baker T, Stuzin J: Personal technique for facelifting. Plast Reconstr Surg 100:502, 1997.

Feldman J: Corset platysmaplasty. Plast Reconstr Surg 85:333, 1990.

Giampapa V, Di Bernardo B: Neck recontouring with suture suspension and liposuction: An alternative for the early rhytidectomy patient. Aesth Plast Surg 19:217, 1995.

Hamra S: The deep-plane rhytidectomy. Plast Reconstr Surg 86:53, 1990.

Miller T: Face lift: Which technique? Plast Reconstr Surg 100:501, 1997.

Owsley J: Lifting the malar fat pad for correction of prominent nasolabial folds. Plast Reconstr Surg 91:463, 1993.

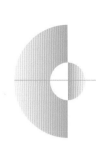

CHAPTER SIX

The Male Patient; Adjunctive Techniques; Complications and Untoward Sequelae

THE MALE PATIENT

Men *are* different, or so it's said—and so they think! In planning for male facial rejuvenation, however, aesthetic goals are no different from those in female facial rejuvenation: replenishing midfacial fullness; softening nasolabial, perioral, cheek, and neck skin folds; eradicating the jowl; restoring a clean, well-contoured jawline; removing any "waddle" under the chin; and creating a well-defined cervicomental angle as close to 120 degrees as possible. The surgical goals are also no different from those for women: cosmetic incisions that result in inconspicuous scars hidden in natural skin lines, an unaltered hairline that requires no unwanted alteration of hairstyling postoperatively, and an aesthetically pleasing ear that can be proudly displayed with a short-cropped haircut after surgery. Even anatomically, the goals of aesthetic plastic surgery in men are no different from those in women: skin tightening, superficial fat repositioning, vertical repositioning of deep layer ptotic soft tissue mass, and correction of musculofascial laxity. Simply stated, the aim of cosmetic facial surgery for men is no different from that for women—to go from the square face of age to the oval face of youth.

Aesthetic Considerations

Where men are different from women is in the distribution and density of their facial and neck hair growth—men are prone to *baldness,* and they are *bearded* (Fig. 6-1). Male pattern baldness begins in affected men in their 20s and 30s and creates individual patterns of temporal recession and coronal hair loss that become well established by the time these men enter their 40s and 50s. Temporal recession creates acute angulation between the frontal forelock and the temporal hairline, as well as a general thinning of the temporal hair. This pattern of hair loss greatly restricts the length of the temporal extension of the preauricular incision and limits the access afforded by this incision. As used in most male patients, this incision is short and serves only to facilitate midfacial flap fixation to the temporal fascia. Fortunately, in the vast majority of men, the temporal tuft of hair and the sideburn are preserved over the entire lifetime. Midfacial access in the male patient is gained primarily through inconspicuously placed extended pretrichal and transverse sideburn incisions. Accordingly, the patient is instructed to grow the sideburns to the level of the tragus for a month prior to surgery. This additional sideburn length allows accommodation for the inevitable rise of the sideburn that occurs after the midfacial flap has been transposed.

Men also have non–hair-bearing strips of skin anterior to the auricle, inferior to the lobule, and in the retroauricular region. Preservation of these non–hair-bearing regions is greatly aided by intraoperative cauterization of hair follicles and by postoperative laser hair removal (Fig. 6-2A and B). In the long run, though, a high rate of patient satisfaction among male rhytidectomy patients is best achieved by careful and thorough preoperative counseling. This means warning them that unwanted hairs may grow in these regions of the face, but that with some minor adjustments in their shaving technique they can easily achieve the cleanly shaven look they desire. Men also have a greater

AESTHETIC CONSIDERATIONS IN MEN

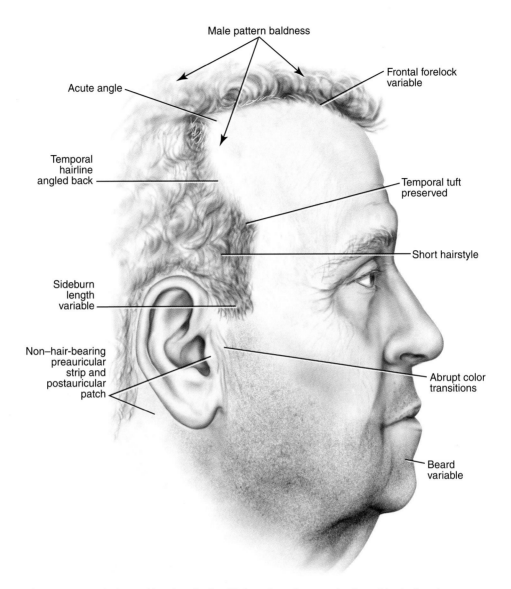

Figure 6-1 *Aesthetic considerations for facelift in male patients are dominated by the fact that men are bearded and they are prone to baldness.*

propensity to exhibit sun-damaged, dyschromic skin, so that color and textural changes are more pronounced with an abrupt transition from bearded cheek or neck skin to bald preauricular or postauricular skin (Fig. 6-3). Switching to a post-tragal incision along the rim prevents abrupt color changes in this region and fools the eye, and the eventual scar is less noticeable. Men also usually wear their hair short and cannot hide occipital incisions as well as women can. In male patients, every attempt should be made to limit the postauricular incision with subsequent scarring, and the usual extension of the posterior incision into the occipital hairline is to be avoided (Fig. 6-4). Nevertheless, in a male patient who exhibits so much cervical skin excess that the postoperative result would be marginalized by constraining the incisions, use of a well-designed retroauricular incision within the sulcus and an occipital hairline incision will result in the least conspicuous of scars (Fig. 6-5).

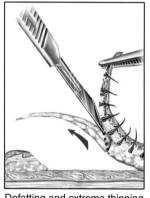

Defatting and extreme thinning of flap by removal of a wedge of subcutaneous fat

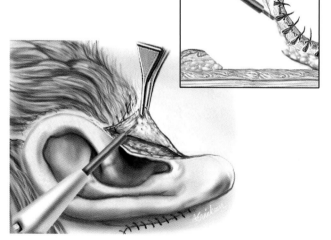

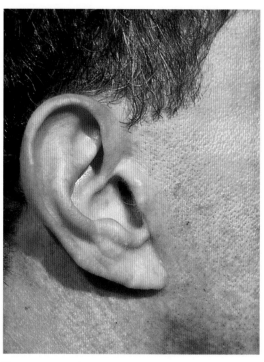

A Intraoperative cauterization of residual hair follicles

Figure 6-2 *Men have non–hair-bearing strips of skin anterior to the auricle, inferior to the lobule, and retroauricularly. This pattern can be preserved by **(A)** intraoperative cauterization of hair follicles. **B,** Postoperative result with this approach.*

B

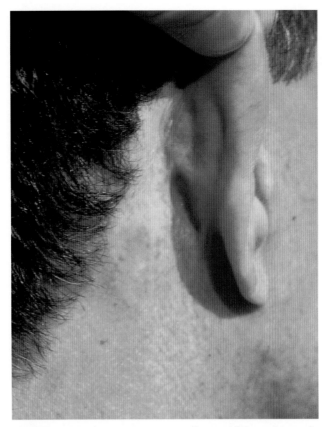

Figure 6-3 *Men have a greater propensity to exhibit sun-damaged, dyschromic skin, so that color and textural changes are more pronounced. There is an abrupt transition from bearded cheek or neck skin to bald preauricular or postauricular skin. Scars can be camouflaged within these regions, as can be demonstrated by the barely detectable occipital hairline scar in this patient.*

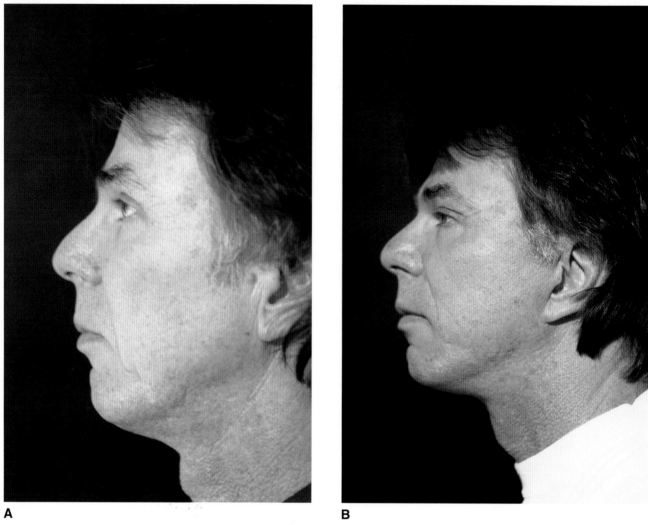

A

B

Figure 6-4 *In male patients, every attempt should be made to limit the postauricular and occipital hairline incisions and subsequent scarring. This 52-year-old man is a good example of a patient in whom a minimal-incision technique can be used.*

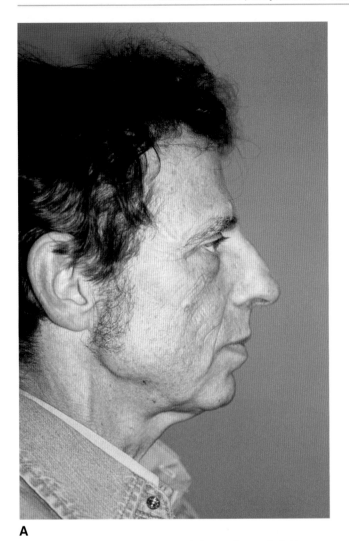

A

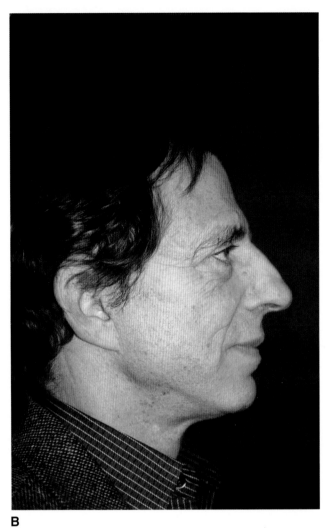

B

Figure 6-5 *In male patients who exhibit excessive cervical skin excess, such as this 58-year-old man, it must be understood that the postoperative result would be marginalized by constraining the incisions to a minimal-incision technique. A retroauricular incision within the sulcus with posterior extension as close as possible to the occipital hairline should be designed for these patients.*

Surgical Considerations

The incisions (Fig. 6-6) used for male rhytidectomy patients generally resemble those used for women, with some minor modifications: (1) the temporal extension of the preauricular incision is shortened considerably and kept low so that sturdy temporal fixation of the midfacial flap is provided by the superficial temporal fascia, and so that the sideburn is not violated; (2) the transverse sideburn incision is generous, transverse, and made at a lower level than for women— a few millimeters above the level of the root of the helix—allowing the sideburn to keep a generous length, to accommodate the shortening that inevitably occurs when the midfacial flap is transposed along a vertical vector (Fig. 6-7); (3) the anterior pretrichal extension of the sideburn incision is kept within the sideburn and made only if anterior temporal soft tissue debulking is judged to be necessary for correction of unsightly temporal bunching occurring with rotation of the midfacial flap; (4) a post-tragal rim incision with a right angle at the conchal notch is the preauricular incision of choice, closed only after thorough defatting, intraoperative cauterization of residual hair follicles, and conservative trimming of skin excess such that the pretragal hollow is replenished without tension; and (5) if at all possible, a minimal-incision postauricular approach is chosen. Of major importance in the minimal-incision approach, the *retroauricular incision is kept short but carried up and onto the auricle well above the sulcus;* it is not kept at the level of the sulcus as it is for women. Carrying the retroauricular incision up and onto the ear makes it far easier to redistribute the retroauricular skin excess into the new sulcus without resultant unsightly bunching up of skin in this aesthetically sensitive and highly visible region of the face and neck in men.

Another major difference between men and women is that the blood supply to the cervicofacial skin is far greater in men than in women. Blood supply is proportional to thickness and depth of the hair follicles. In many men, facial hair follicles are the thickest, coarsest, and deepest follicles on the entire body. Hence, skin flaps are found to be far thicker and more vascular than they are in women. To diminish this skin flap hypervascularity and to minimize its adverse effects, the following measures are recommended. First, 0.2 mg of clonidine hydrochloride is administered 30 minutes preoperatively to level out the blood pressure during surgery and to help prevent spikes in blood pressure in the dangerous immediate postoperative period (<6 hours), when postoperative hematomas can form. In addition, a tumescent anesthetization technique is used after intravenous monitored sedation is accomplished, to create a virtually bloodless operative field and to promote effective hemostasis (see Chapter 4 for details).

Several modifications of surgical technique can assist in reducing bleeding and the incidence and severity of postoperative hematomas in men (Fig. 6-8). In the midface, a deep-plane technique, rather than a two-layer technique, can correct midfacial musculofascial laxity, soften skin folding in the nasolabial and perioral regions, and "lift" a heavy ptotic anterior soft tissue mass, while bleeding from the hypervascular subdermal plane is avoided and postoperative hematoma formation is minimized. Simultaneously, limited lateral skin flap undermining is performed over the lower lateral face and neck regions, and an aggressive lateral platysmaplasty is performed (Figs. 6-9 and 6-10). In the anterior neck, difficult-to-control bleeding can be avoided by limiting the area of closed preplatysmal suction-assisted lipectomy (SAL), using a generous submental incision (2.0 to 2.5 cm) for anterior access, limiting anterior subcutaneous undermining to stay within several centimeters of the anterior platysma borders, using open SAL to remove subplatysmal fat, and performing a limited "corset"-type anterior platysmaplasty with inferior release to contour the cervicomental angle (Figs. 6-11 and 6-12). In extremely difficult necks, important additional aspects of the technique are resection of 1 to 2 cm longitudinal strips of excessive anterior platysma muscle and placement of mastoid-to-mastoid suspension sutures (Fig. 6-13). In the brow region of male patients, endoscopic brow lifts are used exclusively to make certain that even the possibility of unsightly bald scars is kept at an absolute minimum (Fig. 6-14). And for difficult-to-correct, heavy nasolabial folds and deep perioral grooves, direct SAL with primary autologous fat grafting (Fig. 6-15) is used liberally as an adjunctive procedure to avoid excessive undermining into these regions and to improve postoperative results (Figs. 6-16 and 6-17).

MALE INCISIONS

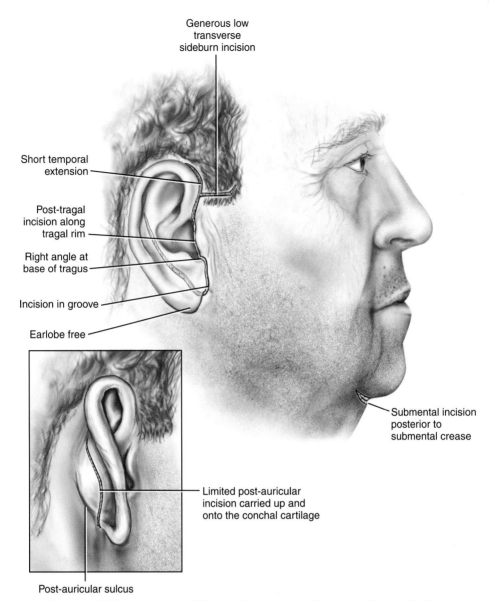

Generous low transverse sideburn incision

Short temporal extension

Post-tragal incision along tragal rim

Right angle at base of tragus

Incision in groove

Earlobe free

Submental incision posterior to submental crease

Limited post-auricular incision carried up and onto the conchal cartilage

Post-auricular sulcus

Figure 6-6   *The incisions of choice used for male rhytidectomy patients generally resemble those used for women, with some minor modifications.*

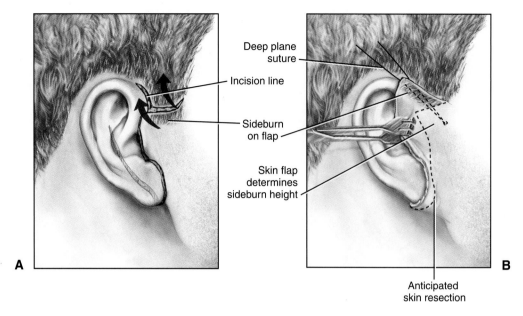

Deep plane
suture

Incision line

Sideburn
on flap

Skin flap
determines
sideburn height

Anticipated
skin resection

A

B

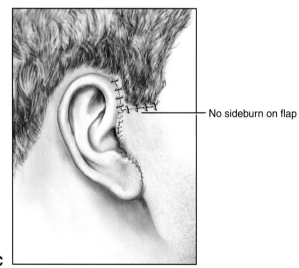

No sideburn on flap

C

Figure 6-7 *The preauricular incision for men is shorter than it is for women. The transverse sideburn incision is also made lower, near the level of the root of the helix, to provide length and to accommodate the shortening that inevitably occurs when the midfacial flap is transposed along a vertical vector.*

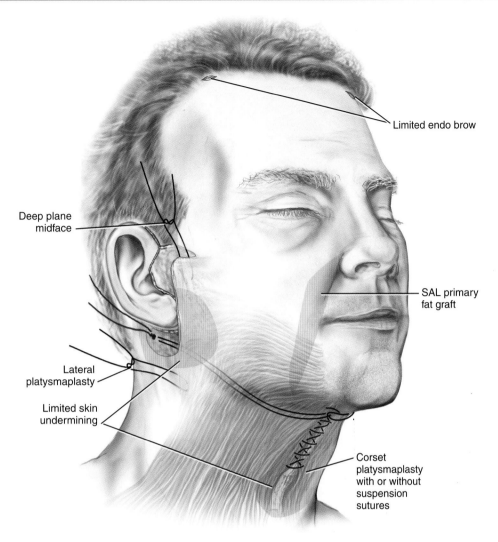

Limited endo brow

Deep plane
midface

SAL primary
fat graft

Lateral
platysmaplasty

Limited skin
undermining

Corset
platysmaplasty
with or without
suspension
sutures

Figure 6-8   *In male patients, bleeding with resultant formation of postoperative hematomas can be reduced by several modifications of the surgical technique: (1) a deep-plane lift, rather than two-layer techniques, in the midface; (2) limited skin undermining to access the deep layer in the lower face and neck; and (3) aggressive use of lateral and anterior platysmaplasty with or without suspension sutures.*

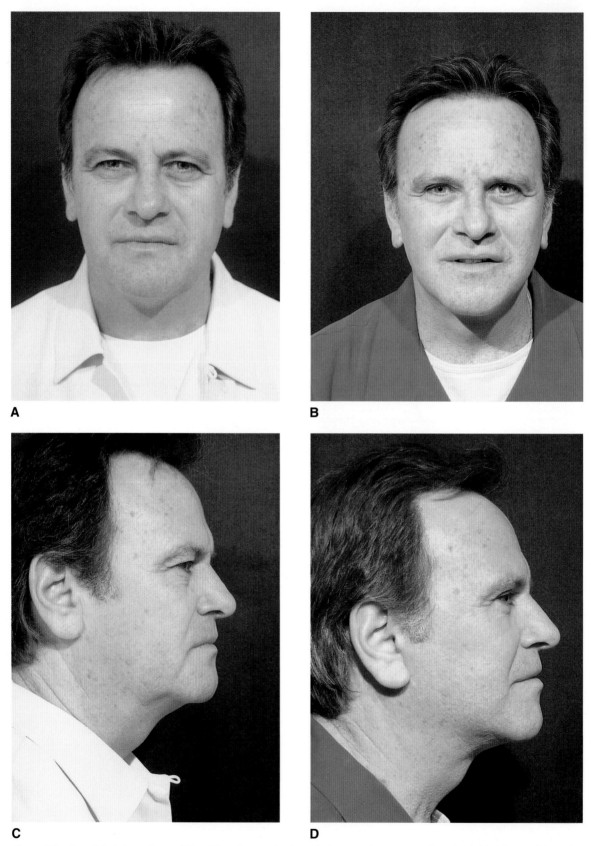

Figure 6-9 **A** *and* **C,** *A deep-plane midface lift and aggressive lateral platysmaplasty corrected much of this 56-year-old man's musculofascial laxity. Conservative upper blepharoplasty was performed as well.* **B** *and* **D,** *His postoperative appearance.*

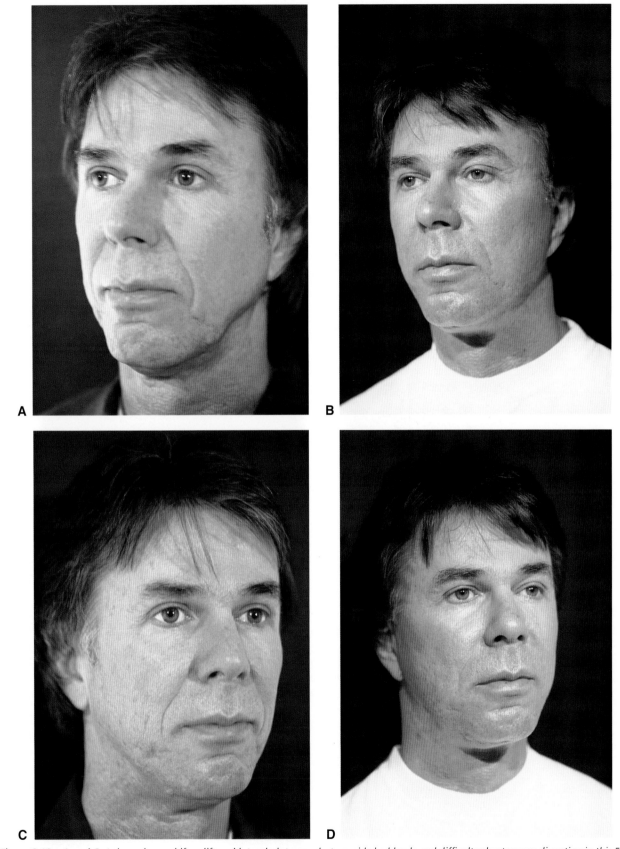

Figure 6-10   **A** and **C,** A deep plane midface lift and lateral platysmaplasty avoided a bloody and difficult subcutaneous dissection in this 50-year-old man's severely acne-scarred skin and provided a good correction of his musculofascial laxity and ptotic anterior soft tissue mass. **B** and **D,** His postoperative appearance.

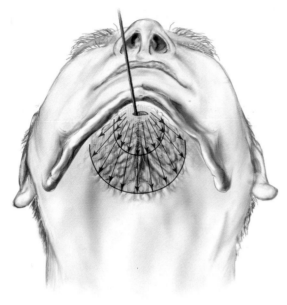

A Area of limited submental liposuction

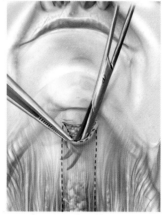

B Limited anterior undermining, 2.0-2.5 cm submental incision

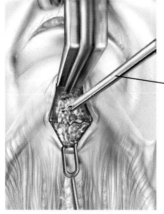

Flat SAL cannula

C Open SAL to remove subplatysmal fat

Figure 6-11 *In the anterior neck, difficult-to-control bleeding can be avoided by limiting the area of closed preplatysmal SAL, using a generous submental incision (2.0 to 2.5 cm) for anterior access, limiting anterior subcutaneous undermining to stay within several centimeters of the anterior platysma borders, and using open SAL to remove subplatysmal fat **(A–C),** and by performing a limited "corset"-type anterior platysmaplasty with inferior release to contour the cervicomental angle **(D–F).***

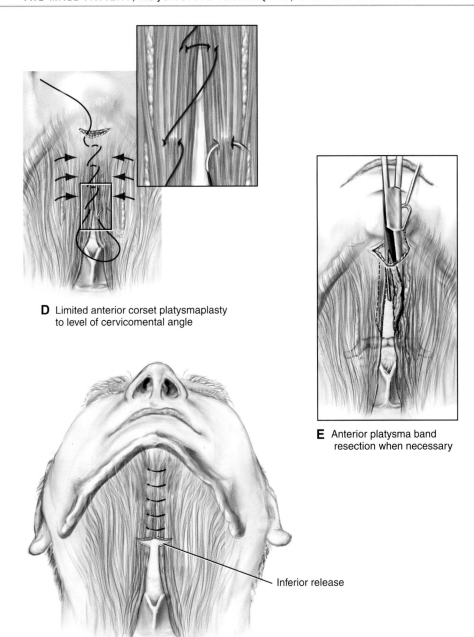

D Limited anterior corset platysmaplasty to level of cervicomental angle

E Anterior platysma band resection when necessary

Inferior release

F Completed anterior neckplasty

Figure 6-11, cont'd

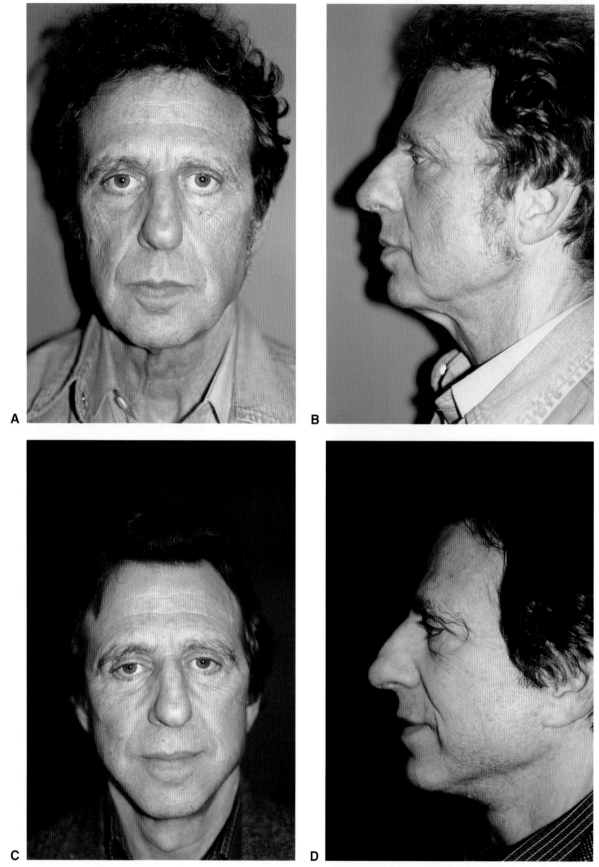

Figure 6-12 *Following the guidelines described in the text for anterior neck cosmetic surgery in men, recontouring of this 57-year-old man's "turkey gobbler" neck was accomplished without incident.* ***A*** *and* ***C,*** *Preoperative photographs.* ***B*** *and* ***D,*** *postoperative appearance.*

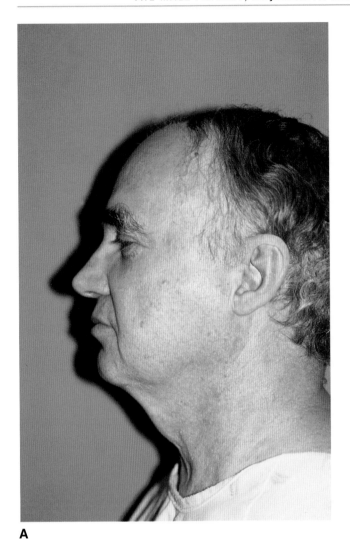

A

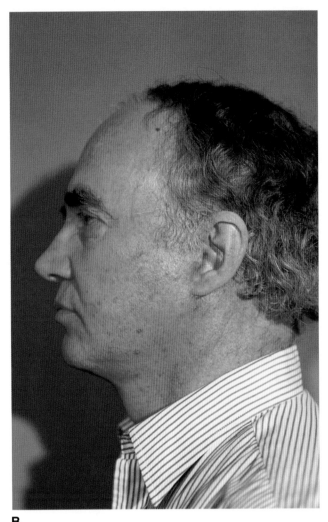

B

Figure 6-13 **A,** *As demonstrated in this 58-year-old man, adding resection of 1 to 2 cm longitudinal strips of excessive anterior platysma muscle and placement of mastoid-to-mastoid suspension sutures greatly aids anterior neck recontouring in patients with difficult necks.* **B,** *His postoperative appearance.*

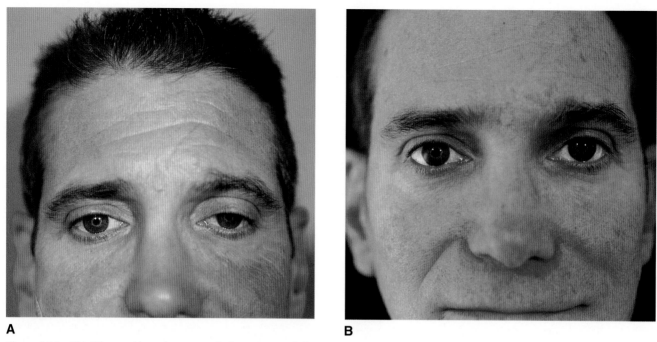

A **B**

Figure 6-14   *This 50-year-old man's asymmetrical post-traumatic brow ptosis **(A)** was improved by an endoscopic brow lift **(B)**.*

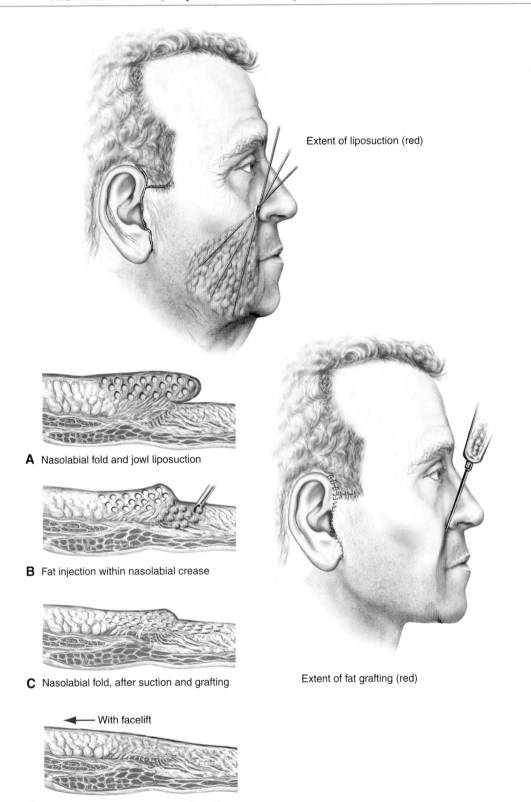

Extent of liposuction (red)

A Nasolabial fold and jowl liposuction

B Fat injection within nasolabial crease

C Nasolabial fold, after suction and grafting

← With facelift

D Nasolabial fold, after suction and grafting and facelift

Extent of fat grafting (red)

Figure 6-15 *For difficult-to-correct heavy nasolabial folds and deep perioral grooves, direct SAL (top) and primary autologous fat grafting (bottom) are used liberally as adjunctive procedures in order to avoid extensive undermining into these regions and to improve postoperative results. Diagrams **A–D** show cross-sectional anatomy at various points in the procedure.*

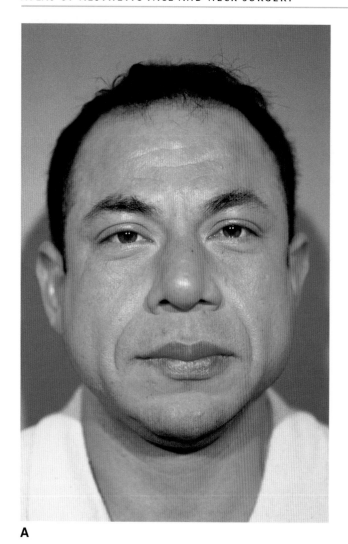

A

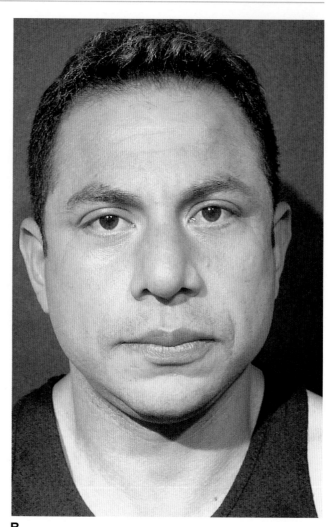

B

Figure 6-16 In this 44-year-old man *(A)*, heavy nasolabial folds were greatly improved by a limited midface lift, direct SAL and primary grafting, and transfacial resection of the fat pad of Bichat *(B)*.

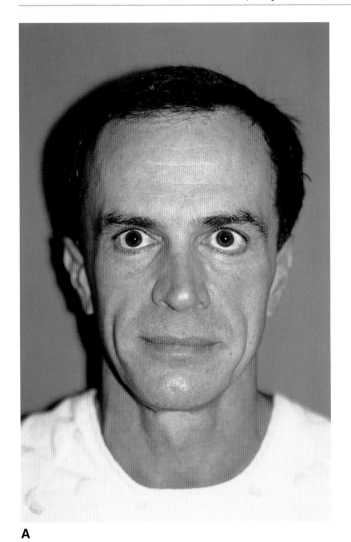

A

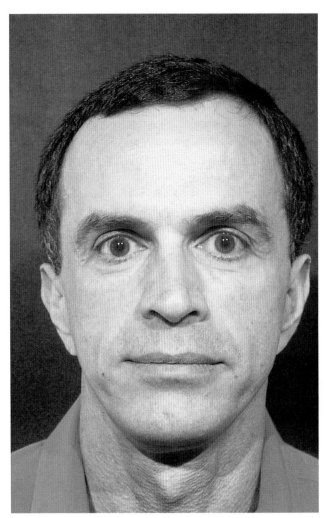

B

Figure 6-17   *In this 50-year-old man* **(A),** *direct SAL and primary extensive autologous fat grafting improved the results that could be achieved by the deep plane midfacial lift alone* **(B).**

Limited Retroauricular Incision Technique

After the skin flaps have been raised, deep-plane midface dissection is completed, hemostasis is performed, and the anterior and lateral platysmaplasty is completed, the midfacial and neck flaps are transposed over the auricle along optimal vectors (Fig. 6-18). The auricle is retracted with a skin hook, and a subdermal buried stitch of 2-0 Vicryl suture is placed in the postauricular sulcus, to provide fixation of the neck flap in optimal position (Fig. 6-19). This maneuver temporarily buries the lobule of the ear under the flap. The postauricular skin is incised and the ear released by making a cut in the anticipated retroauricular sulcus with straight Gorney scissors, extending to the site of the anticipated new lobule site. One must be careful to overcorrect the height of the new lobule site slightly in order to avoid flattening and inferior drag of the lobule.

A Lahey clamp is placed on the deep-plane midfacial flap, and the flap is transposed along a vertical midfacial vector (Fig. 6-20). The anticipated skin resection is drawn on the flaps, the skin excess is resected with straight Gorney scissors, and a buried stitch of 2-0 Vicryl suture is placed into the temporal fascia for fixation of the deep-plane midfacial flap into its anticipated new position (Fig. 6-21). The skin is closed with simple stitches of fine 6-0 nylon suture, the new sideburn height and configuration are established, and the lobule of the ear is inset into a new, slightly overcorrected position with a simple stitch of 5-0 nylon suture (Fig. 6-22). Aggressive defatting of the preauricular flap and cauterization of hair follicles are performed after flipping the flap over, and the preauricular flap is inset with a running stitch of 5-0 nylon suture (Fig. 6-23).

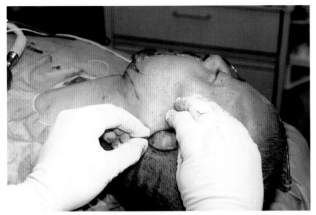

Figure 6-18 *Limited Retroauricular Incision Technique. After the skin flaps have been raised, deep-plane midface dissection is completed, hemostasis is performed, and anterior and lateral platysmaplasty is completed, the facial and neck skin is transposed over the auricle along its optimal vector.*

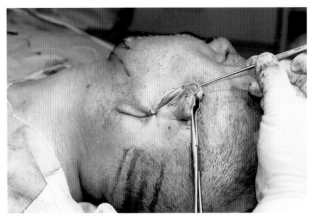

Figure 6-19 *Limited Retroauricular Incision Technique. The auricle is retracted with a skin hook, and a subdermal buried stitch of 2-0 Vicryl suture is placed in the postauricular sulcus to fixate the skin flap into its optimized newly transposed position.*

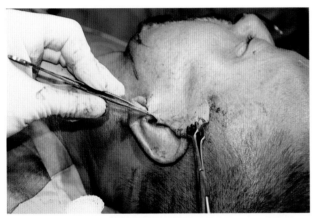

Figure 6-20 *Limited Retroauricular Incision Technique. A Lahey clamp is placed on the deep-plane midfacial flap, and the midfacial flap is transposed along a vertical midfacial vector.*

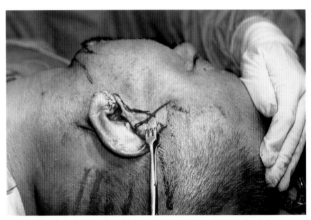

Figure 6-21 *Limited Retroauricular Incision Technique. The anticipated skin resection is drawn roughly on the midfacial flap.*

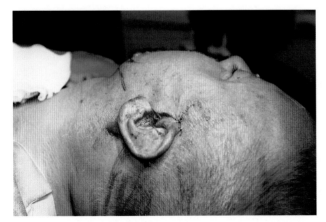

Figure 6-22 *Limited Retroauricular Incision Technique. The skin excess is resected with straight Gorney scissors, and a buried stitch of 2-0 Vicryl suture is placed into the temporal fascia for fixation of the deep plane midfacial flap into its anticipated new position. The new sideburn height and configuration are established, and the lobule of the ear is inset into a new, slightly overcorrected position.*

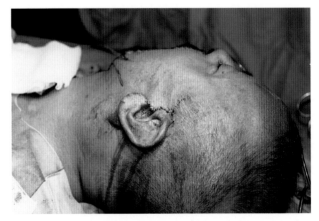

Figure 6-23 *Limited Retroauricular Incision Technique. Aggressive defatting of the preauricular flap and cauterization of hair follicles is performed after flipping the flap over, and the preauricular flap is inset with a running stitch of 5-0 nylon suture.*

The previously placed retroauricular buried stitch of 2-0 Vicryl is removed (Fig. 6-24) and replaced with several buried stitches of 3-0 Vicryl suture placed directly into the base of the conchal cartilage as close as possible to the new lobule site (Fig. 6-25). It is important to emphasize that the postauricular incision should have been made well above the postauricular sulcus and carried onto the conchal cartilage, not in the sulcus as it would be for women. The retroauricular skin excess is then redistributed by a single-tooth Adson forceps into the retroauricular sulcus while a double-tooth skin hook is retracting the ear (Fig. 6-26). Of note, the retroauricular sulcus that requires skin coverage is far larger in men than it is in women because the skin incision has been carried well above the sulcus for men. If skin excess is noted, it is trimmed by straight Gorney scissors (Fig. 6-27). The skin is closed with simple stitches of 4-0 or 5-0 nylon suture after a 7-0 round suction drain has been placed (Fig. 6-28). Unsightly retroauricular skin wrinkling should be kept to an absolute minimum when using the minimal incision technique.

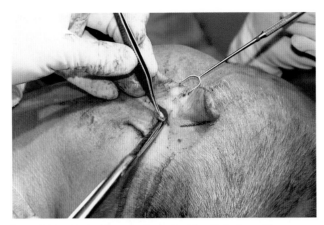

Figure 6-24 *Limited Retroauricular Incision Technique. The previously placed retroauricular buried stitch of 2-0 Vicryl is removed.*

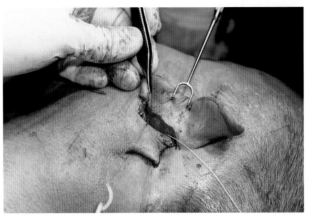

Figure 6-25 *Limited Retroauricular Incision Technique. The neck flap is now fixed into position by several buried stitches of 3-0 Vicryl suture placed directly into the base of the conchal cartilage as close as possible to the new lobule site. Note: The postauricular incision has previously been made well above the postauricular sulcus and onto the conchal cartilage, not in the sulcus as it would have been for women.*

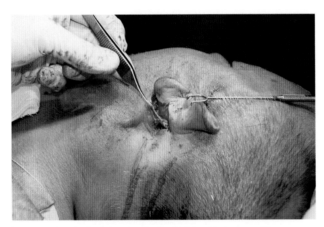

Figure 6-26 *Limited Retroauricular Incision Technique. The retroauricular skin excess is redistributed by a single-tooth Adson forceps into the retroauricular sulcus while a double-tooth skin hook retracts the ear. Note: The retroauricular sulcus that requires skin coverage is far larger for men than it is for women.*

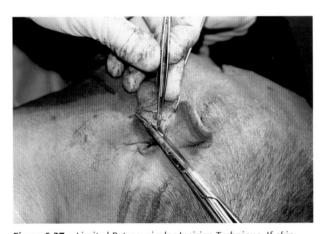

Figure 6-27 *Limited Retroauricular Incision Technique. If skin excess is noted, it is trimmed using straight Gorney scissors.*

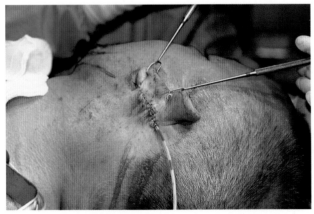

Figure 6-28 *Limited Retroauricular Incision Technique. The retroauricular skin is closed with simple stitches of 4-0 or 5-0 nylon suture after a 7-0 round suction drain has been placed. Note: Unsightly retroauricular skin wrinkling is kept to an absolute minimum with use of the minimal- retroauricular-incision technique.*

ADJUNCTIVE TECHNIQUES

Chin Augmentation

No doubt you remember when you were in medical school and your senior residents would say: "If you're thinking about a spinal tap when evaluating a patient, do it." The same applies to chin implants. During your evaluation of a prospective rhytidectomy patient who is bothered by a poor neckline, you may notice that she also has a "weak" jaw. In such cases it is best to introduce the possibility of simultaneous chin augmentation. Although as a general rule it is unwise to suggest an operation to correct a deformity of which the patient is not aware, chin augmentation is one true exception. Conservatively performed chin augmentation for patients with microgenia will only enhance their rhytidectomy results, especially for the profile. If the patient is reluctant, often just making a simple tracing of the profile, and then demonstrating the added benefit simultaneous chin augmentation will provide, is all that is necessary to convince the patient.

Another general rule is that it is best to perform the chin augmentation *first,* before the anterior and lateral approach rhytidectomy. This sets the bony profile before modulation of the soft tissue profile is performed. Because most patients who require simultaneous chin augmentation will also require significantly detailed anterior neck superficial or deep plane recontouring, it is best to perform the chin augmentation through a generous submental incision (Fig. 6-29). Anterior neck recontouring usually consists of some combination of preplatysmal and subplatysmal fat removal and some type of anterior "corset" platysmaplasty (Fig. 6-30). The usual sequence of surgery in performing simultaneous chin augmentation, then, is submental approach chin augmentation, anterior neck superficial and deep plane recontouring, and lateral approach one- or two-layer rhytidectomy.

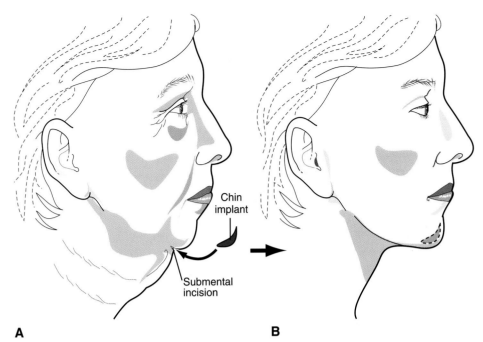

A **B**

Figure 6-29 *Most rhytidectomy patients who require simultaneous chin augmentation also require significantly detailed anterior neck superficial or deep plane recontouring (**A**). It is best to perform the chin augmentation first, and to use a generous submental incision, for an optimal result (**B**).*

And finally, the last general rule in performing simultaneous chin augmentation is to remember that alloplastic augmentation does not correct the soft tissues in a 1:1 ratio; rather, a 0.66:1 ratio of correction is obtained. Hence, in using commercially available chin implants, which usually have a maximal projection of 0.7 to 0.8 cm, no more than 0.5 cm of added chin projection should be expected, regardless of the width of the implant. This added chin projection, although only half a centimeter, can have major benefits for patients suffering from oral incompetence. Many patients with microgenia demonstrate significant perioral muscular strain, even at rest, in a vain attempt to achieve lip closure. Much of this muscular strain can be relieved by simultaneous chin augmentation, contributing to a more relaxed perioral appearance for the rhytidectomy patient who seeks significant cosmetic improvement (see Fig. 6-30).

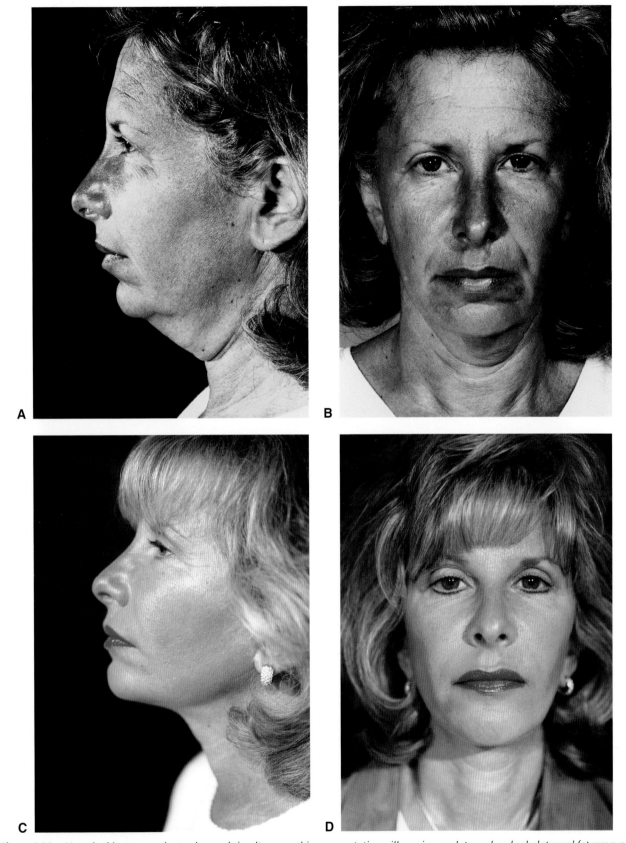

Figure 6-30 Most rhytidectomy patients who need simultaneous chin augmentation will require preplatysmal and subplatysmal fat removal and anterior "corset" platysmaplasty with inferior release, as in this case (**A** and **C**). Note: Many patients who have "weak" chins demonstrate significant perioral muscular strain at rest, which can be relieved by simultaneous chin augmentation, as shown in the postoperative photographs (**B** and **D**).

Technique

The submental incision should be curved and placed in an existing submental crease adjacent to the inner curve of the bony chin (Fig. 6-31A). After the subcutaneous tissue has been incised, the platysma muscle is exposed, and a longitudinal incision of the decussating fascia between platysma muscles is performed (Fig. 6-31B). A ribbon retractor is introduced and subperiosteal dissection of the chin below the labiomental groove is performed with a round-ended subperiosteal elevator (Fig. 6-31C). The pocket for the implant should be made so that the implant sits comfortably over the chin prominence and does not extend higher than the labiomental groove (Fig. 6-31D). A small cut can be made in the midline symmetrically over the chin prominence (Fig. 6-31E). In using wide anatomical chin implants it is vital to make certain that the pocket accurately accommodates the larger size of the implant; otherwise the implant will see-saw over the chin (Fig. 6-31F). If the pocket dissection was overaggressive, the implant can be fixed into a midline position with a simple suture. Otherwise, the platysma muscles and the deep layer should be closed before further anterior neck recontouring is performed (Fig. 6-31G).

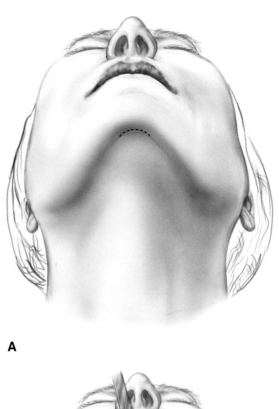

A

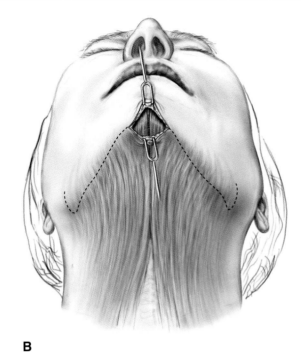

B

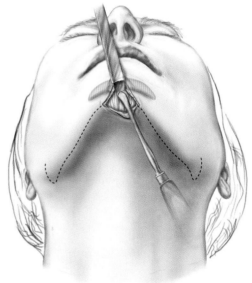

C

Figure 6-31   *Chin Augmentation.* ***A,*** *The submental incision should be curved and placed in an existing submental crease adjacent to the inner curve of the bony chin.* ***B,*** *After the subcutaneous tissue has been incised, the platysma muscle is exposed, and a longitudinal incision of the decussating fascia between platysma muscles is performed.* ***C,*** *A ribbon retractor is introduced, and subperiosteal dissection of the chin below the labiomental groove is performed with a round-ended subperiosteal elevator.*

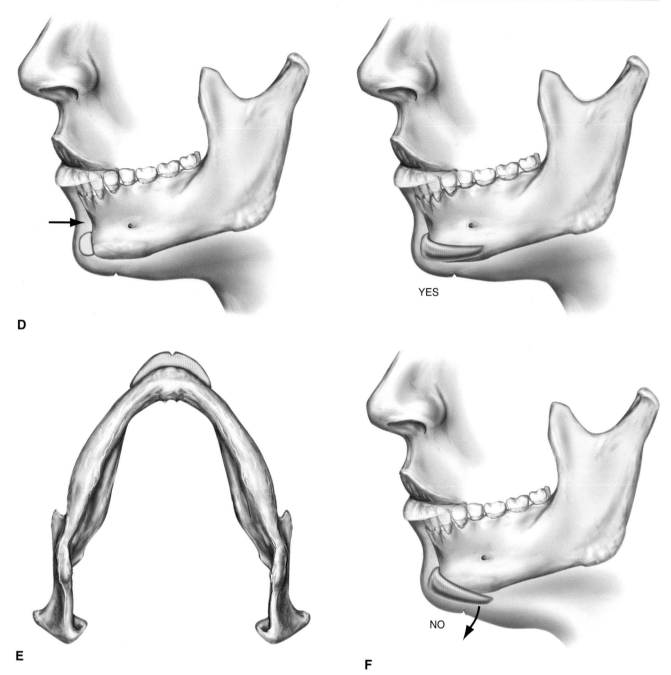

YES

D

E

F

NO

Figure 6-31, cont'd   D, *The pocket for the implant should be made so that the implant sits comfortably over the chin prominence and does not extend higher than the labiomental groove.* **E,** *A small cut can be made in the midline of the implant's anterior surface to allow it to seat squarely and symmetrically over the chin prominence.* **F,** *In using wide anatomical chin implants it is vital to make certain that the pocket accurately accommodates the larger size of the implant (top); otherwise, the implant will see-saw over the chin (bottom).*

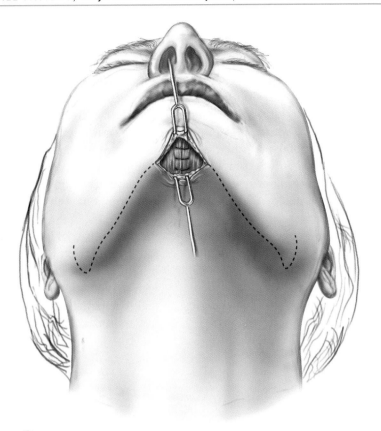

G

Figure 6-31, cont'd ***G,*** *The platysma muscles and the deep fascia layer should be closed before further anterior neck recontouring is performed.*

Laser Resurfacing

Simultaneous CO_2 and/or erbium laser resurfacing is a recent and valuable addition to the plastic surgeon's repertoire. By performing the laser resurfacing at the same time as the rhytidectomy, gravimetric signs of aging as well as fine and coarse perioral, periocular, and forehead rhytides can be improved in one procedure. Whereas prior to the introduction of laser resurfacing, dermabrasion and/or chemical peel was primarily restricted to the upper and lower lip areas when concomitant facelift was performed, the use of the laser allows for resurfacing to be performed in regions that have been surgically undermined. However, despite the initial enthusiasm that followed the introduction of lasers into cosmetic surgery, subsequent studies have found that there are "safe" areas for simultaneous laser resurfacing (Fig. 6-32).

In general, simultaneous laser resurfacing should not be performed within regions of the face where surgical skin-only undermining has been performed—the old adage "Never insult the skin by peeling and undermining in the same area." Accordingly, when simultaneous facial resurfacing is to be performed along with rhytidectomy, it is advisable to perform the midface lift with a deep-plane technique. Simultaneous laser resurfacing should not be performed in the neck when two-layer techniques are to be performed, unless a Skoog-type procedure is to be carried out. Because most surgical undermining in the forehead and brow region is deep to the musculofascial layer, simultaneous laser resurfacing is safe in this region, and spot treatment can be carried out. In fact, laser resurfacing in the forehead and brow region is highly advisable for optimal results in this region, especially because preferential skin tightening is not an integral part of either endoscopic or open brow lift (Fig. 6-33).

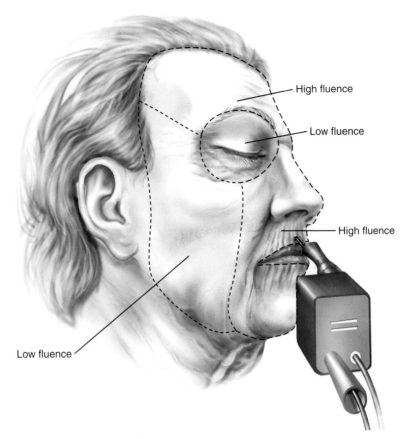

High fluence

Low fluence

High fluence

Low fluence

Figure 6-32 "Safe" areas for simultaneous laser resurfacing correspond to regions of the face in which surgical skin-only undermining has not been performed. Fluence also varies from central and paramedian high fluence zones, where two or more passes of high-watt erbium and high-watt CO_2 are necessary, to paramedian and lateral low fluence zones, where use of high-watt erbium and low-watt CO_2 is advised.

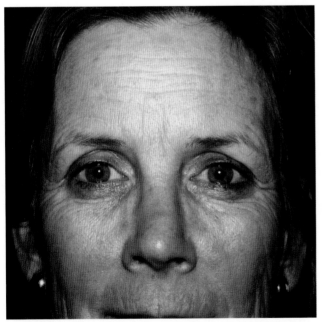

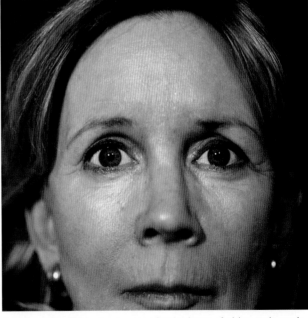

A

B

Figure 6-33 Laser resurfacing in the forehead and brow region is strongly advised, as skin tightening is not an integral part of either endoscopic or open brow lift. **A,** This 53-year-old woman underwent endoscopic brow lift as well as laser resurfacing of the forehead and brow with an ESC Derma K set on high erbium/CO_2 fluence. **B,** Her postoperative appearance.

Of primary importance in performing facial laser resurfacing simultaneously with rhytidectomy is the need for feathering of the CO_2/erbium fluence from medial to lateral (see Fig. 6-32). That is, in the deeper central facial and perioral rhytides regions that are not surgically undermined, far greater fluence is necessary for improvement than in paramedian regions adjacent to the nasolabial, oromandibular, and medial cheek regions. Many of these paramedian rhytides will be greatly decreased by rhytidectomy's deep-plane undermining and tightening alone. The number of passes and watts also vary depending on the region; in high fluence zones, two or more passes of high-watt erbium and high-watt CO_2 are necessary to effect improvement of deep rhytides, whereas in low fluence zones, a single pass of high-watt erbium and low-watt CO_2 may be all that is necessary for reduction of shallower paramedian and lateral rhytides (Figs. 6-33 to 6-36).

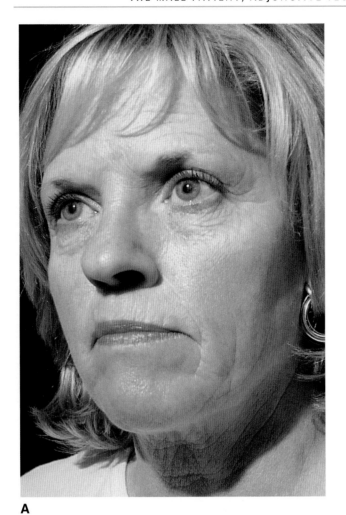

A

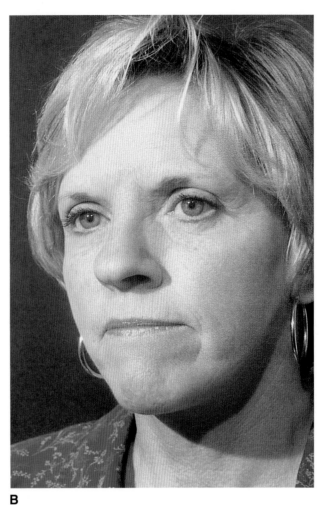

B

Figure 6-34 **A,** *This 58-year-old woman underwent midfacial facelift with a deep-plane technique and simultaneous full-face resurfacing with an ESC Derma K utilizing a feathering technique, with high fluence settings in the central and paramedian regions and low fluence settings laterally.* **B,** *Her postoperative appearance.*

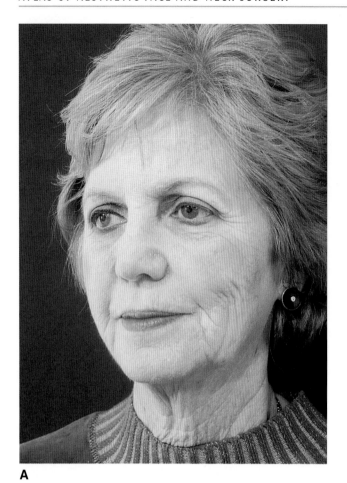

A

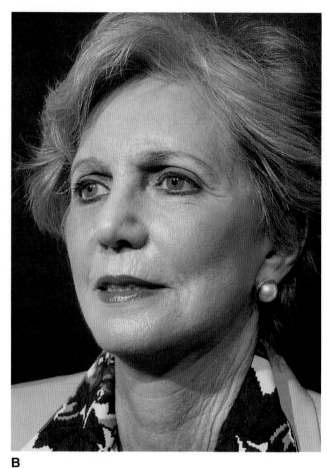

B

Figure 6-35 **A,** *This 66-year-old woman underwent midfacial facelift with a deep plane technique and simultaneous full-face resurfacing with an ESC Derma K also utilizing a feathering technique, with high fluence settings in the central and paramedian regions and low fluence settings laterally.* **B,** *Her postoperative appearance.*

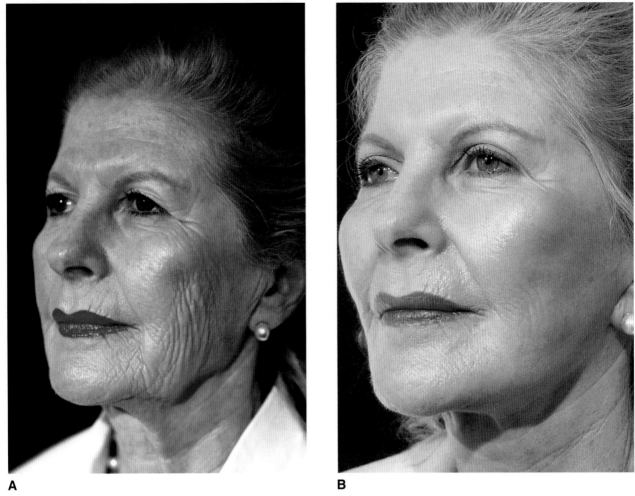

A **B**

Figure 6-36 *A, This 72-year-old woman underwent midface lift with a deep plane technique and simultaneous peri-oral and midfacial resurfacing with an ESC Derma K also utilizing a feathering technique with high fluence settings in the central and paramedian regions and low fluence settings laterally. **B,** Her postoperative appearance.*

COMPLICATIONS AND UNTOWARD SEQUELAE

Complications following rhytidectomy can be divided into two distinct groups: real complications, such as hematoma or infection, and untoward sequelae, such as scarring and patient dissatisfaction.

Hematoma

Hematoma is the most common complication that occurs after rhytidectomy. Hematomas can be divided into those that require operative management and those that can be managed nonoperatively. Hematomas requiring operative management occur in 1.3 % (female) to 4.4% (male) of patients undergoing facelift, whereas hematomas not requiring operative management occur in 4.4% (female) to 6.7% (male) of patients undergoing facelift.

Hematoma formation is related primarily to inadequate operative hemostasis, significant shifts of postoperative blood pressure, and undiagnosed blood dyscrasias. Means to prevent hematomas can be divided into preoperative, operative, and postoperative.

Preoperatively, a bleeding history should be taken and the patient should be instructed to avoid medications that affect platelet adhesion, such as aspirin and nonsteroidal anti-inflammatory medications. A routine complete blood count (CBC) with platelets and determination of prothrombin time/partial thromboplastin time (PT/PTT) are also advised. As a preoperative means to lower blood pressure during the perioperative period, 30 minutes before surgery I administer 0.1 mg of clonidine to each female patient and 0.2 mg of clonidine to each male patient, regardless of the preoperative blood pressure.

Intraoperatively, the head of the bed is kept elevated to prevent venous hypertension, and general inhalational anesthesia is avoided in favor of monitored intravenous sedation. In general, patients have a smoother postoperative course after monitored intravenous sedation, without much of the coughing and gagging that commonly occur with extubation. During the procedure, every effort should be made to obtain adequate hemostasis. Vessels of large caliber should be ligated, and vessels of small caliber coagulated with fine-pointed forceps and cautery. Drains, which do not prevent hematoma, are used to prevent serosanguineous fluid from collecting beneath the flap.

Postoperative methods to avoid hematoma are primarily centered on maintenance of a normotensive state, preventing unwanted postoperative blood pressure spikes, and avoiding inordinate amounts of postoperative pain, anxiety, and nausea. Postoperative administration of medications such as chlorpromazine (Thorazine), ketorolac tromethamine (Toradol), prochlorperazine (Compazine), and dolasetron mesylate (Anzemet) has been found to be vital for preventing rapid-onset (at <12 hours postoperatively) hematomas.

Most hematomas occur within the first 12 hours after surgery, and very few hematomas occur after 2 days. The single most important sign of an expanding hematoma is pain, especially unilateral, in the immediate postoperative period. Pain is common following an uncomplicated facelift, but unrelenting pain is not. Ecchymosis of the buccal mucosa is a sign of hematoma formation within the parotideomasseteric fascia and within the fat pad of Bichat. If there is any question about the existence of a major hematoma, the postoperative dressing must be removed immediately. If a hematoma is present, there is usually a visibly tense swelling noted deep to the facial flap. With evidence of circulatory compromise within the flaps, or if the airway is thought to be compromised, the sutures along the incision line should be snipped to relieve tension. If the airway is still believed to be compromised, the hematoma should be evacuated immediately. Plans should be made for returning the patient to the operating room. General anesthesia is preferable for evacuation of hematomas, but local anesthesia with sedation will also do when necessary.

In the operating room, after adequate sedation and blood pressure control have been established, the sutures are removed and the hematoma is thoroughly evacuated. A fiberoptic retractor is invaluable. After the gross clot is removed, vigorous irrigation with sterile saline will wash away smaller clots. A single bleeding vessel is rarely detected. Hematomas are usually caused by the bleeding of multiple small vessels and in my opinion are related to postoperative blood pressure spikes and bleeding vessels that simply eluded hemostasis.

Smaller hematomas, with blood collections ranging in size from 2 to 20 mL, are usually noted in the retroauricular region on the third to fifth postoperative day (Fig. 6-37). These can be evacuated using local anesthesia in the office, and a small suction drain placed for a day or two to prevent seroma formation. Very small hematomas can simply be aspirated with a large-bore needle after the clot liquefies, which generally occurs between postoperative days 7 and 14. It may be necessary to repeat the procedure on two to four successive days to ensure removal of as much of the accumulated blood as possible.

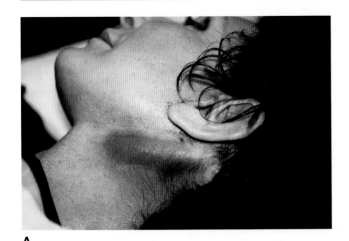
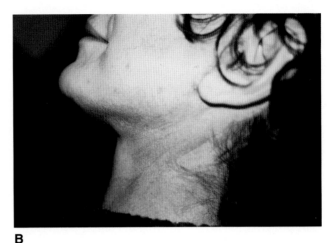

A   **B**

Figure 6-37   *Small hematomas, with blood collections ranging in size from 2 to 20 mL, are usually noted in the retroauricular region on the third to fifth postoperative day* **(A).** *These can be evacuated using local anesthesia in the office, and a small suction drain placed for a day or two to prevent seroma formation without untoward sequelae* **(B).** *Very small hematomas (<2 mL of blood) can simply be aspirated with a large-bore needle after the clot liquefies, which generally occurs between postoperative days 7 and 14.*

With proper care, patients who develop hematomas after rhytidectomy do not experience any long-term sequelae; however, failure to evacuate collections of blood at the proper time can result in organization of the clot with resultant discoloration, hyperpigmentation, retraction, and skin puckering. If this occurs, it can take several months to up to a year before the skin regains its normal texture and appearance.

Skin Slough

Skin slough is the most annoying of complications after facelift. In a recent survey of plastic surgeons, this complication was noted in 1.86% of patients. Minor degrees of slough occur most often in the retroauricular region, because the mastoid skin is the thinnest, is often placed under maximal tension, and is farthest from the blood supply of the flap (Fig. 6-38). Fortunately, these sloughs are rarely extensive, and the resulting scar is behind the ear, where it can easily be hidden by appropriate hairstyling. Occasionally, however, a slough can extend below the lobule of the ear, so that after it heals the scar is visible and noticeable (Fig. 6-39). Hypertrophic scar revision inevitably becomes necessary in such cases. If the patient can be reassured and management temporized with serial Kenalog injections, then after 6 months, scar revision can be performed with a retroauricular "hike" type of procedure. This procedure elevates and transposes the scar into the inconspicuous location of the retroauricular sulcus.

During the early phases of necrosis, a dark bruise is noted that eventuates in a black eschar. This lesion should be treated conservatively and débrided only if extremely unsightly. Aggressive débridement and skin grafting have no place here, for the eschar is an excellent biological dressing. The patient should be educated and reassured. If infection occurs, which it rarely does, then antibiotics are, of course, indicated.

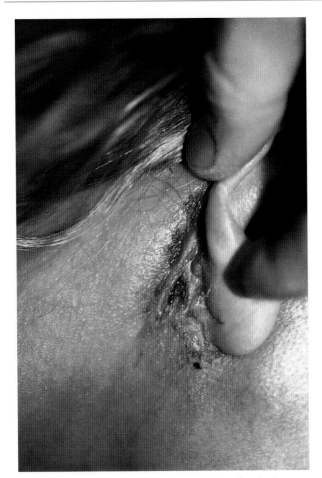

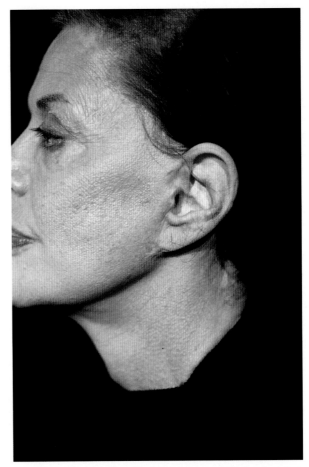

Figure 6-38 *Minor degrees of slough occur most often in the retroauricular region, because the mastoid skin is the thinnest, is often placed under maximal tension, and is farthest from the blood supply of the flap.*

Figure 6-39 *Occasionally skin sloughs can extend below the lobule of the ear and be visibly noticeable after they've healed. Hypertrophic scar revision inevitably becomes necessary for these patients.*

The causes of skin slough after rhytidectomy include streptococcal infection, undrained and tense hematomas, excessive thinning of skin flaps during undermining, excessive tension placed on the flaps during transposition, and cigarette smoking. There is no question that cigarette smoking has a significant impact on the risk of skin slough. All facial skin sloughs, regardless of the location or the extent, are treated conservatively and not surgically. The necrotic areas contract dramatically, even when in preauricular locations. Although it is difficult to watch the region of skin slough resolve, the resultant scar is far preferable. The patient should become "bored with care" during this difficult and trying time, which can often last 4 to 6 weeks. Depending on the size of the residual scar, it may be possible to readvance the facial flap after 4 to 6 months and excise the region of the resultant scar. Unfortunately, it is usually years before sufficient skin laxity allows such a procedure and even then the amount of skin that can be excised secondarily is surprisingly small. In general, scars that are farther than a centimeter from the previous incision cannot be excised at the time of secondary facelift.

Major skin sloughs are rare. They may be the result of massive hematoma that has been neglected. Occasionally, a large slough occurs for undetermined reasons. Such sloughs are undoubtedly the result of a marginal circulation in the skin flap, or localized thrombosis or ischemia. It is actually somewhat surprising that such problems are not encountered more often in facelifting because the skin flaps are very thin and the undercutting is often extensive. When these sloughs occur in the preauricular area, the resulting scar can be unsightly and may require secondary excision and repair as soon as the elasticity of the skin permits.

As with many of the complications that can follow rhytidectomy, preventive measures are of the utmost importance. Every effort should be made to prevent hematomas by adequate hemostasis at the time of surgery. Skin flaps must be handled as gently as possible, using skin hooks, T clamps, or thimble hooks on the flap margins and avoiding traction with sharp retractors or the fingertips. Tension on retractors under a skin flap during dissection or while hemostasis is obtained should be carefully controlled, as excess tension can severely damage the flap. Care should be taken to slightly retract the guarded forceps when cautery is applied, thereby preventing small cautery burns, which can mar an otherwise excellent postoperative result (Fig. 6-40).

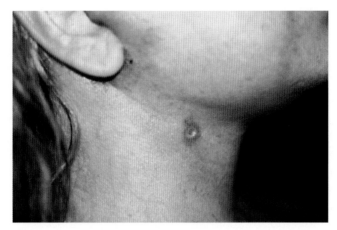

Figure 6-40   *Care should be taken to slightly retract the guarded forceps when cautery is applied, thereby preventing small cautery burns. These small burns inevitably heal well.*

Infection

Infection requiring hospitalization is exceedingly rare (occurring in <0.1% of cases). The face and hair are not sterile and cannot be "sterilized" with any known chemical agent. Infection is rare because of the rich blood supply to the head and neck. If cellulitis and small localized abscesses are noted, they are treated by evacuation, open drainage, and appropriate antibiotics. Although there is little or no evidence to support the use of antibiotics for rhytidectomy patients, most surgeons report using them prophylactically.

The possibility of two rare infections should be heeded. Group B streptococcal infection is a rapid-onset cellulitis infection that can result in slough of the facial flap if not treated rapidly with intravenous antibiotics, and appropriate débridement, if indicated. Another rare but equally devastating infection is *Pseudomonas* chondritis of the conchal cartilage. *Pseudomonas aeruginosa* is a normal contaminant of the ear canal. Chondritis is most often associated with deep suturing in the retroauricular region. A plug of povidone-iodine (Betadine)-saturated cotton placed in the external ear during surgery, as well as gentle handling of the conchal cartilage if fixation is deemed necessary, can be helpful in avoiding chondritis. Chondritis is an indication for hospitalization, wound drainage, and intensive antibiotic therapy to minimize cartilage destruction and subsequent ear deformity.

Sensory Nerve Injury

The most frequently injured nerve after rhytidectomy is not a motor nerve but a sensory nerve—the greater auricular nerve. It is common for many patients to complain about transient numbness in the preauricular areas, especially in the lateral cheek directly anterior to the lobule of the ear. This is a watershed region for the sensory nerve supply in this region, and usually the last region in the face and neck to undergo reinnervation following rhytidectomy. Delayed reinnervation should not be confused with greater auricular nerve injury. If the greater auricular nerve is injured, permanent loss of sensation and/or paresthesia over the lower portion of the ear will result. Injury to this nerve occurs when dissection is too deep over its course along the anterior border of the sternocleidomastoid muscle. When injury to this nerve is recognized during surgery, it should be repaired immediately by microneurovascular technique.

Sensory loss after brow lift varies depending on use of either the open (0.1%) or the endoscopic (0.6%) technique. Some degree of sensory loss will occur with any open brow lift procedure above the area of the suture line, especially in the temporoparietal region of the scalp. This region of the scalp is innervated by the deep branch of the supraorbital nerve. Use of the gull-wing modification of the coronal brow lift minimizes this complication. Sensory loss after endoscopic brow lift can be reduced by using the subperiosteal approach for undermining, employing meticulous and gentle dissection technique around the supraorbital and supra-trochlear nerve roots, using endoscopes and video cameras with high-quality optics, and switching to blunt rather than sharp depressor myotomies.

Motor Nerve Injury

Facial nerve injury is the most dreaded complication of rhytidectomy. It is also, quite fortunately, one of the rarest. The incidence of all intraoperative motor nerve injuries after rhytidectomy is reported to be 0.4%, specifically reported as 0.3% for "altered expression" and 0.1% for permanent facial nerve injury. The temporal branch is the most commonly injured, with the mandibular branch running a very close second in incidence. The vast majority of temporal and mandibular nerve injuries resolve within 3 to 6 months. In fact, the vast majority of zygomatic, buccal, and cervical branch injuries resolve within 3 to 6 months. The temporal branch, however, if injured, has the greatest probability for permanent injury. The major problem with temporal and mandibular nerve injuries is that they result in obvious deformity. Injury to the frontal branch results in paralysis of the ipsilateral frontal muscle and an inability to elevate the eyebrow. The result is ptosis of that eyebrow. Injury to the marginal mandibular nerve results in an inability to depress the ipsilateral side of the lower lip. During the period of resolution, if the cosmetic deformity caused by the nerve injury has caused the patient significant alarm, selective use of botulinum toxin (Botox) for symmetrization purposes can alleviate concern in selected patients.

It behooves the surgeon performing rhytidectomy to have an intimate knowledge of the usual course and common variations of the facial nerve. The facial nerve is deep laterally but moves into a more superficial and vulnerable position as it branches medially. By keeping this knowledge in mind and by careful dissection technique, especially when performing anterior and deep subcutaneous plane techniques, the surgeon can keep the incidence of facial nerve injury to an absolute minimum.

Following infiltration of the face with anesthetic solution, temporary partial or total paralysis of muscles supplied by the facial nerve may occur. Complete return of muscular function occurs over the next 4 to 8 hours as the anesthetic solution is metabolized and its effect on the nerve branches is resolved. Occasionally, a patient may have lingering paresis until the first morning after surgery. Weakness, as long as it is not complete paralysis, is little cause for alarm, and full function generally returns within a few days to a few weeks

If it becomes obvious during the surgical procedure

that a branch of the facial nerve has been transected, immediate surgical approximation of the nerve ends with microneurovascular technique yields the most fruitful recovery of function.

During the preoperative consultation, it is imperative for the surgeon to inspect the patient for facial nerve function and to document with photographs any deficiency in function. This aspect of evaluation becomes especially vital when a secondary rhytidectomy is to be performed on a patient for whom the surgeon did not perform the first procedure (Fig. 6-41). For that matter, any facial asymmetry or facial muscle weakness noticed during the preoperative examination should be pointed out to the patient before surgery and photographically documented so that it cannot later be ascribed to the operative procedure.

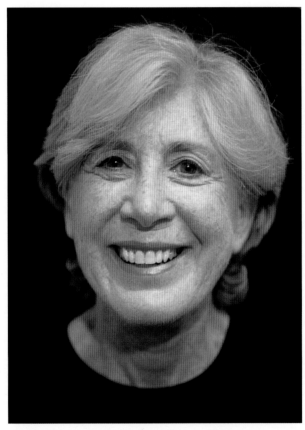

Figure 6-41 *During the preoperative consultation it is imperative for the surgeon to inspect the patient for facial nerve function and to document with photographs any deficiency in function. This aspect of the evaluation becomes especially vital when a secondary rhytidectomy is to be performed on a patient for whom the surgeon did not perform the first procedure, as can be demonstrated in this prospective 59-year-old secondary facelift patient with a permanent left marginal mandibular palsy.*

Hair Loss

Hair loss can occur in any hair-bearing region where incisions are made or where surgical undermining has been performed. Postoperative hair loss is most often found in patients with thin hair who have a tendency toward alopecia. The incidence of hair loss after rhytidectomy is <0.1 %, but after brow lift it is 4.0% for open approaches and 2.9% for endoscopic approaches. Temporary hair loss is far more common than permanent loss (Fig. 6-42). The vast majority of patients should be reassured that their hair will grow back within a few months. When hair loss is severe, however, it can take up to 6 months to replenish a given area.

When hair loss appears unusually extensive, a dermatologic consultation should be obtained. Often, suitable medication such as topical minoxidil (Rogaine) or injectable steroids can reverse the trend. Localized hair loss adjacent to incisions or from spreading of scars can occasionally be improved by scar excision and revision, as long as undue tension is not placed on the region.

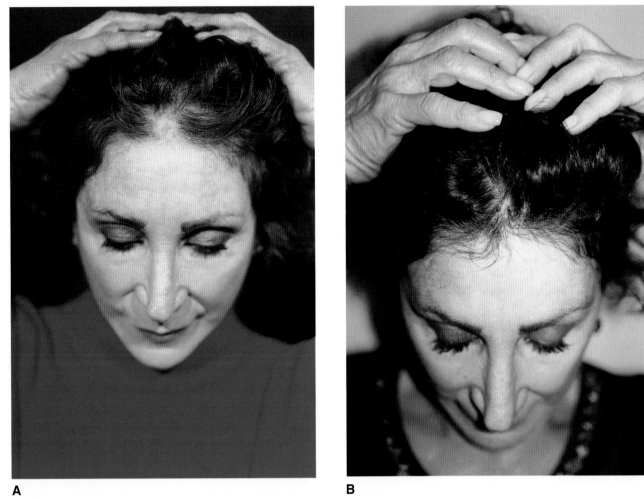

A   **B**

Figure 6-42   *The incidence of hair loss after rhytidectomy is <0.1 % but after brow lift is 4.0% for open approaches and 2.9% for endoscopic approaches. The vast majority of patients should be reassured that their hair will grow back within a few months. When hair loss is severe, however **(A)**, it can take up to 6 months to replenish a given area, as it did for this patient who underwent endoscopic brow lift **(B)**.*

Untoward Sequelae

Scars

Unsightly scars can mar an otherwise excellent result. The most obvious and troublesome scarring is that which occurs in the preauricular and lobular area (Fig. 6-43). Conspicuous scarring following rhytidectomy is caused by excessive tension on suture lines and vascular compromise of the flaps. Skin flaps must approximate easily and must be sutured with minimal tension; otherwise, the scar will migrate and widen during the postoperative course. All necessary tension should be exerted on the deep subcutaneous suture lines and at the key temporal and retroauricular suture sites. Excessive tension in the temporal and mastoidal areas, however, may cause bald scars that are difficult to camouflage. Should such scarring occur, it may be possible after several months to revise these defects by approximating hair-growing follicles. If excessive tension is placed on the earlobe, it will ultimately be pulled downward and result in a "pixie ear" deformity (Fig. 6-44). This deformity may require a secondary retroauricular "hike" procedure for correction after a year of healing, or ultimately a secondary rhytidectomy may be needed for full correction.

Occasionally, however, unsightly scarring can simply result. After all, scar formation and resolution is still a biological "black box." Hypertrophic scars, if they occur, usually appear in the postauricular area within 2 to 4 months postoperatively. Small doses of intralesional steroids, such as 0.2 to 0.4 mg triamcinolone, will aid significantly in resolution of such scars. Often, two or three injections spaced 3 to 4 weeks apart will be necessary. Hypertrophy of the preauricular or temporal scars is uncommon but can occur. True keloids are exceedingly rare.

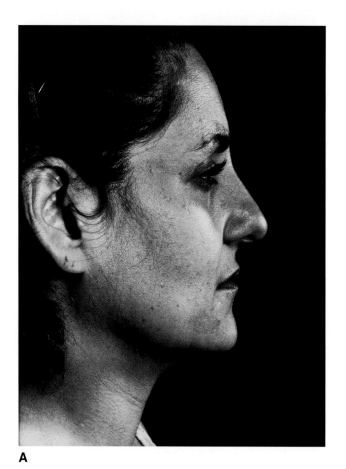

A

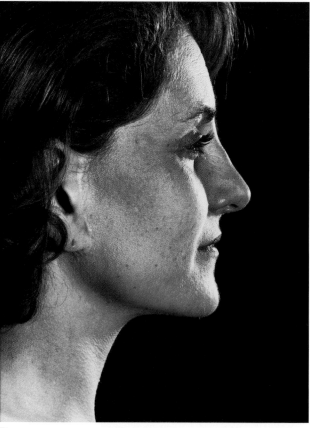

B

Figure 6-43   *Unsightly scars can mar an otherwise excellent result. The most obvious and troublesome scarring is that which occurs in the preauricular and lobular area, as in this patient (**A,** preoperative photograph; **B,** postoperative appearance). Conspicuous scarring following rhytidectomy is caused by excessive tension on suture lines and vascular compromise of the flaps. Skin flaps must approximate easily and must be sutured with minimal tension; otherwise, the scar will migrate and widen during the postoperative course.*

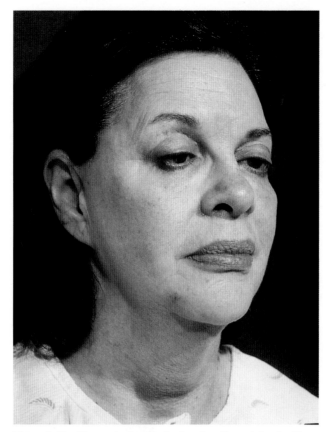

Figure 6-44   *If excessive tension is placed on the earlobe, it will ultimately be pulled downward, resulting in a "pixie ear" deformity, as exhibited by this prospective secondary rhytidectomy patient. This deformity may require a secondary retroauricular "hike" procedure for correction after a year of healing, or ultimately a secondary rhytidectomy may be needed for full correction.*

Pigmentary Alteration

Pigmentation sequelae are more common in Fitzpatrick III to VI skin types. The "two-scoop look"—characterized by sharp contrast between long-term hypopigmented facial skin and hyperpigmented sun-damaged neck skin—can occasionally result after injudicious use of CO_2 full-face laser resurfacing (Fig. 6-45). Probably the most helpful means of managing these difficult long-term problems is for the physician to have the patient make an appointment with a cosmetic make-up professional.

Hyperpigmentation can result from hemosiderin deposition from small undrained hematomas and areas of extensive postoperative ecchymosis. Patients with a preoperative history of bruising also have a greater tendency to postoperative hyperpigmentation. Proper use of skin bleaches (i.e., hydroquinones) is the best available solution for these difficult-to-manage long-term sequelae.

Telangiectasia of the facial skin may be aggravated after rhytidectomy simply because of the skin flap undermining and operative hemostasis. This problem can be confused with acne rosacea. In addition, an increase in the incidence of small vascular lesions is occasionally found. In general, appropriate vascular laser treatment by trained professionals is best for eradicating these difficult problems.

Contour Irregularity

Probably the most common untoward sequelae after rhytidectomy, especially after surgery of the deep subcutaneous layer, are minor asymmetries and contour irregularities. These can be noted especially along the course of fascia and mimetic muscle transection, near areas of deep suture fixation, and across regions of deep subcutaneous flap transposition. These irregularities and asymmetries are rarely noted by the patient, except perhaps during periods of animation. Permanent asymmetry and contour irregularity have been noted in 1.2% of rhytidectomy patients and 1.0% of brow lift patients. Patients should be reassured that with most asymmetries and minor contour irregularities, improvement over time is the rule.

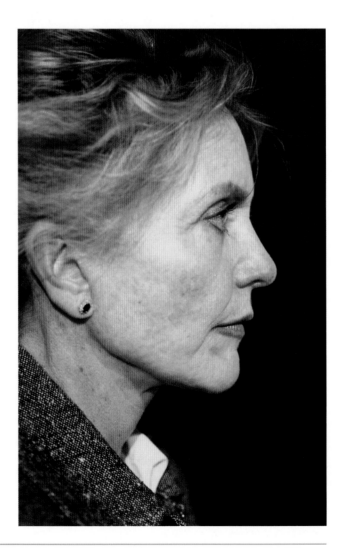

Figure 6-45 *Pigmentation sequelae are more common in Fitzpatrick III to VI skin types. The "two-scoop look"—in which long-term hypopigmented facial skin sharply contrasts with hyperpigmented sun damaged neck skin—occasionally arises after injudicious use of CO_2 full-face laser resurfacing, whether performed simultaneously with the rhytidectomy or not. Probably the most helpful means of management of these difficult long-term problems is for the physician to have the patient make an appointment with a cosmetic make-up professional.*

REFERENCES

The Male Patient

Bell T: Facelift incisions in men. Aesthet Surg J 23:53-55, 2003.
Connell B: Male face lift. Aesthet Surg J 22:385-396, 2002.
Lawson W, Naidu R: The male facelift. Arch Otol Head Neck Surg 119:535-539, 1993.

Adjunctive Techniques

LaTrenta GS: Facial contouring. In Rees T, LaTrenta GS: Aesthetic Plastic Surgery, 2nd ed. Philadelphia, WB Saunders, 1994, pp 784-889.

Laser Resurfacing

Achauer BM, Adair S, VanderKam V: Combined rhytidectomy and full-face laser resurfacing, Plast Reconstr Surg 106:1608, 2000.

Dingman D, Hartog J, Sieminow M, et al: Simultaneous deep plane facelift and trichloroacetic acid peel. Plast Reconstr Surg 93:86, 1993.

Complications and Untoward Sequelae

Elkwood A, Matarasso A, Rankin M, et al: National Plastic Surgery Survey: Brow lifting, techniques and complications. Plast Reconstr Surg 108:2143, 2001.
Matarasso A, Elkwood A, Rankin M, Elkowitz M: National Plastic Surgery Survey: Face lift techniques and complications. Plast Reconstr Surg 106:1185, 2000.
Rees T, Aston S, Thorne C: Postoperative Considerations and Complications. In Rees T, LaTrenta GS: Aesthetic Plastic Surgery, 2nd ed. Philadelphia, WB Saunders, 1994, pp 740-756.

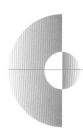

Index

Page numbers followed by f indicate figures.

A

Adjunctive techniques
    chin augmentation in. *See* Chin
        augmentation.
    laser resurfacing in. *See* Laser resurfacing.
Aging (face and neck), 46-67. *See also* Facelift.
    anatomic region affected in, 62-66, 63f,
        65f, 67f
        lower face and neck, 66, 67f
        midface, 64, 65f, 69f-71f
        upper face, 62, 63f
    areolar planes role in, 58-60, 59f-61f
    basic mechanisms of, 46-47
    key points for, 47
    laser resurfacing treatment of, 321f, 323f-
        325f
    lines in. *See* Lines.
    skin folds in. *See* Skin folds.
    soft tissue foundations affected by, 52-56,
        53f, 55f, 57f
    theories of, 46-47, 61f, 188
    wrinkles and furrows in, 48-50, 49f, 51f,
        321f, 323f-325f
Anesthetization
    clinical pearls for, 152
    one-layer facelift role of, 150-152, 151f,
        153f
    solution used for, 150, 152
Angle, cervicomental. *See* Cervicomental
    angle.
Angular artery, 42, 43f
Anterior techniques. *See* Facelift, anterior
    (neck) approaches in.
Areolar planes, 58-60, 59f-61f
    aging process role of, 58-60, 59f-61f
    anatomy of, 58-60, 59f-61f
    key points on, 60
Artery(ies)
    angular, 42, 43f
    facial, 42, 43f
    facial zone divisions of, 42, 43f
    inferior labial, 42, 43f
    infraorbital, 42, 43f
    jugal, 42, 43f
    masseteric, 42, 43f
    mental, 42, 43f
    nasal, 42, 43f
    SMAS dissection role of, 42, 43f
    submental, 42, 43f
    superficial temporal, 42, 43f

Artery(ies) *(Continued)*
    superior labial, 42, 43f
    supraorbital, 43f
    supratrochlear, 42, 43f
    transverse facial, 42, 43f
    zygomaticoorbital, 42, 43f
Atrophy
    protease inhibitors causing, 2, 3f
    subcutaneous fat loss in, 2, 3f
Auricle. *See also* Platysma-auricular ligament.
    male facelift and, 288-290, 289f-291f
    non-hair bearing margins of, 288-290,
        289f-291f
Auriculotemporal nerve, 44, 45f

B

Bags
    eyelid, 60, 61, 61f, 64, 65f
    malar, 60, 61, 61f, 64, 65f
Baldness pattern, in male patient, 288-290,
    289f
Basic metabolic rate, aging effects role of, 46
Beard hair, male patient with, 288-290, 289f,
    291f
Bichat fat pad, 6, 6f
    dissection of SMAS and, 24, 25f, 26
    resection of, 306f
    temporal extension of, 30, 31f
Bleeding
    hematoma due to, 326-328, 327f
    male patient hypervascularity role in, 294,
        297f
Bone loss
    aging changes related to, 47, 50, 51f, 60,
        61f, 64, 65f
    cheekbone affected by, 64, 65f
    submalar hollow due to, 60, 61f, 64, 65f
    wrinkles, furrows and folds due to, 47, 50,
        51f
    zygoma with, 61f
Botulinum therapy, 72-74, 72f, 73f, 75f
    indications for, 72-74, 72f, 73f, 75f
    limitations of, 74, 75f
"Bowstring" deformity, 264, 271f, 272f, 276f
Brow. *See also* Facelift.
    aging effects in, 62, 63f
    anatomic region of, 63f, 69f-71f
    botulinum therapy in, 72-74, 72f, 73f, 75f
    laser resurfacing in, 321f, 323f-325f
    muscles controlling, 36, 37f

Brow *(Continued)*
    surgical techniques for
        aesthetic considerations in, 80-81,
            82f
        anatomical considerations in, 78, 79f
        choice of, 76, 77f
        coronal lift in, 106-116
            clinical pearls for, 116
            ideal candidate for, 76, 77f, 106,
                107f-109f
            operative procedures for, 110-116,
                111f, 113f, 115, 117f
            results of, 77f, 106, 107f-109f
        endoscopic lift in, 92-104
            clinical pearls for, 104
            hair loss following, 334, 335f
            ideal candidate for, 76, 77f, 92, 93f-
                97f
            male patient in, 294, 304f
            operative procedures for, 98-104,
                99f, 101f, 103f, 105f
            results of, 77f, 92, 93f-97f
        key points on, 78, 80
        temporal lift in, 82-92
            clinical pearls for, 92
            ideal candidate for, 76, 77f, 82, 83f-
                85f
            operative procedures for, 86-90,
                87f, 89f-91f, 92
            results of, 77f, 82, 83f-85f
Buccal fat, 4f, 6f
    dissection of SMAS and, 22, 22f, 25f
    temporal extension of, 30, 31f
Buccal nerve, 44, 45f
Buccal-labial nerve, 44, 45f
Buccal-maxillary ligament, 8, 9f, 10, 11f, 12,
    14, 15f
    aging of, 53f, 54, 55f, 57f
    dissection and, 18, 19f, 22f, 27f
    perioral muscles and, 41f
Buccinator muscle, 40, 41f

C

Canthal bowing, 64, 65f
Cervicomental angle
    loss of, 67f
    male patient facelift and, 294, 297f, 300f-
        303f
    platysmaplasty affecting, 276, 276f-279f,
        280, 281f

Cervicomental angle (Continued)
    suspension sutures for, 282-284, 283f,
        285f, 286f
Cheek
    aging effects in, 61f, 64, 65f, 66, 67f
    anatomic regions of, 69f-71f
    anterior bunching in, 60, 61f
    fat of, 4, 5f, 6, 61f, 64, 65f, 66, 67f
Chin
    anatomic region of, 61f, 66, 67f
    lines of, 50, 51f
Chin augmentation, 312-319
    indications for, 312, 313f
    sequencing of other procedures with, 312-
        314, 315f
    surgical technique for, 316, 317f-319f
Clonidine, hematoma prevention using, 326
Combination facelift techniques, 236-238,
        237f, 239f-241f
    before and after photographs for, 237f,
        239f-241f
    clinical pearls for, 238
    indications for, 236, 237f, 239f-241f
    key points for, 236
    surgical techniques for, 236, 237f, 239f-
        241f
Complications
    contour irregularity in, 338
    hair loss in, 334, 335f
    hematoma in, 326-328, 327f
    infection in, 332
    nerve injury in
        motor, 332-333, 333f
        sensory, 332
    pigmentary alteration in, 338, 338f
    "pixie ear" deformity in, 336, 337f
    scars in, 336, 336f, 337f
    skin slough in, 328-330, 329f, 331f
Contour irregularity, 338
Coronal brow lift, 106-116
    clinical pearls for, 116
    ideal candidate for, 76, 77f, 106, 107f-109f
    operative procedures for, 110-116, 111f,
        113f, 115, 117f
    results of, 77f, 106, 107f-109f
Corrugator muscle, 36, 37f
"Crow's feet," 50, 51f, 61f

D

Deep plane technique, 242-254
    before and after photographs for, 245f-
        247f
    clinical pearls for, 254
    closure tension of, 253f, 254, 255f
    dissection in, 248-252, 249f, 251f
    indications for, 242-244, 243f, 245f-247f
    keypoints for, 244
    male patient in, 294, 297f-299f
    platysmaplasty required for, 248, 249f,
        252, 253f
    surgical procedure for, 248-254, 249f,
        251f, 253f, 255f
Deformity
    "bowstring," 264, 271f, 272f, 276f
    "pixie ear," 336, 337f
    turkey gobbler, 47, 50, 66, 67f, 302f

Depressor anguli oris muscle, 38, 39f
    attenuation and lengthening of, 66, 67f
Depressor labii inferioris muscle, 40
Depressor supercilii muscle, 36, 37f
Dermal elastosis
    aging effects due to, 46-47, 48, 49f, 57f
    wrinkles, furrows, and folds due to, 46-47,
        48, 49f
Drain placement, one-layer lift with, 168,
        168f, 182, 184f

E

Ear
    male patient lift role of, 289f-291f, 308-
        310, 309f, 311f
    one-layer lift role of, 165f, 167f, 178, 179f,
        180, 181f
    "pixie" deformity affecting, 336, 337f
Endoscopic brow lift, 92-104
    clinical pearls for, 104
    hair loss following, 334, 335f
    ideal candidate for, 76, 77f, 92, 93f-97f
    male patient with, 294, 304f
    operative procedures for, 98-104, 99f, 101f,
        103f, 105f
    results of, 77f, 92, 93f-97f
Extended lateral SMAS/platysma flap, 222-
        235
    before and after photographs for, 224f-
        227f
    clinical pearls for, 234
    closure of, 234, 235f
    dissection for, 230, 231f, 233, 233f, 235f
    incision for, 228, 229f
    indications for, 222-224, 223f, 224f-227f
    key points for, 224
    limitations of, 222-224, 223f
    surgical procedure for, 223f, 228-234,
        229f, 231f, 233f, 235f
Eyebrow
    aging effects in, 58, 60, 61f, 62, 63f
    canopy effect in, 58
    muscles controlling, 36, 37f
    ptosis of, 58, 60, 61f, 62, 63f, 304f
Eyelid
    aging effects in, 60, 61f, 62, 63f
    hooding of, 60, 61f, 62, 63f
    muscles controlling, 36, 37f
    pseudoptosis of, 60, 61f

F

Face
    aging process of. See Aging (face and
        neck).
    anatomy of, 2-45
        arterial supply in, 42, 43f
        fascia in, 16-27, 17f, 19f, 21f-25f, 27f.
            See also Fascia.
        fat in, 2-7, 3f-7f. See also Fat.
        key points for, 70
        lower region in, 63f, 66, 67f, 69f-71f
        midface region in, 64, 65f, 69f-71f. See
            also Midface.
        muscle(s) in, 36-41. See also Muscle(s).
        key points for, 40, 62

Face (Continued)
        periocular, 36, 37f
        perioral, 38-40, 39f, 41f
    neck region in, 69f-71f. See also Neck.
    nerve(s) in. See also Nerve(s).
        facial, 28-35, 28f-31f, 33f, 35f, 44,
            45f
        key points on, 44
        sensory supply by, 44, 45f, 332
        watershed zones for, 44, 45f
    regions in, 62-65, 63f, 65f, 67f, 69f-
        71f
    retaining ligaments in, 8-15, 9f, 11f,
        13f, 15f. See also Retaining
        ligaments.
    SMAS in, 16-27, 17f, 19f, 21f-25f, 27f
    surgical units in, 68-70, 69f-71f
    upper region in, 62, 63f, 69f-71f
    atrophy of. See also Bone loss.
        aging changes with, 46-67
        fat loss in, 2, 3f, 46-67
    complications affecting. See
        Complications.
Facelift. See also Brow.
    anterior (neck) approaches in, 254-286
        clinical pearls for, 260, 264, 270, 280,
            284
        full "corset" platysmaplasty in, 276,
            276f-279f, 280, 281f
        hierarchy of procedures in, 256
        key points for, 256
        lateral platysmaplasty alone in, 256,
            256f-259f
        limited "corset" platysmaplasty in, 264,
            265f-269f, 271f, 272f
        male patient in, 294, 300f, 301f
        plication of anterior platysma in, 260,
            261f-263f
        prior over-resection corrected in, 254,
            255f
        resection of anterior platysma in, 270,
            271f-275f
        subplatysma fat resection for, 260,
            261f-263f
        superficial submental liposuction in,
            256, 256f-259f
        suspension sutures in, 282-284, 283f,
            285f, 286f
    complications following. See
        Complications.
    deep plane technique in, 242-254
        before and after photographs of, 245f-
            247f
        clinical pearls for, 254
        closure tension of, 253f, 254, 255f
        dissection in, 248-252, 249f, 251f
        indications for, 242-244, 243f, 245f-
            247f
        keypoints for, 244
        platysmaplasty required for, 248, 249f,
            252, 253f
        surgical procedure for, 248-254, 249f,
            251f, 253f, 255f
    male patient in. See Male patient facelift.
    one-layer approach to, 118-185
        key points for, 118, 119
        middle-age patient refusal of, 138f

Facelift (Continued)
  operative strategies analysis for, 120-147
  secondary facelift patient in, 136-144, 139f, 141f-143f, 145f-147f
  surgical techniques of, 148-185
    anesthetization in, 150-152, 151f, 153f
    closure sequence in, 162, 163f, 165f, 168, 168f, 172, 173f, 179f, 180, 181f, 182, 183f, 184f
    drain placement in, 168, 168f, 182, 184f
    earlobes in, 165f, 167f, 178, 179f, 180, 181f
    flap fashioning in, 162-184, 166f-169f, 171f, 173f-177f, 179f, 181f
    hemostasis in, 162, 163f
    key anchor sutures in, 164, 165f, 170, 171f, 174, 175f
    liposculpture in, 154, 154f, 155f
    lipostructure in, 164, 182, 185f
    marking the incisions for, 148, 149f
    midface in, 162, 163f, 169f, 171f
    neck skin in, 162, 163f, 166, 166f, 167f
    postauricular "dog ears" in, 167, 167f
    scalp bunching in, 176, 176f-177f
    sideburns in, 165f, 169f, 171f, 172, 173f, 176
    temporal region in, 174, 174f-177f, 176
    tension vectors in, 163f, 166, 167f, 169f, 173f, 175f
    undermining in, 156-160, 156f-161f
  thick vs. thin flap indications in, 119
  vs. two-layer, 188-190, 189f
  youthful patient in, 120-137, 121f-125f, 127f-135f, 137f
  two-layer approach to, 186-286
    basic overview of, 186-187
      deep vs. superficial layers in, 186-187
      key points for, 187, 200
      retaining ligaments role in, 187
      SMAS and platysma role in, 187
    combination techniques in, 236-238, 237f, 239f-241f
      before and after photographs for, 237f, 239f-241f
      clinical pearls for, 238
      indications for, 236, 237f, 239f-241f
      key points for, 236
      surgical techniques for, 236, 237f, 239f-241f
    extended lateral SMAS/platysma flap in, 222-235
      before and after photographs of, 224f-227f
      clinical pearls for, 234
      closure of, 234, 235f
      dissection for, 230, 231f, 233, 233f, 235f
      incision for, 228, 229f

Facelift (Continued)
      indications for, 222-224, 223f, 224f-227f
      key points for, 224
      limitations of, 222-224, 223f
      surgical procedure for, 223f, 228-234, 229f, 231f, 233f, 235f
    goals of, 190-199, 191f, 194f, 195f, 197f, 199f
      key points for, 198
      square vs. oval face in, 190, 191f
    indications for, 190-199, 191f, 194f, 195f, 197f, 199f
      key points for, 198
      musculofascial laxity in, 192, 194, 194f, 195f
      ptotic soft tissue in, 192, 193f, 196, 197f
      simple test for, 194-196, 194f, 195f, 197f
      skin folds in, 192, 198, 199f
    lateral SMAS/platysma-ectomy in, 212-221
      before and after photographs of, 215f-217f
      clinical pearls for, 220
      indications for, 212-214, 213f, 215f-217f
      key points for, 214
      "lateral sweep" avoidance in, 214, 218
      surgical procedure for, 213f, 218-220, 219f, 221f
    limited lateral SMAS/platysma flap in, 200-208
      before and after photographs for, 202f-204f
      clinical pearls for, 208
      indications for, 200, 201f, 202f-204f
      key points for, 200
      surgical technique for, 201f, 205-208, 205f-207f, 209f-211f
    one-layer vs., 188-190, 189f
    plication/imbrication in, 200-208, 201f-207f, 210f, 211f
      before and after photographs of, 202f-204f
      clinical pearls for, 208
      indications for, 200, 201f, 202f-204f
      key points for, 200
      surgical procedure for, 201f, 205-208, 205f, 209f, 210f, 211f
    resective techniques in
      anterior, 260, 261f-263f, 270, 271f-275f
      lateral, 212-221
Facial artery, 42, 43f
Facial expression. See also Lines.
  "sad eyes," 94f
  "sad mouth," 66, 67f
  smile as, 38
  snarl as, 36
Facial nerve, 28-35, 44
  anatomy of, 28-35, 28f-31f, 33f, 35f, 44, 45f
  buccal branch of, 28

Facial nerve (Continued)
  cervical division of, 28, 35f
  deep plane technique risk to, 248, 249f
  dissection of SMAS role of, 18, 19f, 27f
  extended lateral SMAS/platysma flap and, 230, 231f
  frontal branch of, 28-30, 28f, 29f, 37f
  key points on, 34
  lateral SMAS/platysma-ectomy risk for, 219f, 221f
  marginal mandibular branch of, 28, 32-34, 33f, 35f
  periocular muscle innervated by, 36, 37f
  prior injury to, 333, 333f
  sentinel vein for, 28, 29f
  temporal division of, 28-30
  two-layer facelift risk for, 206, 207f, 208, 211f
Fascia. See also SMAS (superficial musculoaponeurotic system).
  aging effects role of, 52-54, 53f, 55f, 57f, 58
  areolar planes in, 58-60, 59f-61f
  cervical investing, 60, 60f
  double layering of, 58-60, 60f
  facial anatomy role of, 16-27, 17f, 19f, 21f-25f, 27f
  key points on, 26, 56, 60
  parotid-masseteric
    areolar plane of, 60, 60f
    dissection of SMAS role of, 22, 22f, 23f, 24, 24f
  ptotic. See Ptotic soft tissue.
  temporoparietal
    areolar plane of, 60, 60f
    dissection of SMAS role of, 18, 19f, 21f
    facial nerve in, 28-30, 28f-31f
Fat
  aging effects role of, 46-48
  areolar plane role of, 58-60, 59f-61f
  Bichat, 6, 6f
    dissection of SMAS and, 24, 25f, 26
    resection of, 306f
    temporal extension of, 30, 31f
  buccal, 4f, 6f
    dissection of SMAS and, 22, 22f, 25f
    temporal extension of, 30, 31f
  cheek, 4, 5f, 6, 61f, 64, 65f, 66, 67f
  facial aesthetic anatomy role of, 2-7, 3f-7f
  galeal, 4, 4f-6f
    brow region with, 37f, 62, 63f
  grafting with. See Lipostructure.
  jowl, 4, 4f, 5f, 60, 61f, 66, 67f
  malar, 4f-6f, 63f, 65f
  nasolabial, 4, 4f, 5f, 61f, 65f
  orbital, 6f, 61f, 63f, 65f
  premental, 4, 5f
  preplatysmal, 4f, 5f, 67f
    aging effects in, 67f
    neck dissection showing, 33f
  removal of. See Liposculpture.
  suborbicularis oculi (SOOF), 6, 6f
    aging effects in, 64, 65f
    dissection of SMAS role of, 22f, 24, 25f
  subplatysmal, 4f, 6f
    aging effects in, 67f
    neck dissection showing, 35f

Fat (Continued)
    resection of, 260, 261f-263f, 300f
    temporal, 4, 6f
        dissection of SMAS and, 22, 22f, 27f
        facial nerve near, 28f, 30f, 31f
Festoons, aging face with, 64, 65f
Fixation screws, endoscopic brow lift use of, 102, 103f
Flaps
    extended lateral. See Extended lateral SMAS/platysma flap.
    limited lateral. See Limited lateral SMAS/platysma flap.
    male patient facelift with, 294, 297f, 308-310, 309f, 311f
Folds. See Grooves; Lines; Skin folds; Wrinkles and furrows.
Forehead. See also Facelift.
    aging effects in, 62, 63f
    anatomic region of, 63f, 69f-71f
    botulinum therapy in, 72-74, 72f, 73f, 75f
    muscles controlling, 36, 37f
    surgical techniques for
        aesthetic considerations in, 80-81, 82f
        anatomical considerations in, 78, 79f
        choice of, 76, 77f
        coronal lift in, 106-116
            clinical pearls for, 116
            ideal candidate for, 76, 77f, 106, 107f-109f
            operative procedures for, 110-116, 111f, 113f, 115f, 117f
            results of, 77f, 106, 107f-109f
        endoscopic lift in, 92-104
            clinical pearls for, 104
            hair loss following, 334, 335f
            ideal candidate for, 76, 77f, 92, 93f-97f
            operative procedures for, 98-104, 99f, 101f, 103f, 105f
            results of, 77f, 92, 93f-97f
        temporal lift in, 82-92
            clinical pearls for, 92
            ideal candidate for, 76, 77f, 82, 83f-85f
            operative procedures for, 86-90, 87f, 89f-91f, 92
            results of, 77f, 82, 83f-85f
         tightening sequence vectors for, 70f, 71f
Frontalis muscle, 36, 37f
    "worry" lines due to, 62, 63f
Furrows. See Wrinkles and furrows.

G

Galea
    areolar planes associated with, 58-60, 59f
    fat associated with, 4, 4f-6f, 37f, 62, 63f
Glabella
    aging effects of, 62, 63f
    botulinum therapy in, 72-74, 72f, 73f, 75f
    frown lines in, 50, 51f
    muscles affecting, 36, 37f
Gland(s)
    aging effects related to, 47
    parotid
        dissection of SMAS and, 22f, 27f

Gland(s) (Continued)
        extended lateral SMAS/platysma flap and, 231f, 233f
        lateral SMAS/platysma-ectomy role of, 219f, 221f
        neck dissection showing, 35f
        two-layer facelift dissection and, 205f, 207f
    submandibular, ptosis of, 67f
Glide plane space, obliteration of, 58, 59f
Gravimetric soft tissue descent theory, 46, 61f, 188
Greater auricular nerve, 44, 45f
    neck dissection showing, 32, 33f, 35f
Grooves. See also Lines; Skin folds; Wrinkles and furrows.
    fat grafting for, 294, 305f-307f
    nasolabial, 38, 61f, 64, 65f, 305f-307f
    oromandibular, 51f, 67f

H

Hair follicles
    cauterization of, 288, 290f
    laser hair removal and, 288, 290f
Hair loss
    facelift followed by, 334, 335f
    male pattern baldness causing, 288-290, 289f
Hair-bearing skin. See also Sideburns.
    male patient facelift role of. See Male patient facelift.
    one-layer facelift role of
        postauricular, 167f, 168, 168f
        sideburn, 169f, 171f, 172, 173f
        temporal region, 174, 174f-177f
Hairline, male patient, 288-290, 289f, 291f, 292f
Hematoma, 326-328, 327f
    prevention of, 326-328
    treatment of, 326-328, 327f
Hemostasis
    one-layer facelift role of, 162, 163f
    skin slough related to, 330, 331f
Hyoid bone
    anterior platysma resection to, 271f
    limited "corset" platysmaplasty to, 265f

I

Imbrication. See Plication/imbrication.
Incision
    clinical pearls related to, 148
    extended lateral SMAS/platysma flap with, 228, 229f
    male patient facelift role of, 294, 295f, 296f
        retroauricular incision and, 293f, 294, 295f
        surgical technique and, 308-310, 309f, 311f
    one-layer facelift marking for, 148, 149f
Infection, 332
Inferior labial artery, 42, 43f
Inferior release
    male patient facelift role of, 300f, 301f
    platysmaplasty with, 264, 265f-269f, 271f, 272f, 300f, 301f

Infraorbital artery, 42, 43f
Infratrochlear nerve, 44, 45f

J

Jowls, fat of, 4, 4f, 5f, 61f, 66, 67f
Jugal artery, 42, 43f
Jugular vein(s)
    anterior, 35f
    external, 33f, 35f
    neck dissection showing, 33f, 35f

L

Lacrimal nerve, 44
Langer's lines, facial muscles related to, 36
Laser hair removal, 288, 290f
Laser resurfacing, 320-325
    before and after photographs of, 321f, 323f-325f
    indications for, 320
    pigmentary alteration due to, 338, 338f
    precautionary areas for, 320-322, 321f
    procedure for, 320-322, 321f
    "safe" areas for, 320-322, 321f
Lateral flaps
    extended. See Extended lateral SMAS/platysma flap.
    limited. See Limited lateral SMAS/platysma flap.
Lateral SMAS/platysma-ectomy, 212-221
    before and after photographs of, 215f-217f
    clinical pearls for, 220
    indications for, 212-214, 213f, 215f-217f
    key points for, 214
    "lateral sweep" avoidance in, 214, 218
    surgical procedure for, 213f, 218-220, 219f, 221f
Levator anguli oris muscle, 38, 39f, 40, 41f
Levator labii superioris alaeque nasi muscle, 39f, 40
Levator labii superioris muscle, 38, 39f, 40, 41f
Ligament(s)
    buccal-maxillary, 8, 9f, 10, 11f, 12, 14, 15f
        aging of, 53f, 54, 55f, 57f
        dissection and, 18, 19f, 22f, 27f
        perioral muscles and, 41f
    facial anatomy role of, 8-15, 9f, 11f, 13f, 15f
    mandibular, 8, 9f, 10, 11f
        aging of, 53f, 57f
        dissection of SMAS role of, 21f
        neck dissection showing, 35f
    masseteric, dissection of SMAS role of, 20, 21f, 22f, 27f
    masseteric-cutaneous, 9f, 12, 13f
        aging of, 54, 55f
        extended lateral SMAS/platysma flap and, 233f
        perioral muscles and, 41f
    maxillary, 10, 11f
    orbital, 8, 9f, 10, 11f
        aging of, 53f
        dissection of SMAS role of, 21f
        key points on, 78

Ligament(s) *(Continued)*
  platysma-auricular, 9f, 12, 13f
    aging of, 54, 55f, 57f
    deep plane technique role of, 250, 251f
    dissection of SMAS role of, 18f, 20, 21f
    extended lateral SMAS/platysma flap
      and, 231f, 233f
    neck dissection showing, 33f
    two-layer facelift and, 206, 206f, 207f
  retaining, 8-15, 9f, 11f, 13f, 15f
    aging effects role of, 52-54, 53f, 55f,
      57f
    dissection of SMAS role of, 16-24, 19f,
      21f, 22f, 27f
    false, 8, 9f, 12-14, 13f, 15f, 187
    key points for, 14, 56
    true, 8-10, 9f, 11f, 14, 187
    two-layer facelift role of, 187
  zygomatic, 8, 9f, 10, 11f
    aging of, 53f, 57f
    dissection of SMAS role of, 18, 19f, 20,
      21f
Limited auricular incision technique, 308-310,
  309f, 311f
Limited lateral SMAS/platysma flap, 200-208
  before and after photographs for, 202f,
    203f, 204f
  clinical pearls for, 208
  key points for, 200
  surgical technique for, 201f, 205-208,
    205f-207f, 209f-211f
Lines. *See also* Grooves; Skin folds; Wrinkles
    and furrows.
  "cheek," 50, 51f, 65f
  "chin," 50, 51f
  "commissural," 50, 51f
  "crow's feet," 50, 51f, 61f
  "frown," 50, 51f, 62, 63f
  key points related to, 50, 62, 64, 66
  laser resurfacing and, 321f, 323f-325f
  "lip," 50, 51f, 64, 65f, 66, 67f
  "marionette," 50, 51f, 66, 67f
  "mimetic," 48, 50, 51f
  "nasolabial," 50, 51f, 64, 65f
  "neck," 50, 51f
  "preauricular," 50, 51f
  "smile," 50, 51f
  "worry," 50, 51f, 62, 63f
Liposculpture
  male patient in, 294, 300f, 305f-307f
  one-layer lift procedure with, 119, 154,
    154f, 155f
    before and after of, 121f-124f, 128f-
      134f
  overaggressive cervical, 254, 255f
  patient who refused facelift getting, 136,
    137f, 138f
  superficial submental
    anterior platysmaplasty with, 294,
      300f-303f
    lateral platysmaplasty with, 256, 256f,
      257f
Lipostructure
  key points for, 136
  male patient in, 294, 305f-307f
  one-layer lift procedure with, 119, 164,
    182, 185f

Lipostructure *(Continued)*
  before and after of, 122f-125f, 130f-
    134f
  patient who refuses facelift getting, 136,
    138f
  secondary facelift patient getting, 136,
    139f, 141f-143f, 145f
Lips
  aging effects in, 64, 65f, 66, 67f
  muscles controlling, 38-40, 39f, 41f
Lower face, anatomic region of, 63f, 66, 67f,
  69f-71f

M

Malar fat, 4f-6f, 63f, 65f
Male patient facelift, 288-311
  aesthetic considerations for, 288-290,
    289f-293f
  auricular non-hair bearing margins in,
    288-290, 289f-291f
  baldness pattern and, 288-290, 289f
  beard in, 288-290, 289f, 291f
  blood supply elevation in, 294, 297f
  deep plane technique for, 294, 297f-299f
  endoscopic brow lift in, 294, 304f
  fat grafting in, 294, 305f-307f
  fat resection for, 294, 300f
  hair follicle cauterization for, 288, 290f
  hairline in, 288-290, 289f, 291f, 292f
  incisions of choice for, 294, 295f, 296f
  laser hair removal in, 288, 290f
  platysmaplasty with, 294, 297f-303f
  retroauricular incision for, 293f, 294, 295f
    surgical technique using, 308-310,
      309f, 311f
  sideburns in, 288, 289f, 290f, 295f, 296f
  submental liposuction for, 294, 300f
  surgical considerations for, 294, 295f-307f
  suspension sutures in, 294, 297f, 303f
  tragus in, 295f, 296f
Mandibular ligament, 8, 9f, 10, 11f
  aging of, 53f, 57f
  dissection of SMAS role of, 21f
  neck dissection showing, 35f
Marginal mandibular nerve, 28, 32-34, 33f,
  35f
"Marionette" lines, 50, 51f, 66, 67f
Masseter muscle
  neck dissection showing, 35f
  perioral muscles and, 41f
Masseteric artery, 42, 43f
Masseteric ligament, 20, 21f, 22f, 27f
Masseteric-cutaneous ligament, 9f, 12, 13f
  aging of, 54, 55f
  extended lateral SMAS/platysma flap and,
    233f
  perioral muscles and, 41f
Mattress suture, buried, 211f
Maxillary ligament, 10, 11f
McGregor's patch
  dissection of SMAS and, 18, 19f
  zygomatic retaining ligaments of, 9f, 10,
    11f
Menopause, aging effects associated with, 46-
  47
Mental artery, 42, 43f

Mental nerve, 44, 45f
Mentalis muscle, 39f, 40
Midface. *See also* Facelift.
  anatomic region of, 64, 65f, 69f-71f
  deep plane technique indicated for, 242-
    244, 243f, 245f-247f
  extended lateral SMAS/platysma flap for,
    222-224, 223f, 224f-227f
  laser resurfacing in, 321f, 323f-325f
  male patient facelift role of, 294, 305, 308,
    309f, 311f
  tightening sequence vectors for, 70f, 71f
    key points for, 190
    one-layer lift procedure with, 162,
      163f, 169, 169f, 171f
    two-layer lift procedure with, 188-190,
      189f
Motor nerve injury, 332-333, 333f
Mouth
  corner seal of, 38
  laser resurfacing around, 321f, 323f-325f
  muscles controlling, 38-40, 39f, 41f
  oromandibular grooves of, 51f, 67f
  smile expression of, 38, 40
Muscle(s)
  aging effects associated with, 62-66, 63f,
    65f, 67f
  buccinator, 40, 41f
  corrugator, 36, 37f
  depressor anguli oris, 38, 39f
    attenuation and lengthening of, 66, 67f
  depressor labii inferioris, 40
  depressor supercilii, 36, 37f
  facial anatomy role of, 36-41, 37f, 39f, 41f
  frontalis, 36, 37f
    "worry" lines due to, 62, 63f
  levator anguli oris, 38, 39f, 40, 41f
  levator labii superioris, 38, 39f, 40, 41f
  levator labii superioris alaeque nasi, 39f,
    40
  masseter
    neck dissection showing, 35f
    perioral muscles and, 41f
  mentalis, 39f, 40
  orbicularis oculi, 36, 37f
    deep plane technique role of, 250, 251f
    lengthening and attenuation of, 63f,
      65f
  orbicularis oris, 38-40, 41f
    attenuation and lengthening of, 66, 67f
  periocular, 36, 37f, 64
  perioral, 38-40, 39f, 41f, 66
  platysma. *See also* Platysmaplasty.
    aging effects in, 60, 61f, 66, 67f
    attenuation and banding in, 61f, 67f
    fat pads associated with, 4, 4f-6f, 67f
    mouth effects of, 38, 39f
    neck dissection showing, 33f, 35f
    plication of, 260, 261f-263f
    resection of, 270, 271f-275f
    transverse creasing in, 61f
  procerus, 36, 37f
    frown lines due to, 62, 63f
  risorius, 38, 39f
  zygomaticus, 38
  zygomaticus major, 205f, 210f
    deep plane technique role of, 250, 251f

Musculofascial laxity
  simple test for assessment of, 192, 194, 194f, 195f
    two-layer facelift indicated for, 192, 194, 194f, 195f
    postoperative results of, 201f, 202f

N

Nasal artery, 42, 43f
Nasal nerve, 44, 45f
Nasolabial crease
  aging effects in, 61f, 64, 65f
  fat grafting for, 294, 305f-307f
  formation of, 38
Nasolabial fat, 4, 4f, 5f, 61f, 65f
Neck. See also Aging (face and neck); Facelift.
  aging effects in, 50, 51f, 61f, 66, 67f
  anatomic regions of, 69f-71f
  areolar plane of, 60, 61f
  lateral SMAS/platysma-ectomy role of, 212-214, 213f, 215f-217f
  lines in, 50, 51f
  one-layer facelift role of, 162, 163f, 166, 166f, 167f
  surgical units of, 69f-71f
  tightening sequence vectors for, 70f, 71f, 163f, 188-190, 189f
  turkey gobbler deformity in, 47, 50, 66, 67f, 302f
  two-layer facelift role of, 189f
Nerve(s)
  auriculotemporal, 44, 45f
  buccal, 44, 45f
  buccal-labial, 44, 45f
  facial, 28-35, 44
    anatomy of, 28-35, 28f-31f, 33f, 35f, 44, 45f
    buccal branch of, 28
    cervical division of, 28, 35f
    deep plane technique risk to, 248, 249f
    dissection of SMAS role of, 18, 19f, 27f
    extended lateral SMAS/platysma flap and, 230, 231f
    frontal branch of, 28-30, 28f, 29f, 37f
    key points on, 34
    lateral SMAS/platysma-ectomy risk for, 219f, 221f
    marginal mandibular branch of, 28, 32-34, 33f, 35f
    periocular muscle innervated by, 36, 37f
    prior injury to, 333, 333f
    sentinel vein for, 28, 29f
    temporal division of, 28-30
    two-layer facelift risk for, 206, 207f, 208, 211f
  facial anatomy role of, 28-35, 28f-31f, 33f, 35f, 44, 45f
  greater auricular, 44, 45f
    neck dissection showing, 32, 33f, 35f
  infratrochlear, 44, 45f
  injury to, 332-333, 333f
  lacrimal, 44
  marginal mandibular, 28, 32-34, 33f, 35f
  mental, 44, 45f
  nasal, 44, 45f

Nerve(s) (Continued)
  supraorbital, 28f, 37f, 44, 45f
  supratrochlear, 28f, 37f, 44, 45f
  transverse cervical, 44, 45f
  trigeminal, 44, 45f
  zygomaticofacial, 28, 37f, 44, 45f
  zygomaticotemporal, 44, 45f
Nose, "droopy," 47

O

One-layer facelift. See Facelift, one-layer approach to.
Orbicularis oculi muscle, 36, 37f
  deep plane technique role of, 250, 251f
  lengthening and attenuation of, 63f, 65f
Orbicularis oris muscle, 38-40, 41f
  attenuation and lengthening of, 66, 67f
Orbital fat, 6f, 61f, 63f, 65f
Orbital ligament, 8, 9f, 10, 11f
  aging of, 53f
  dissection of SMAS role of, 21f
  key points for, 78
Orbital rim, facial nerve near, 28f
Oromandibular groove, 51f, 67f

P

Pain, following facelift, 326
Parotid gland
  dissection of SMAS and, 22f, 27f
  extended lateral SMAS/platysma flap and, 231f, 233f
  lateral SMAS/platysma-ectomy role of, 219f, 221f
  neck dissection showing, 35f
  two-layer facelift dissection and, 205f, 207f
Periocular muscle, 36, 37f, 64
Perioral muscle, 38-40, 39f, 41f, 66
Periosteum
  areolar planes associated with, 58-60, 59f
  dense vs. loose, 58-60, 59f
Pigmentation alteration, 338, 338f
  laser resurfacing role in, 338, 338f
"Pixie ear" deformity, 336, 337f
Platysma muscle. See also Facelift.
  aging effects in, 60, 61f, 66, 67f
  attenuation and banding in, 61f, 67f
  fat pads associated with, 4, 4f-6f, 67f
  mouth effects of, 38, 39f
  neck dissection showing, 33f, 35f
  plication of, 260, 261f-263f
  resection of, 270, 271f-275f
  transverse creasing in, 61f
Platysma-auricular ligament, 9f, 12, 13f
  aging of, 54, 55f, 57f
  deep plane technique role of, 250, 251f
  dissection of SMAS role of, 18f, 20, 21f
  extended lateral SMAS/platysma flap and, 231f, 233f
  neck dissection showing, 33f
  two-layer facelift and, 206, 206f, 207f
Platysmaplasty
  "bowstring" deformity of, 264, 271f, 272f, 276f
  deep plane procedure requiring, 248, 249f, 252, 253f

Platysmaplasty (Continued)
  fat resection for, 260, 261f-263f, 300f
  full "corset," 276, 276f-279f, 280, 281f, 297f
  lateral alone, 256, 256f-259f
  limited "corset" with inferior release, 264, 265f-269f, 271f, 272f, 300f
  male patient facelift with, 294, 297f-303f
  plication of anterior platysma in, 260, 261f-263f
  resection of anterior platysma in, 270, 271f-275f, 301f, 303f
  secondary facelift patient with, 142f-143f, 145f-147f
Plication/imbrication, 200-208, 201f-207f, 210f, 211f
  anterior platysma in, 260, 261f-263f
  before and after photographs of, 202f-204f
  clinical pearls for, 208
  indications for, 200, 201f, 202f-204f
  key points for, 200
  surgical procedure for, 201f, 205-208, 205f, 209f, 210f, 211f
Procerus muscle, 36, 37f
  frown lines due to, 62, 63f
Protease inhibitors, facial atrophy due to, 2, 3f
Ptotic soft tissue
  combination lift techniques for, 236-238, 237f, 239f-241f
  extended lateral SMAS/platysma flap for, 222-224, 223f-227f
  simple test for assessment of, 194-196, 194f, 195f, 197f
  two-layer facelift indicated for, 192, 193f, 196, 197f
    postoperative results of, 204f

R

Resective techniques
  anterior, 260, 261f-263f, 270, 271f-275f
  lateral, 212-221
Resurfacing. See Laser resurfacing.
Retaining ligaments, 8-15, 9f, 11f, 13f, 15f
  aging effects role of, 52-54, 53f, 55f, 57f
  dissection of SMAS role of, 16-24, 19f, 21f, 22f, 27f
  false, 8, 9f, 12-14, 13f, 15f, 187
  key points for, 14, 56
  true, 8-10, 9f, 11f, 14, 187
  two-layer facelift role of, 187
Risorius muscle, 38, 39f

S

"Sad eyes" appearance, 94f
"Sad mouth" appearance, 66, 67f
SAL (suction-assisted lipectomy). See Liposculpture.
Scalp bunching, avoidance of, 176, 176f-177f
Scars, 336, 336f, 337f
  prevention of, 336, 336f
Screws, endoscopic brow lift use of, 102, 103f
Sensory nerves. See also Nerve(s).
  facial aesthetic anatomy role of, 44, 45f
  injury to, 332

Sideburns
female facelift role of, 165f, 169f, 171f, 172, 173f, 176
male facelift role of, 288, 289f, 290f, 295f, 296f
one-layer facelift role of, 165f, 169f, 171f, 172, 173f, 176
Skeletonization. *See* Bone loss.
Skin
actinic damage to, 46
aging effects in, 46-48, 49f, 51f, 57f
sloughing of, 328-330, 329f, 331f
prevention of, 328-330
trampoline effect in, 56, 57f
Skin folds, 49f, 50, 64, 65f, 67f. *See also* Grooves; Lines; Wrinkles and furrows.
aging face and neck with, 49f, 50, 64, 65f, 67f
deep plane technique indicated for, 242-244, 243f, 245f-247f
extended lateral SMAS/platysma flap for, 222-224, 223f, 224f-227f
key points related to, 50, 62
laser resurfacing and, 321f, 323f-325f
lateral SMAS/platysma-ectomy for, 212-214, 213f, 215f-217f
male patient with, 294, 305f-307f
two-layer facelift indicated for, 192, 198, 199f
postoperative results of, 203f
SMAS (superficial musculoaponeurotic system). *See also* Facelift; Fascia.
anatomy of, 16-27, 17f, 19f, 21f-25f, 27f
areolar plane of, 60, 60f
dissection of, 16-27, 17f, 19f, 21f-25f, 27f
key points on, 26, 56, 60
ptotic. *See* Ptotic soft tissue.
two-layer facelift role of, 187
SMAS/platysma flap
extended lateral. *See* Extended lateral SMAS/platysma flap.
limited lateral. *See* Limited lateral SMAS/platysma flap.
Soft tissue. *See* Fascia; Ptotic soft tissue.
SOOF (suborbicularis oculi fat), 6, 6f
aging effects in, 64, 65f
dissection of SMAS role of, 22f, 24, 25f
Squinting, aging effects related to, 47
Submalar hollow, 63f, 64, 65f
Submandibular gland, ptosis of, 67f
Submental artery, 42, 43f
Suborbicularis oculi fat (SOOF), 6, 6f
aging effects in, 64, 65f
dissection of SMAS role of, 22f, 24, 25f
Subplatysmal fat, 4f, 6f
aging effects in, 67f
neck dissection showing, 35f

Subplatysmal fat *(Continued)*
resection of, 260, 261f-263f, 300f
Suction-assisted lipectomy (SAL). *See* Liposculpture.
Superficial temporal artery, 42, 43f
Superior labial artery, 42, 43f
Supraorbital artery, 43f
Supraorbital nerve, 28f, 37f, 44, 45f
Supratrochlear artery, 42, 43f
Supratrochlear nerve, 28f, 37f, 44, 45f
Suture(s)
mattress, buried, 211f
suspension
cervicomental angle role of, 282-284, 283f, 285f, 286f
male patient facelift with, 294, 297f, 303f
zygomatic, 41f
zygomaticofrontal, 9f, 11f

T

Telangiectasia, following facelift, 338
Temporal crest, 28f
Temporal fat, 4, 6f
dissection of SMAS and, 22, 22f, 27f
facial nerve near, 28f, 30f, 31f
Temporal lift, 82-92
clinical pearls related to, 92
ideal candidate for, 76, 77f, 82, 83f-85f
operative procedures for, 86-90, 87f, 89f-91f, 92
results of, 77f, 82, 83f-85f
Temporal region
aging effects of, 62, 63f
areolar planes of, 60, 61f
atrophy of, 61f
definition of, 30
facial nerve in, 28, 28f, 29f. *See also* Facial nerve.
hollowing of, 62, 63f
one-layer facelift role of, 174, 174f-177f
Thyroid cartilage, platysmaplasty to, 276f
Tragus, male patient facelift incision at, 295f, 296f
Trampoline effect, 56, 57f
Transverse cervical nerve, 44, 45f
Transverse facial artery, 42, 43f
Trigeminal nerve, 44, 45f
Turkey gobbler neck deformity, 47, 50, 66, 67f
male patient with, 302f
Two-layer facelift. *See* Facelift, two-layer approach to.

U

Undermining, one-layer facelift role of, 156-160, 156f-161f

Upper face. *See also* Brow; Forehead.
anatomic region of, 62, 63f, 69f-71f
key points for, 78, 80
tightening sequence vectors for, 70, 71f
one- vs. two-layer facelift with, 188-190, 189f

V

Vectors
key points for, 190
one-layer facelift role of, 163f, 166, 167f, 169f, 173f, 175f, 189f
surgical tightening sequence with, 70, 70f, 71f
two-layer facelift role of, 188-190, 189f, 207f, 253f, 265f, 276f, 283f
Vein(s)
anterior jugular, 35f
external jugular, 33f, 35f

W

Wrinkles and furrows. *See also* Grooves; Lines; Skin folds.
aging face and neck with, 48-50, 49f, 51f, 61f, 64f, 65f, 67f
key points for, 50, 62
laser resurfacing treatment of, 321f, 323f-325f
mechanisms of, 48-50, 49f, 51f, 64, 66
mimetic wrinkles in, 49f, 50
skin changes in, 48-50, 49f, 51f, 64f, 66f
types and sites of, 48-50, 49f, 51f, 63f, 65f, 67f

Z

Zygoma, bone loss affecting, 61f
Zygomatic arch
dissection of SMAS role of, 19f
facial nerve relation to, 28, 28f, 253f
Zygomatic body, deep plane sutures in, 252, 253f
Zygomatic ligament, 8, 9f, 10, 11f
aging of, 53f, 57f
dissection of SMAS role of, 18, 19f, 20, 21f
Zygomaticofacial nerve, 28, 37f, 44, 45f
Zygomaticoorbital artery, 42, 43f
Zygomaticotemporal nerve, 44, 45f
Zygomaticus major muscle, 205f, 210f
deep plane technique role of, 250, 251f
Zygomaticus muscle, 38